SLAVERY AND MEDICINE

Enslavement and Medical Practices in Antebellum Louisiana

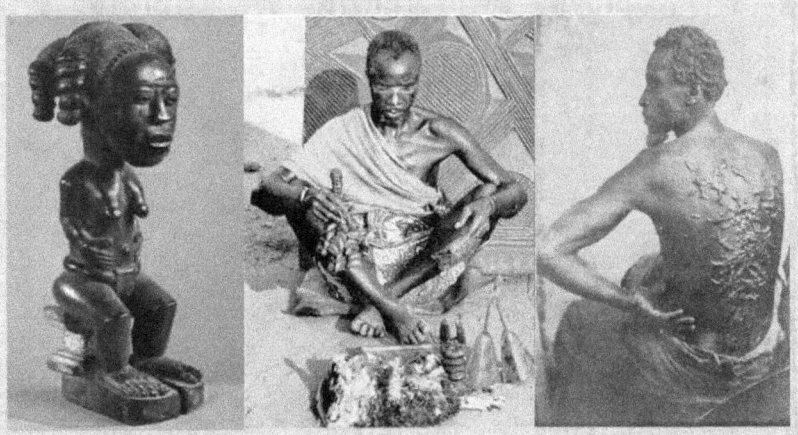

Katherine Bankole-Medina

Liberated Scholars Press publishes classic and influential works in History and Africana Studies.

We are pleased to commemorate the publishing (reprinting) of *Slavery and Medicine: Enslavement and Medical Practices in Antebellum Louisiana*. Over the past two decades this work has contributed significantly to the area of slavery and medicine, within the history of science, medicine and technology field; and has influenced countless scholars across disciplines.

Liberated Scholars Press independently presents this publication in recognition of the United Nations International Decade for People of African Descent (2015-2024)

Liberated Scholars Press
liberatedscholarspress@mail.com
(formally LSA Press)
Washington, D.C.

Copyright © 1998-2017 Katherine Bankole-Medina

All rights reserved. No part of this book may be reproduced or utilized in any form or by any means, electronic or mechanical, including photocopying, recording, or by any information storage and retrieval system, without permission in writing from the publisher.

First published by Garland Publishing, Inc., New York, 1998

First issued as a Liberated Scholars Press paperback, 2017

ISBN-13: 978-0692895290
ISBN-10: 0692895299

Slavery and Medicine
Enslavement and Medical Practices in Antebellum Louisiana

by Katherine Bankole-Medina, Ph.D.

© 2017

DEDICATION

To my great-grandparents Annie and Frank Rosebud, formerly enslaved, who lived to know freedom; to Anarcha and all of the Africans who learned to endure, survive and ultimately break free from the labyrinth of the Holocaust of Enslavement; the ancestors who guided this work; my daughter, Zamaniya Baderinwa Bankole; and especially to Virginia Lee Rosebud Garner, Ruby Bell Garner Allen, Todd Greathouse Allen, Sr., and Thunder Mountain who cared about it all.

PREFACE TO THE LIBERATED SCHOLARS PRESS REPRINT

In the many years since I researched and wrote the first edition of *Slavery and Medicine: Enslavement and Medical Practices in Antebellum Louisiana*, many new and exciting developments have occurred in the area within the disciplines of history and Black Studies. The academic field of slavery and medicine solidified, and various historians and Africana Studies scholars pursued the subject with enthusiasm and vigor. During this time countless scholars and graduate students contacted me about using the book for their own research; and over the years, several adopted the book for advanced courses. Since the book's release I have continued the research into slavery and medicine, and this has produced three scholarly articles (two published) and another book (unpublished). Moreover, the book *Slavery and Medicine: Enslavement and Medical Practices in Antebellum Louisiana* has been in the processes of revision (intermittently) and this important enterprise continues. However, to accommodate those still seeking the now out-of-print book, I am grateful that Liberated Scholars Press was able to reprint the original text of the manuscript with very few changes. This area of research and scholarship continues to be my passion, and I am pleased to say that I was always undeterred in its pursuit. For those who championed the book, know that it has rather humbly withstood the test of time. I also acknowledge the support of many individuals and organizations (some of whom are cited in the book); and I thank them profusely—especially the following: Dr. Michael White, Dr. Abena Lewis-Mhoon, Dr. Kokahvah Zauditu-Selassie, Dr. Claudia Nelson, Dr. Molefi Kete Asante, and Dr. Elizabeth Clark-Lewis. And, as always, I truly appreciate the support of Carlos Medina-Montes and Zamaniya Bankole. This research has been the undertaking of a lifetime, one which constantly reminds me of at least two cardinal virtues of scholarship: always ask the right question and tell the truth.

Katherine Bankole-Medina
Baltimore, Maryland
January, 2017

TABLE OF CONTENTS

Dedication

Preface to the Liberated Scholars Press Reprint

Acknowledgments   i

List of Tables   ii

Introduction   iii

PART ONE—OVERVIEW OF ENSLAVEMENT AND MEDICINE

1. The History and Scholarship of Enslavement and Medicine   1
2. "Slave Medicine": The Extent of Medical Care of Enslaved Africans   31
3. Brutality/Punishment and the Issue of Medical Health Care   37
4. Protection of Property and Legislation   49
5. Labor and Medical Health Care   57

PART TWO—AFRICANS, MEDICAL THEORIES AND PRACTICES

6. Human/Subhuman Issue: Physiological and Pseudo-Scientific Theories   81
7. Medical Management, Practices and the Hospital Experience   89
8. Medical Experiments, Treatments, Surgical Procedures and Post-Mortem Examinations   111
9. "Negro/Slave Diseases" and other Illness Attributed to or Affecting Enslaved Africans   123

PART THREE—AFRICAN MATERIA MEDICA AND ENSLAVEMENT

10	Characterizations of African Medicine	139
11	African Perceptions of Slaveocracy Medicine	145
12	The Traditional African Worldview and Medicine	149
13	African Agency in the Care and Treatment of Illness/Disease	161
	Summary and Conclusion	175
	Bibliographic Essay	183

APPENDICES

A—A List Of Related Risk Factors To Medical Health Among Enslaved Africans Of Southeastern Louisiana	205
B—Admission Book Of The Touro Infirmary 1855-1860, Enslaved Africans	207
C—Selected Pharmacopoeia Used By Enslaved Africans In The Southeastern Parishes Of Antebellum Louisiana	271
D—Glossary: Common Definitions For Selected Maladies	275
Bibliography	287
Index	317
About the Author	323

ACKNOWLEDGMENTS

I am very grateful to faculty members of Temple University's Department of African American Studies: Dr. Molefi Kete Asante, Dr. Abu Abarry, Dr. Nilgun Okur, and Dr. Emeka Nwadiora of Temple University's School of Social Administration. While I am indebted to numerous individuals and institutions, I would like to thank Ms. Catherine Kahn, Archivist at the Touro Infirmary Archives, New Orleans, Louisiana; the Amistad Research Center and the Howard Tilton Library, Louisiana Collection, of Tulane University; the libraries of Southern University at New Orleans, the University of New Orleans, and the Louisiana State University in Baton Rouge, Louisiana. I am also indebted to Ms. Nakia Laurie of Atlanta, Georgia; Ms. Sekai Adero and Mrs. Doris Clowney, both of Temple University, Philadelphia; and Ms. Colleen McMullen of the University of Pittsburgh.

LIST OF TABLES

Table		Page
1	Touro Infirmary Pregnancy, Abortion and Uterine Conditions of Enslaved African Women 1855–1860	76
2	Touro Infirmary Place of Birth of Enslaved Africans 1855–1860	97
3	Touro Infirmary Recorded Deaths of Enslaved Africans 1855–1860	99
4	Touro Infirmary Enslaved Africans Age at Time of Admission 1855–1860	101
5	Touro Infirmary Account Holders Named for Enslaved Africans 1855–1860	102
6	Touro Infirmary Maladies Attributed to Enslaved Africans 1855–1860	106
7	Touro Infirmary Marital Status of Enslaved Africans 855–1860	107
8	Touro Infirmary Enslaved Africans Gender 1855–1860	107
9	Touro Infirmary Surgical Procedures Performed upon Enslaved Africans 1855–1860	108
10	General Conceptual Components of the African Living Belief System	153

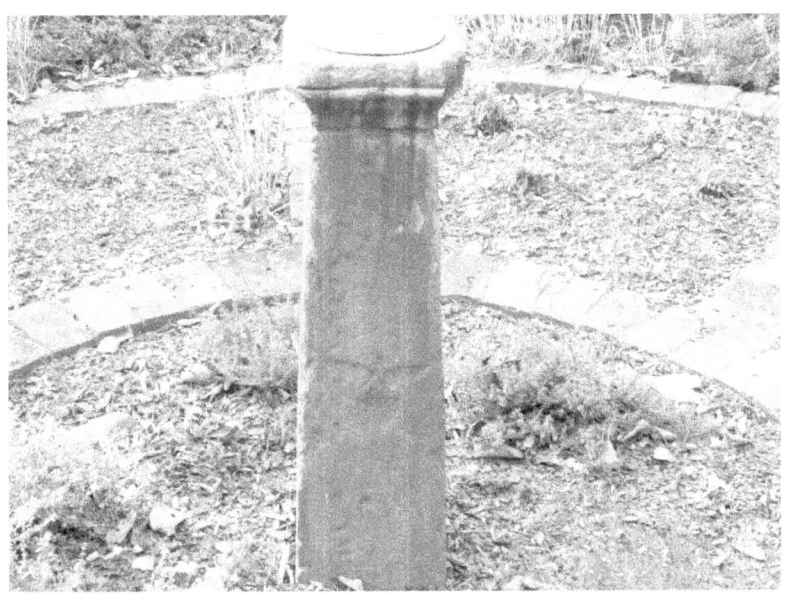

African herb garden, The Hampton Estate, Hampton National Historic Site, National Park Service. Photo by Katherine Bankole-Medina

INTRODUCTION

Enslavement and medicine historiography has not addressed the African's proactive participation in, and development of, medicine in the United States. The scholarly literature largely focuses on "Negro/Slave Medicine" and the efforts of slaveowners to acquire adequate care for the enslaved African. Enslavement and medicine scholars have contended that Africans were incapable of fostering a medical universe that was reflective of their indigenous African culture and different from the European medical legacy left to Whites. This research Afrocentrically addresses the African's proactive management of medical care; and the neglect of scholars to include brutality and punishment, and its arbitrary nature, in the enslaved African's constant need for medical attention. In addition, slave labor (particularly that involving agriculture) was found to be an important medical health risk factor, including two overlooked labor tasks of enslaved African women—breeding and concubinage. Enslaved Africans in the southeastern parishes of antebellum Louisiana retained a significant Africanism in their medical universe which was the sustained pursuit of holistic healing. Enslaved Africans operated as agents of their own medical care, and not always as dependent recipients of care from slaveowners as the literature suggests. Africans participated as diviners and dispensers of medical care (in the Babalawo and Onishegun sense, representative of the West African Yoruba tradition). However, antebellum observers and contemporary scholars have characterized the African materia medica in the institution of enslavement in the United States as "superstitious" legacies from the continent of Africa. Due to many external factors, and because of their enslavement status, Africans had a higher medical health risk (mortality and morbidity) than other members of antebellum society. Through the necessity to respond immediately to medical care issues, enslaved Africans in the diaspora demonstrated the persistence of the traditional African worldview regarding holistic well-being.

PART ONE

OVERVIEW OF ENSLAVEMENT AND MEDICINE

The enslavement of Africans and medical care in the southeastern parishes of Louisiana was influenced by four main factors: the extent of medical care provided to Africans, the impact of brutality and punishment, the protection of property and legislation, and the influence of labor upon medical health. Enslavement and medicine scholars have not reviewed the data with attention to the extent of medical care, brutality/punishment, property status and labor. Moreover, the work on the extent of medical care provided to enslaved Africans often supports the "good master" thesis—which seeks to provide a positive value judgement on the intent and actions of slaveowners in providing care. The extent of medical care is often discussed in the absence of the inherent brutality of the system; and to suggest that the existence of enslaved Africans was not as challenging as the slave narratives and oral histories suggest.

CHAPTER 1

THE HISTORY AND SCHOLARSHIP OF ENSLAVEMENT AND MEDICINE

Slavery was the worst days that was ever seed in the world. They was things past tellin', but I got the scars on my old body to show to this day. I seed worse than what happened to me. I seed them put the men and women in the stock with they hands screwed down through holes in the board and they feets tied together and they naked behinds to the world. Solomon the overseer beat them with a big whip and Massa look on. The niggers better not stop in the fields when they hear them yellin'. They cut the flesh 'most to the bones, and some they was, when they taken them out of stock and put them on the beds, they never got up again. . .I sets and 'members the times in the world. I 'members now clear as yesterday things I forgot for a long time. I 'members 'bout the days of slavery and I don't 'lieve they ever gwine have slaves no more on this earth.

Mary Reynolds
[from James Mellon's *Bullwhip Days*]

By the time the French settlement La Nouvelle Orleans (New Orleans) was founded in 1718 there were approximately 172 enslaved Africans. The city itself underwent monumental changes as the Louisiana Territory changed rulers. First, as a French colony in the "new world"; then as a holding of the Spanish from 1763; and then briefly back to French rule in 1802 until finally sold to the

SLAVERY AND MEDICINE: ENSLAVEMENT AND MEDICAL PRACTICES IN
ANTEBELLUM LOUISIANA

United States in 1803. Not long after the first Africans were brought to Louisiana, the territory's Black Code, known as Le Code Noir under the French, was brought from the French colonial holdings of the West Indies and officially outlined the rights of slaveowners and the restrictions upon African people. With each subsequent change of leadership in Louisiana the Black Code followed. In fact, each new regime in Louisiana made their own modifications to the preexistent Black Code (Wall 1990, 96).

The history of enslavement in southeastern Louisiana, and especially New Orleans is considered complex, and at times, very different from the other southern cities. Most of the various interpretations of New Orleans enslavement include the intense French, Spanish and American occupation, the phenomena of les gens de la couleur libre (free people of color some-times known as "creoles de couleur") living in close proximity to enslaved Africans; and the existence of a Black Code which applied to both enslaved Africans and the gens de couleur libre. These phenomena have caused some scholars and historians to suggest that the enslavement of Africans under French and/or Spanish domination was less harsh than under the Americans. But the gens de couleur libre enjoyed many privileges as well as many outrages to their own dignity—all tied to their quasi-free status (Ingersoll 1991, 173–200). Yet it was the enslaved African who cleared the land, performed the intensive agriculture and built the infrastructures of the city of New Orleans and southeastern Louisiana.

The unique character of southeastern Louisiana history also extend to the interpretation of the medical health care status of enslaved Africans. The various schools of thought offer analysis along a broad spectrum. There is the theory that most slaves were well cared for, especially with reference to disease and illness. The research in this arena attempts to demonstrate that, despite the inherent cruelty of the system, slaveowners possessed a sense of

SLAVERY AND MEDICINE: ENSLAVEMENT AND MEDICAL PRACTICES IN
ANTEBELLUM LOUISIANA

compassion and humanity toward enslaved Africans. Other scholars posit that slave care was a simple issue of efficient management and that medical/health care was only a priority when the health of chattel property threatened the slaveowners' investment or future earnings. In addition, there persists in southern folklore, the notion that enslaved Africans learned any medical knowledge and/or healing skills they possessed from the White slaveowners or Native American peoples.

Enslavement and medicine is a central research area for understanding the extent of illness, physical trauma and how enslaved Africans and slaveowners responded to medical/health care conditions. There is significant contention regarding the extent of medical care provided by slaveowners. There are also various interpretations of the role of enslaved Africans in providing medical care. For the purposes of this study the term "medicine" refers to any activity which engages diagnoses, treatment, or the prevention of disease, injury and other damage to the physical body or mind. This includes surgical and non-surgical treatment such as drugs, herbs, diet and other activities intended to control the physical body and to effect a cure. This research does not attempt to argue the effectiveness of the medical cures and remedies used by Africans or European Americans.

In this study the term enslavement will be used. The term enslavement "Refers to an individual who has been made a slave or reduced to servitude. . .Enslavement includes physical subjugation; (and) the exploitation of labor (means of production)" (Bankole 1995, 76). The term is a response to the neutrality and ambiguity implicit in the word "slavery" as noted by C. Tsehloane Keto (Keto 1989, 26). The term enslavement is also a response to the contemporary intellectual phenomena of equating the word "slave" with only one group of people, "Africans." The term enslavement more accurately describes a class of people (Africans)

SLAVERY AND MEDICINE: ENSLAVEMENT AND MEDICAL PRACTICES IN ANTEBELLUM LOUISIANA

subject to forced migration, bondage and involuntary labor (Slavery). As Asante notes, part of the issue with enslavement historiography is the "mental orientation" of traditional scholars who must ultimately learn to "view the people not as 'slaves' but as 'Africans'" (Asante 1993, 21). In Africology the term also refers to the mental and psychological abuse fundamental to the European trade in enslaved Africans and the Holocaust of Enslavement in general (Karenga 1993, 115–116). This study also refers to the subjects at hand, "enslaved Africans in southeastern Louisiana" as Africans, or people of African descent. In the antebellum literature Africans were often referred to as "negroes" or "niggers"; occasionally as "Ethiopes," or "blacks," and sometimes the African ethnic group was identified (Congo, Bambara, etc.). Yet collectively, especially when referring to ship's cargoes, they were referred to as Africans ("Salt Water," "Raw," or "Fresh" Africans). The masses of enslaved people were of African descent. Many of those Africans who possessed significant European admixture (designated as mulatto, quadroon, octoroon or "white niggers") were also enslaved; not because of their European (White) blood, or physical features, but ultimately because of their Africanity.

The existing scholarship examines enslavement and medicine in terms of how the slaveowner was affected by the development of the field of medicine and the health management of enslaved Africans. There are no in-depth attempts to view the African as the subject of the examination. The concerns of enslavement and medicine scholars includes such issues as: "slave diseases," "slave health," "African physiology," "surgical cases," "medical management of slaves," "racial theories," "medical experimentation," "medical costs," "slave mortality," and the "diet/nutrition" of enslaved Africans. In addition, scholars are also interested in fertility patterns, the impact of contagions and epidemics on the African population; and the belief that some slaveowners held that Africans were prone to feigning illness.

SLAVERY AND MEDICINE: ENSLAVEMENT AND MEDICAL PRACTICES IN
ANTEBELLUM LOUISIANA

The three main areas of enslavement and medicine in the antebellum period are: theory, management and experimentation. First, enslavement and medicine theories center upon the attempt at classifying African people as a race or species and the study of African physiology. Southern leaders in the study of race and the physiology of African people in the South, included antebellum physician Samuel A. Cartwright and journalist J.D.B. De Bow. These authors, and many others, believed in the idea of innate African biological inferiority and the physical and intellectual superiority of the White race.

Second, an abundance of scholarship focuses on the management of enslaved Africans and medical care. This medical management dealt with general health, disease, diet/nutrition, clothing, mortality and the medical costs incurred by slaveowners. Of the three main areas regarding enslavement and medicine, the medical management of enslaved Africans was extremely essential to the successful running of a farm or plantation. Slaveowners recognized the importance of maintaining optimal medical care of Africans because it was linked to their labor and profit potential. Antebellum society supported the needs of slaveowners by offering medical care, hospitalization and cures at a reduced cost to slaveowners. The management of enslaved Africans also included the development and dissemination of medical and scientific journals, almanacs, pamphlets and treatise.

Finally, the historical record also documents the experimental side of enslavement and medicine, including: surgical cases, experimental treatments and procedures. These studies provide the perspective of the medical doctors, expressly how they developed their practices and careers relying heavily on enslaved Africans as their subjects. The research represents the continued view of Africans as marginal beings in the White antebellum world. Africans did indeed serve as "guinea pigs" in the development of

Slavery and Medicine: Enslavement and Medical Practices in Antebellum Louisiana

surgical procedures; often subject to painful operations performed against their free will.

Surgery and experimental treatments/procedures were performed without the consent of the African. It was only necessary that the slaveowner gave consent. Surgery and experiments were risks to the slave property, but provided some cost benefit to the slaveowner. If a slaveowner consented to surgery/experiments, it was usually with an agreement that the attending physician pay for the African's food, lodging, clothing, medicine—everything associated with the procedure. This freed the slaveowners resources somewhat, and still allowed him to retain title to the slave property. The scholarship fails to acknowledge the African contribution to the development of medicine in the antebellum United States. The use of enslaved Africans in medical experiments advanced some medical careers and took many White physicians in new directions. This was during a time when the culture of White society shunned the idea of, and often refused to submit to, experimental medical treatments and surgical procedures.

In the general interpretation of these three main areas, the enslaved African is an object in relationship to his own medical experience. In each area the enslaved African is actually the central figure of the issue, yet the African's position is altered and their significance is diminished within their own history. Therefore, antebellum and contemporary studies of enslavement and medicine focus on the thoughts, feelings, ideas and experiences of the slaveowning class. The African is a victim of the slaveowner's history and experiences, especially when it comes to medical care issues. Notwithstanding this phenomena few historians acknowledge the gross victimization of the African and rarely analyze the European's motivation and rationales (Ani 1994, 95–100).

SLAVERY AND MEDICINE: ENSLAVEMENT AND MEDICAL PRACTICES IN ANTEBELLUM LOUISIANA

There is little, almost no discussion and/or analysis of the African's position regarding medicine. It is significant to note that in the general literature regarding enslavement, scholars debate and affirm the perceived quasi-human status of the African. The notion that people of African descent were not human, or at least were not the same human species as the White race permeates antebellum medical thought. In addition, Most studies do not provide discussion as to the Africans response to the medical care/treatment that he received. Furthermore, African illnesses/diseases were "separated"—categorized and made different—from the same illnesses/diseases experienced by Whites. Slaveowners, through the medical journals read by plantation physicians, were alerted to the relationship between diet/nutrition and well-being, yet because of racial beliefs and economic priorities, they rarely acted upon this knowledge.

The general health of enslaved Africans was influenced by numerous external forces (See Appendix A: A List of Related Risk Factors to Medical Health Among Africans of Southeastern Louisiana). In Louisiana, as elsewhere in the slaveocracy, the maintenance of the general health of enslaved Africans was, in a very limited sense, stated or implied in the Black Codes of the French, Spanish and American regimes. Plantations usually had their own systems for providing medical care which often rested on the report of the overseer or plantation manager. On the plantation the slaveowner, his wife, and the overseer had the final say about the care enslaved Africans received. The slaveowner made the final determination when a licensed, trained physician was consulted. However, it became quite common for large plantations to have a "plantation doctor" in residence, an infirmary or at least a "sickhouse." The slaveowners weighed the cost of medical care against the value of the enslaved African. Often physicians were called in too late to save the patient. A slaveowner might surmise that his best alternative would be to forgo medical care and work

Slavery and Medicine: Enslavement and Medical Practices in Antebellum Louisiana

the slave for the unknown number of years he or she had left. Furthermore, slaveowners often relied on ineffective home and folk remedies to cure enslaved Africans.

Mortality and morbidity were important issues to the slaveowner as death and disease affected his investment in the slave property. However, mortality is a difficult issue to accurately examine in the general scheme of the existence of the African, since so many life threatening factors presented themselves. According to John Duffy, the life of an enslaved African was precarious in that h/she:

> Suffered from their native African disorders and were brought into contact with a host of European ailments. Add to these factors, hard manual labor, a restricted diet, and the psychological impact of slavery, and it is easy to see why the slave population had to be constantly replenished (Duffy 1967, 6).

The babies of enslaved Africans had the highest mortality rate, due to poor pre-natal care, the ravages of disease and accidental (or intentional) death (Kiple and Kiple 1977, 284–306; Steckel 1986, 721–741) and in general the high mortality rate of the 1800s. For adults, mortality risks were also dictated by the behavior of the African. Capital punishment (execution) was a legal means of responding to attempts the African made to gain freedom or to retaliate against Whites through such activities as striking a White person, murder, insurrection, conspiracy and running away.

Regarding African retentions of medicine, whenever the voice of the African is presented, it is generally characterized as nothing more than the anecdotal ramblings of a largely illiterate people. The testimonies of formerly enslaved Africans are often described

SLAVERY AND MEDICINE: ENSLAVEMENT AND MEDICAL PRACTICES IN ANTEBELLUM LOUISIANA

as the "quaint folkways" of bondsmen who were the backbone to the development of the antebellum South. The narratives of former enslaved Africans are often questioned regarding their significance and validity in scholarly research (Phillips 1929, 219). A concern among historiographers is that since many of the accounts were given years after enslavement officially ended, Africans probably exaggerated the reality of the institution or were otherwise less than truthful in their testimonies and recollections.

Because of their social status, and the limited access of education to many members of White American society, the enslaved African was not educated. In the Louisiana testimonies John McDonald stated that he couldn't read or write because "if my boss-man catch me with a pencil or paper, it was twenty-five lashes" (Clayton 1990, 164–165). There were harsher penalties for Africans attempting to acquire literacy skills and there are notable exceptions regarding the educational efforts on the part of enslaved Africans and some slaveowners. However, the majority of Africans were, of course, not able to keep written records of their lives as slaves. Conversely, slaveowners kept numerous detailed records regarding the life of Africans. Many slaveowners kept birth and death records, medical records, food and supplies issued to the slave, insurance and mortgage documents, inventories of slaves (sometimes called slave rolls), bills of sale and whipping logs. The Last Will and Testament of the slaveowners, their bequest and succession documents, detailed their property holdings which included their slave property. In addition, slaveowners—largely males and the few sole White female owner/managers of slaves (Webb 1983, 49)—often kept journals and diaries and wrote letters which provide an insight into their attitudes, feelings and perspectives about enslaved Africans and often about the machinery of control which operated the institution of enslavement. Slaveowners and their families kept private and official (public) documents on transactions involving enslaved

SLAVERY AND MEDICINE: ENSLAVEMENT AND MEDICAL PRACTICES IN
ANTEBELLUM LOUISIANA

Africans; and in addition to the letters to their families, friends and colleagues, they also produced advertisements and announcements of slave sales which offer their impressions on the lot of enslaved Africans.

Years after the institution of enslavement was formally abolished, the voice of the African regarding enslavement was still not reckoned with. Some early White scholars responded to the institution of enslavement with apologist analysis and "objective" interpretations which supported the traditional views of Africans in American historiography. By 1924, the editor of the *Louisiana Historical Quarterly* commented on the study of slavery: ". . . the present generation has never been concerned with it, in any shape or form. It is for us purely a matter of history and it does not seem amiss to begin to study it now" (Dart 1924, 332). Henry P. Dart was speaking largely to the White historians who would research and record the system of enslavement in the United States, particularly the experiences of Louisiana and the old South. Dart's perspective is apologetic in tone as he acknowledges "The generations that tolerated the evil" of enslavement, further noting that the descendants of the original slaveowners "were at the worst only the innocent victims of a system created by their forefathers and scarcely to be held responsible for its errors" (Dart 1924, 333). In addition, Howard Mahorner, in "The History of Medicine in Louisiana" stated:

> One may shudder with horror at the treatment of the slaves, particularly by the slavers who imported them. But it was not only that which characterized the behavior of mankind at that particular time. Looking at it in retrospect, there is a good deal to emphasize the constancy of the prevalence of human suffering and death, which was more or less casually accepted. It was a cruel

and brutal age, as compared to the twentieth century, our recent period (Mahorner 1973, 55–56).

Therefore, enslaved Africans were denied their voice during enslavement; and after slavery formally ended, Africans were still relegated to quasi-enslavement, vis-a-vis the peonage system. Africans were confined to the status of a footnote when the histories were first being compiled and written by White scholars and historians. The descendants of these enslaved Africans, however, always made attempts to reconstruct the lives of their foreparents. For example in the case of Louisiana, Marcus B. Christian directed the Works Progress Administration's Dillard Project at a time when African American historians were routinely denied access to libraries, research institutions, and publishing houses. The Dillard Project included the oral histories of enslaved Africans of Louisiana and the efforts to collect relevant published newspaper accounts (Johnson 1979, 113–115). By the time the Works Progress Administration began comprehensive oral history projects among some of the last ex-slaves, African American scholars such as W.E.B. DuBois, Carter G. Woodson, Luther Porter Jackson and Zora Neale Hurston had already laid the foundation for bodies of knowledge which attempted to document the institution of enslavement, post-enslavement society for African Americans, and African American culture and folklore.

From an African centered perspective the institution of enslavement represented a constant threat to the medical health of enslaved Africans. The risks of enslavement included physical trauma (punishment, brutality and injuries from labor), mortality, morbidity and psychological damage. From the very beginning, the process of enslavement proved dangerous, and fatal for millions of Africans. The Africans who were captured and marched in coffles to the slaveholding factories were taken by force and those who

SLAVERY AND MEDICINE: ENSLAVEMENT AND MEDICAL PRACTICES IN ANTEBELLUM LOUISIANA

fought against enslavement escaped the fate of others only through death. The slaveholding factories, castles and slave houses along the African coast presented its own risks to the health and well-being of Africans, who were crammed into the small, damp holding cells. Subjected to these conditions, enslaved Africans were provided meager diets and exposed to contagious disease and infection.

If the African survived capture s/he had the Maafa (Middle Passage) to endure. The horrors of the Maafa are systematically well-documented (Ani 1994, 290–294; Karenga 1993, 115–142; Keto 1989, 25–31). Enslaved Africans, often chained, were packed into the holds of ships which provided little ventilation or drinkable water. Africans suffered the suffocating fecal environment, and communicable diseases. Enslaved Africans and non-African participant-observers give similar accounts of the conditions on-board slave ships which would give rise to the need for medical care. Olaudah Equiano, in *The Interesting Narrative of the Life of Olaudah Equiano, or Gustavus Vassa, The African*, recounted the following:

> The stench of the hold, while we were on the coast, was so intolerably loathsome, that it was dangerous to remain there for any time, and some of us had been permitted to stay on the deck for the fresh air; but now that the whole ship's cargo were confined together, it became absolutely pestilential. The closeness of the place, and the heat of the climate, added to the number in the ship, being so crowded that each had scarcely room to turn himself, almost suffocated us. This produced copious perspirations, so that the air soon became unfit for respiration, from a variety of loathsome smells, and brought on a sickness

Slavery and Medicine: Enslavement and Medical Practices in Antebellum Louisiana

> among the slaves, of which many died, thus falling victims to the improvident avarice, as I may call it, of their purchasers. This deplorable situation was again aggravated by the galling of the chains, now become insupportable; and the filth of necessary tubs, into which the children often fell, and were almost suffocated. The shrieks of the women, and the groans of the dying, rendered it a scene of horror almost inconceivable (Gates 1987, 35).

Ships crews, usually a ships physician, were responsible for a minimum of care to maximize the profit of the cargo. According to the account of one slave ship surgeon:

> fluxes and fevers among the negroes resulted. While they were in this situation, my profession requiring it, I frequently went down among them, till at length their apartments became so extremely hot as to be only sufferable for a very short time. But the excessive heat was not the only thing that rendered their situation intolerable. The deck, that is the floor of their rooms, was so covered with the blood and mucus which had proceeded from them in consequence of the flux, that it resembled a slaughterhouse (d'Auvergne 1933, 27).

They expected a high mortality rate among Africans under these circumstances which accounts for the over-packing of slaving vessels. Under guarded conditions, Africans were required to move their limbs on deck and present themselves for inspection. There are documented cases where Africans took advantage of the forced exercised and mutinied, but more often jumped overboard and drowned accidentally (or intentionally) or were attacked by sharks in the surrounding waters. Slave ship crews often removed the bodies of Africans (men, women and children) who "mysteriously" died during the night and dumped their bodies overboard. Removing the corpses was a mandatory health requirement; as was exercising and supplying water to the bodies of Africans. In addition, African women were, very early on, the victims of shipboard sexual exploitation from the White crew before they were sold at the various auction blocks.

When slave ships docked in the Caribbean Islands, enslaved Africans began the process of "seasoning." Seasoning was often a necessary requirement in making slaves. This process involved the physical, and accompanying psychological, indoctrination/abuse in order to "break" the African's spirit of resistance to enslavement. On the hot and humid plantations of the Caribbean, the African was introduced to the arduous agricultural requirements of enslavement. The intensive labor of the West Indies also brought enslaved Africans an introduction to the plantation punishments which would be a significant feature of the North American system of enslavement. The seasoning process continued throughout the life of the slave, where every opportunity to remind the African of h/her enslavement status was taken.

Plantation punishments were important factors to the health care status of enslaved Africans because, despite some legally stated restrictions, they were wholly arbitrary. Slaveowners determined how Africans would be punished, for what reasons and the frequency and duration of the punishment. The slaveowner's wife also provided punishment at her own, or her husband's discretion. Another key person, often responsible for the most consistent form of punishment and the cruelest brutality, where the largest groups of Africans were concerned, was the plantation overseer. For research purposes, plantation punishments are challenging to study because some slaveowners kept records of punishments,

SLAVERY AND MEDICINE: ENSLAVEMENT AND MEDICAL PRACTICES IN
ANTEBELLUM LOUISIANA

such as "whipping logs," while many others did not. Africans such as Olaudah Equiano, Solomon Northup, and Frederick Douglass describe some of the punishment meted out to enslaved Africans. Some White chroniclers have noted that even if a slaveowner objected to the punishment practices of another he was more than reluctant to report his neighbor to territorial governing bodies. In addition, while some states said that a slave could press charges against the slaveowners for cruelty, significant numbers of enslaved Africans almost never exercised this option. Given the threat of retaliation and the socialization process of Africans, it was impossible for appreciable numbers of Africans in the institution of enslavement to do so.

Plantation punishments included: whipping/ beatings, branding, ridicule, isolation, field-work, prison, stockades, rape and mutilation. Africans who continued to present problems to the slaveowner could expect an increase in the severity of the punishments, to be placed in the city jails, or to be sold away. Plantation punishments cannot be dismissed as the result of a few overzealous slaveowners; especially since they also served another important purpose—controlling the general slave population. On large plantations, slaves were rarely punished in private in the old South and certainly if so, the results of their infraction was made known to other enslaved Africans. This served to instill fear and obedience in the masses of enslaved Africans.

When a slave committed a crime (and resistance activities were always considered criminal), a supplemental set of rules augmented those of the slaveowner to punish the slave. Slaves who primarily inhabited the urban areas were most subject to criminal prosecution. Enslaved Africans who were accused and found guilty of theft, rape and murder could expect the chain gang, torture, and very often, capital punishment. Enslaved Africans involved in both the agricultural and domestic occupations were subject to criminal

Slavery and Medicine: Enslavement and Medical Practices in Antebellum Louisiana

prosecution for conspiracy to commit murder and for murdering the slaveowner, overseer or some other White person. If found guilty of conspiracy or murder, the African could be executed. The execution of Africans for these crimes did not necessarily reflect the loss of the financial investment made by the slaveowner. There was a system of compensation by many governing bodies if a slave was executed for insurrection or conspiracy. Further, if an enslaved African was maimed or killed by another person, for example, through a "secondary slaveowner" who hired the slave from his original owner, the secondary slaveowner could be sued to pay the value of the slave to the original slaveowner.

Enslaved Africans who ran away from bondage also jeopardized their health status in a number of ways. Many enslavement historians note among the reasons Africans ran away was the poor living conditions of slaves. Historians often cite poor diet, physical abuse, etc. as the main reasons for Africans running away (Wall 1990, 174); very little analysis posits that a main motivation was the African's desire for freedom. Despite the literature praising the slaveowners efforts in caring for his slaves, some did not provide adequate diets, shelter, clothing or medical care. In conjunction with dire nutrition, slaves also ran to escape cruel slaveowners and their overseers who physically abused them. Before running away, Africans often took provisions. When they ran out, they supplemented their diet with what the swamps, forests and hills provided, and they often went back to their former plantations for more provisions. Another important legacy of the African under slavery was the establishment of maroon communities. The more successful maroon communities provided for the nutritional needs of its members and some have been known to trade goods with poor Whites. Those Africans who did not become part of the maroon societies, and who were not successful living in isolation (in the swamps, marshes, caves, forests and hills) until the Jubilation, were captured and subjected to severe consequences. If

Slavery and Medicine: Enslavement and Medical Practices in Antebellum Louisiana

not sold away, a runaway was summarily punished. One slaveowner stated that he could tolerate almost any behavior from a slave except running away. Runaways were usually stripped, bound and whipped (the laws varied, but often included a specified number of lash strokes to be administered) and then their backs were washed in brine, a salt solution, to intensify the pain. Chronic runaways would be locked in plantation prisons each night and on weekends after laboring in the fields. Other chronic runaways were permanently consigned to the prisons of the towns and cities often labeled "the old ball and chain." In Louisiana an acceptable punishment for runaway slaves was branding them with the fleur-de-lis, a three-petal iris which represented the King of France, also known as the Bourbon Lily (Dunbar-Nelson 1916, 364).

Punishments for insurrections planned and carried out by Africans were covered by the Black or Slave Codes. Insurrection activities usually mandated capital punishment (execution) and had an impact on Africans in general. The word of slave insurrections travelled far and near and usually resulted in a harsher implementation of the slave codes and plantation punishments. Africans indirectly involved in insurrections (for example, having knowledge but refusing to report it to the slaveowner) were also punished. All enslaved Africans could look forward to insurrection punishments being used as examples of what could happen to them if they tried this avenue of self-liberation. Punishment for insurrections and rumors of rebellion added to the mortality risk of enslaved Africans and caused overseers to remind the African population of who controlled them physically and psychologically.

The occupational health hazards rooted in the institution of enslavement were numerous. Regardless of whether enslaved Africans labored in the fields or in the "big" house; in the cities or the plantations, they were all subject to slaveowner punishments, diseases of the time and ailments specific to certain regions, crops

Slavery and Medicine: Enslavement and Medical Practices in Antebellum Louisiana

and types of labor. In Louisiana cotton and sugar were major crops to the agricultural slaveowners, and the sugar industry was an indicator of swift mortality among enslaved Africans. Slaveowners gave Africans a life expectancy of approximately five years once they began sugar labor (Moody 1924, 232–253). Whenever machinery was used in labor, there was the increased chance of injury. The long hours and backbreaking labor kept Africans in peril of work related ailments and injuries. If an African was fortunate he or she got permission, after an eighteen hour day, to cultivate a small garden "patch" ("kitchen garden," "nigger grounds") next to the slave quarters. While this provided a meager vegetable (vitamin C) supplement to the diet, the extra time it took to maintain added to the physical stress on the enslaved African.

Enslaved Africans contracted the same diseases and ailments as the White descendants of Europeans, yet Africans were purported to have their own special pathology, labeled "negro diseases," "African fevers," etc. Africans proved to be more immune to certain diseases of Europeans than Native American people, yet Africans also died from these diseases. While the yellow fever epidemic of 1853 devastated the White European population of Louisiana, statistics suggest that Africans suffered less from the ravages of the disease because of the immunity they brought from Africa. But regardless of their occupation, enslaved Africans suffered from a myriad of health ailments. In addition to fractures, puncture wounds and general injuries, hospital records and the research of area scholars indicate that enslaved Africans also suffered significantly from yellow fever (labeled "Vomito Negro," "Black Vomit," and the "Saffron Scourge"). Enslaved Africans were considered to be relatively immune to malaria and yellow fever because of their exposure to these diseases on the continent of Africa; antebellum statistics reinforce this belief in African immunity, however, some scholars disagree with the idea of a significant African immunity to these diseases. However, in

SLAVERY AND MEDICINE: ENSLAVEMENT AND MEDICAL PRACTICES IN ANTEBELLUM LOUISIANA

addition to malaria and yellow fever, a host of other "maladies" affecting Africans included: yaws, fevers, cholera, scrofula, dysentery, typhoid pneumonia, syphilis, gonorrhea, bronchitis, catarrh, hernias, convulsions, worms, diarrhea, consumption, urinal retention, eczema, constipation, necrosis, small pox, hemorrhoids, gastric problems, pellagra (Black Tongue), asthma, measles and the common cold. Furthermore, African women also had difficult births, cesarian sections, vaginal/uterine fistulas, premature abortions (miscarriages), irregular discharges, tumors, amenorrhea, dysmenorrhea, menorrhea and prolaspsis of the uterus (falling of the womb). Enslaved Africans were also treated for hysteria, indisposition, "rascality," dirt-eating (Cachexia Africana), and running away (Drapetomania).

The latter conditions, Cachexia Africana and Drapetomania, are significant because they are accompanied by detailed racial theories citing the "inferiority of the African race." The racist thought of the antebellum period sought to justify the institution of enslavement and to respond aggressively to the anti-slavery movement. The racist ideas expounded upon the following premises. First, that the White race was intellectually and physiologically superior to the Black race; second, the African (Black) race was in fact the most inferior among all the races of men; third, that African people possessed a unique physical body which (while inferior to Whites) allowed them to work like beasts of the field; fourth, because of this unique African physiology and innate inferiority, Africans required special medical care/treatment; finally, the very humanity of the African was questionable, such that (given all of the above), the White man and the African would never be equal in mind, body or spirit. Some of the prominent medical doctors and researchers of the time go on to assert that certain illnesses were selective to the White European race, and because of the inferiority of Africans, such "superior race" diseases would never enter the body of the African and cause illness.

SLAVERY AND MEDICINE: ENSLAVEMENT AND MEDICAL PRACTICES IN ANTEBELLUM LOUISIANA

Notwithstanding the racist theories about African humanity, slaveowners, concerned about their investment and the future labor the African would accomplish, provided medical care after it could be determined whether or not the African was feigning illness and if the condition was serious and persisted beyond a certain period of time. A better indicator of illness was when several slaves contracted the same disease and were sick at the same time which was quite common. Normally, slaveowners made the determination of the health status of the African, yet the mistress of the plantation, the plantation manager and the overseer also made major health care decisions for the African.

Enslaved Africans were subject to mutilations as evidenced in the antebellum advertisements regarding the sale of slaves and to inform the public about the distinguishing characteristics of some runaway slaves. Specifically, these mutilations included: the loss of digits, scars, burns, loss of ears or pieces, missing teeth, a lost eye, branding, knife wounds, and crippled or missing limbs (Weld 1839, 77–84). The advertisements almost never indicate that the slaveowner or overseer mutilated the slave. The descriptions are for identification purposes only, however, the advertisements for the sale of Africans also served to provide clues as to the physical health status, and perhaps even the demeanor of the enslaved African. The advertisements do not tell us whether there is any evidence of self-mutilation, overseer punishments or altercations with other enslaved Africans. Like plantation punishments, mutilations were arbitrary and would not be questioned by outsiders except for the most extreme cases.

The legislated Black Codes allowed each slaveholding state to prescribe their own set of rules governing slave and slaveowner conduct, and the rules and regulations regarding the punishment of slaves. In the Louisiana territory the rules regarding enslaved Africans were detailed under the governance of the French, the

SLAVERY AND MEDICINE: ENSLAVEMENT AND MEDICAL PRACTICES IN ANTEBELLUM LOUISIANA

Spanish and the Americans. In 1724 the French colonizers adopted the 1685 Code Noir (Black Code or Edict of the King of France) which outlined the obligations and rights of slaveowners regarding their slaves and included provisions with reference to punishments (Riddell 1925, 321–329). For example, in 1728 an enslaved African called Biron, from the Bambara ethnic group who had come to Louisiana on the slave ship "L'Aurore," was brought before the Superior Council of Louisiana on charges of being a runaway and for taking his master's gun. Biron was found in "rebellion against his master; all the more punishment from the fact that the number of negroes is increasing in this colony, and that one would not be in safety on the distant plantations." In accordance with the Code Noir, Biron was sentenced to be "whipped at the foot of the gallows and sent back to his master, forbidding him to repeat the offense under penalty of corporal punishment" (Cruzat 1925, 24–25).

While the gens de la coleur libre (free people of color) were also included in the Code Noir, the Louisiana Code Noir and Police Codes were introduced largely to address the movement and behavior of Africans. The Spanish controlled Louisiana from 1763 and by 1769 they had made small changes to Code Noir. The Spanish version was included in Las Siete Partidas (the Code of Seven Parts) which originated in 1348 and included the elements of Roman and Cannon Law (Oppenheim 1973, 1–9). It was called "O'Reilly's Code," named after General Alejandro O'Reilly who brought the Louisiana government under Spanish control. In 1785 the Spanish Black Code became more stringent for enslaved Africans and the gens de la coleur libre. It was not long after the Louisiana Territory was sold to the Americans, that an even more rigid Black Code was established. By the early 1800s a plantation manager or overseer was mandatory for every plantation. The Americans adopted the Black Codes of the French and Spanish colonizers and added them to their territorial acts, which were used

SLAVERY AND MEDICINE: ENSLAVEMENT AND MEDICAL PRACTICES IN ANTEBELLUM LOUISIANA

by the slave patrols and police juries in disciplining enslaved Africans.

It is difficult to discern from antebellum records what Africans thought about the European's practice of medicine. To be sure, slave narratives indicate that some Africans believed their slaveowners to be "good masters" because they seemed to provide adequate medical care in a timely manner. On the other hand, since no one kept detailed records of what the slaves thought of their condition or treatment, we do not know much about those Africans who refused treatment or who hid maladies to keep from being administered treatment. The folklore of the post-bellum period indicates that some Africans expressed a significant fear of doctors and hospitals. There is documentation and the persistence of legends regarding "night doctors" who allegedly paid slaves and/or poor Whites to dig up freshly buried corpses. There are additional myths which suggest that Africans feared the Night Riders for reasons other than punishment for being caught off the plantation without a pass (Fry 1975, 170–197). The idea here is that some doctors might have paid people to murder unsuspecting Africans and then their bodies were used for medical demonstration and dissection. However, these extreme measures were not always necessary since there is evidence of compliance in securing bodies for dissection. After the execution of Nat Turner on November 11, 1831 "His body, after death, was given over to the surgeons for dissection" (Ducas et al. 1970, 123).

We do know that Africans were used for medical experimentation and administered treatment and procedures which would not have been performed on the general White population at the time. Slaveowners allowed Africans to be used for such purposes in a first attempt to cure the slave and, hopefully, make h/she ready to return to labor. In these cases, doctors took the responsibility for feeding, housing and providing the necessary

Slavery and Medicine: Enslavement and Medical Practices in Antebellum Louisiana

medication for the slave in exchange for the opportunity to perform, what was oftentimes, risky treatments and procedures. Doctors also sustained the risks of being sued by the slaveowner if the slave died as a result of the experimental medical care/treatment. Physicians such as J. Marion Sims performed surgical experiments upon enslaved African women and left a record of his use of them. The slave women were not able to tell their side of the story, yet Sims noted in one case: "Lucy's agony was extreme. She was much prostrated and I thought that she was going to die. . .It took Lucy two or three months to recover entirely from the effects of the operation" (Sims 1884, 238–239). With reference to Louisiana and other areas of the lower South, these medical experiments, surgical procedures and treatments have been discussed extensively in *De Bow's Review*, the *New Orleans Medical and Surgical Journal* and other antebellum medical, scientific and agricultural/industrial journals.

Experiments upon enslaved Africans ranged from procedures regarding vaginal/uterine disorders to amputations, and all were important to the development of medicine in the United States territory and especially to the old South. Physicians kept detailed records regarding the number of surgical procedures required to facilitate a successful recovery. However, we do not know how the African responded to the surgical procedures and/or if h/she was given a choice as to certain treatments; or if h/she even understood the experimental nature of certain procedures. Nonetheless, Africans made prime candidates for medical experimentation because of their restricted social status and because, ultimately, no permission from the African was legally required. And in the case of an unsuccessful treatment or procedure, generally the physician only had to answer to the slaveowner.

In the antebellum South "slave medicine" constituted a collection of plantation procedures and apparatus, visiting physicians, physicians-in-residence or physicians on retainer (or on call), and the use of plantation and/or city hospitals and infirmaries. Since the primary goal was to re-establish the health of the African so that h/she could continue to labor on behalf of the slaveowner, precautions were put in place to save the slaveowner money; and records indicate that enslaved Africans were provided medical care in some consistent manner:

> since slave owners had an economic stake in the health of their "chattel," it was not unknown for a Louisiana owner to provide medical care for his slaves. Some owners contracted with physicians for routine visits to the slave quarters (though most care was much less systematic and based on the economic bottom line). Other owners provided yearly physical examinations for the plantation's slaves. Some owners transported slaves to doctors on an as-needed basis. Owners considered preventive health maintenance a simple matter of economy—it made good business sense to protect one's investment. A sick slave could not work or could not work as efficiently as desired. And a dead slave represented a total loss on the owner's financial investment (Bodin 1990, 13–14).

Large plantations usually had hospitals or infirmaries (sometimes known as "sickhouses") which were usually staffed by enslaved African women even though the preference was for a White person. Some physicians found a career in servicing plantations on a regular basis, while city hospitals and infirmaries hosted Africans as patients for very serious illnesses. Generally, an enslaved African who was ill reported or had the illness reported to the overseer, plantation manager, the slaveowner or his wife.

SLAVERY AND MEDICINE: ENSLAVEMENT AND MEDICAL PRACTICES IN ANTEBELLUM LOUISIANA

Overseers had the responsibility of identifying ill slaves and reporting them himself. The slaveowner had the ultimate say as to when medical care would be provided to the slave since it was his expense. Yet when the slaveowner was not available, the determination of treatment and cost had to be made by the next in charge which was usually the plantation manager and/or the mistress of the house. A major question regarding enslavement and medicine is how long was the slave ill before actual care was sought? An enslaved person may not come forward immediately with an illness. Furthermore, such a person may not recognize an illness from, for example, fatigue from labor or pregnancy. It is difficult to determine, yet some hospital records indicate that slaves could be sick for weeks or months before being brought to the hospitals. On isolated plantations and farms, slaveowners had some difficulty and lengthy travel which affected their ability to respond to the illnesses of Africans in a timely manner, which was why plantation hospitals were so important.

Slaveowners, of course, did not find it difficult to differentiate the African as a member of human society from chattel property. The African represented a significant investment in moveable personal property. Records left do not indicate that slaveowners took any serious interest in African knowledge of medicine and healing unless African practitioners were unusually successful in cases where they had failed. Certainly such knowledge was often considered more evidence of "African savagery." Slaveowners perceived African attitudes toward healing as representative of "native" or "negro superstitions." Slaveowners were concerned about the spread of African spiritual beliefs, which all have been generically labeled as "Voodoo," and sometimes "Hoodoo." However, much of the structure and ritual of Voodoo involved healing. Slave narratives highlight the use of Voodoo and the African materia medica used to effect cures for illnesses. Voodoo is an important example of the diasporan African's worldview regarding medicine. This African worldview is dependent upon the premise that human prosperity was inextricably intertwined to physical and psychological well-being.

The narratives of former slaves are filled with information about the medical treatment provided by the slaveowners and their own efforts to utilize folk knowledge and African retentions in healing. Many of these Africans gave testimony of their lives as slaves sixty-five to seventy-five years after enslavement had ended in the 1930s and 1940s. A large portion of these narratives were from people who were born on the eve of or during the Civil War and therefore recounted the life, experiences and traditions of their parents, relatives and other elders who survived the Holocaust of Enslavement. Survivors of enslavement remembered the stories and songs of their ancestors. They recounted their experiences as children and young adults in the institution of enslavement. They describe the herbal medicine and belief system of the enslaved African. Yet even the narratives themselves, especially those conducted by the Louisiana Writers Project, were carried out with a measure of bias that the project director and the participants did not discern. For example, the Louisiana Writer's Project interviewers (only two were African American) were encouraged to gather as much information as possible on slavery and folk beliefs with reference to "superstitions." Yet on their questionnaire they failed to ask any questions regarding the African's heritage and how such knowledge could inform the interview. There were participants in the study who were between 80 and 100 years old or more who might have provided more insight on their African origins and the ancestral origins of their parents. In addition, the interviews indicate that many of the participants were suspicious of the interviewers, as most of them were living very frugal lives in their old age and felt that the White ("government") interviewers might somehow threaten their meager incomes.

SLAVERY AND MEDICINE: ENSLAVEMENT AND MEDICAL PRACTICES IN ANTEBELLUM LOUISIANA

In the literature related to the early African experience in America, Africans are perceived as passive participants in a cruel and brutal (yet necessary) economic system which would, eventually, make them better beings and elevate them to the scale of human. This view still permeates today, especially in the area of enslavement and medicine. The Eurocentric historiography on enslavement and medicine continues to exploit the themes of slaveowner as victim of a system which he inherited; and the African as beneficiary of the brutality, conflicts and challenges inherent in the "peculiar institution."

The primary source documents of the antebellum South detail the inhuman treatment of Africans, yet recent scholarly studies fail to acknowledge any relationship, or even an attempt at a correlation between, brutality and the medical care needs of Africans. Further, in the effort to show that enslaved African's ideas of medical cures were wholly rooted in delusional fears, researchers included those aspects which seemed to demonstrate this phenomena. The victimization of Africans in medicine is not well documented and is rarely acknowledged in the contemporary interpretive scholarship.

Yet the spiritual folklore of enslaved Africans cites the belief, even among the most oppressed of the Africans, that h/she could look forward to an afterlife of peace. The attempt at spiritual redemption (Tate 1991, 213–222) was necessary to surviving enslavement. The enslaved Africans who were taught selected portions of the Bible (while largely distorted to support the slaveowner's position) could envision for themselves the necessity of "heaven," "going home," and the "promised land." In that realm of life after death, the African would be far removed from slavery. And it was the African's hope that they would not be "buried in the land of slaves," as Frances Ellen Watkins Harper wrote. This transplanted African spirituality was often a major component of the African's medical universe during the antebellum period.

For many enslaved Africans, even death offered no peace or comfort for those who were left to remember the departed. We know from the previous research in the field of "slave medicine" in the United States that many enslaved Africans were used as subjects for experimental treatments and medicines; and that the corpses of Africans were used for demonstration purposes at medical schools. Knowledge of this use of Africans after death had a profound impact upon the African community and is demonstrated in the slave narratives and in African American folklore. This field of American medicine has left a body of knowledge which has been largely uncovered and in need of scholarly critique. There are numerous reasons why this study is significant to the discourse in the area of enslavement and medicine. There are issues of antebellum ethics, the African's contribution to medical development, further "proof" to Whites that Africans were inferior beings, and the incidence of "slave medicine," with respect to the use of African corpses, as another mechanism to control and contain the enslaved population.

The system of enslavement was consistently harmful to the physical existence of African people. The African could never achieve optimal physical (or psychological) health under the institution of enslavement. Despite their experience in and contribution to the European American world of medicine, Africans garner little historical and intellectual respect, and even less scholarly acknowledgement. The African voice regarding the development of medical knowledge and care in the United States is largely ignored by Eurocentric scholarship. The findings of enslavement and medicine research provide evidence of the strength and fortitude of African people who survived the system of enslavement, and whose voices speak, not only to the reality of victimization, but also to the African's desire to be heard, remembered and respected as a member of humanity..

CHAPTER 2

"SLAVE MEDICINE": THE EXTENT OF MEDICAL CARE OF ENSLAVED AFRICANS

>We ain't had no doctor. Our missus and one of the slaves would attend the sick.
>
>*Adele Frost*

>The medicine I remember was castor oil and dogwood and cherry bark, which they put in whiskey and give you. They give you this to keep your blood good. Dogwood will bitter your blood; it good medicine, I know.
>
>*Amy Perry*

>Our master and missus was good to us when we was sick. They send for the doctor right off and the doctor do all he could for us, but he ain't had no kind of medicine to give us 'cepting spirits of turpentine, castor oil and a little blue mass. They ain't had all kinds of pills and stuff then, like they has now.
>
>*Fannie Griffin*

Major issues regarding the extent of medical care of enslaved Africans include: the extent of illness, the type of illness, the quality of medical care provided, and the congruency of the medical maintenance theory in reference to enslaved African people. Scholarly interpretations vary, however, slaveowners perceived a slaveocracy where enslaved Africans were continuously and consistently cared for. Enslaved Africans confirm that they were provided care by the slaveowners, that slaveowners also denied care when they thought Africans were feigning illness, and they relate the various circumstances which led to medical health conditions. Characteristics of extent of medical care include: 1) the

Slavery and Medicine: Enslavement and Medical Practices in Antebellum Louisiana

slaveowners' perspective; 2) the enslaved Africans perspective; 3) the differing medical care roles of Whites and enslaved Africans; 4) critical/acute care of enslaved Africans; and 5) general health maintenance.

The interest in the health status of enslaved Africans began in the slave holding factories of West Africa, continued on to the seasoning process of the Caribbean and subsequently can be found in the slave trading pens of the South. Often slaveowners equate the care they provided to enslaved Africans to the care provided to horses or other farm/plantation animals. According to Solomon Northup, who was kidnapped into the system of enslavement and brought to Louisiana, ". . .many customers called to examine Freeman's 'new lot'. . .He would make us hold up our heads, walk briskly back and forth, while customers would feel of our hands and arms and bodies, turn us about, ask us what we could do, make us open our mouths and show our teeth, precisely as a jockey examines a horse. . .Sometimes a man or woman was taken back to the small house in the yard, stripped, and inspected more minutely. Scars upon a slave's back were considered evidence of a rebellious or unruly spirit, and hurt his sale" (Eakin and Logsdon 1968, 52–53). Numerous enslaved Africans from various parts of the lower south speak to the general maintenance of Africans held in slave pens before slave sales. Mr. Chapman, a former enslaved African of Memphis, Tennessee noted:

> Me and my brother was in the trading yard before the Civil War. We stayed in there three or four weeks. They would fix us all up and carry us in a great big old room and circle us all around every morning and every evening. They would have us up in the show room to show us to the people. They would hit us in the breast to see if we was strong and sound. Monkeys would play with us and see if any boogies was in our heads. They would do pretty well if they found any, but if

> they didn't they would slap us. They had the monkeys there to keep our heads clean. They made us dance and made us take exercise all the time we was there (Johnson 1945, 33).

Slaveowners' perspectives regarding medical care for Africans varied. While most slaveowners emphasized the medical care they provided to enslaved Africans, a few among their ranks (notably women) provided another perspective. Frances Ann Kemble, mistress of Butler's Island in 1839 described several chronic and acute care cases among enslaved Africans, noting that the physician "visits the estate whenever medical assistance is required" (Rose 1976, 421). New Orleans served as an important gauge for the socio-economic status of the old South, and of course significantly influenced southern Louisiana. Medical historians emphasize the general status of health care coupled with the environmental factors of Louisiana:

> The immigrants—the newcomers—were more prone to develop infectious diseases. Yellow fever, smallpox, dysentery, were all highly contagious to them, and the mortality was extremely high. Part of this was due to the lack of knowledge of sanitation and public health measures. The first people of New Orleans got their water from the Mississippi River. This was clean and unpolluted at that time; after standing, it became clear and was fit for drinking. As time passed, there are repeated stories of poor sanitation and the failure to proper disposal of human refuse, carrion, dead dogs and cats, and stagnant water, which was customarily found up to about 1861 (Mahorner 1973, 55).

Enslaved Africans were at a higher risk of suffering significant medical health conditions. As forced immigrants they suffered numerous infections on slave ships (Mahorner 1973, 55). In the antebellum hospitals enslaved Africans were treated for yellow fever, cholera, small pox and dysentery in significant numbers. Their living conditions, especially on the developing plantations and farms, exposed them, much more than Whites, to the poor sanitation of the slave "quarters" and the necessity for potable water.

Slave planters provided specific details and observations on the "care of negro slaves." Louisiana planters offered advice on feeding and cleanliness as a regiment to good health care. For example, a Louisiana planter in 1856, who possessed a large force of enslaved Africans, noted:

> See that the negroes are regularly fed, and that their food is wholesome, nutritious and well cooked, and that they keep themselves clean. At least once in every week, a visit each of their houses, and see that they have been swept out and cleaned; examine their bedding, &c. . .The manager will, every Sunday morning after breakfast, visit and inspect every quarter, see that the houses and yards are kept clean and in order, and that the families are dressed in clean clothes . . . The negroes will not be permitted (and it is here particularly enjoined on the overseers not to suffer them) to have barrels, ashes, chicken-coops, or trash, or filth of any kind under or about their houses (Acklen 1856, 617–20).

Many enslaved Africans were reminded of the plantation policies on cleanliness. Formerly enslaved in Louisiana, Elizabeth Ross Hite recalled:

> We slept on wooden beds wid fresh moss mattress. Our bed was kept clean, much cleaner

SLAVERY AND MEDICINE: ENSLAVEMENT AND MEDICAL PRACTICES IN ANTEBELLUM LOUISIANA

> den de beds of today. Dey was scrubbed every Saturday. Dere wasn't a chinch [bug] on a one of dem. Better not see a chinch on a bed. De master would sure fuss about it. I remember one day another master brought one of his slaves over wid him when he came to see my master's daughter. And de first thing my master wanted to know was did dat darky have any fleas, bugs, or chinches on him (Clayton 1990, 99).

Slaveowners knew that seemingly innocuous insects and creatures could cause health problems for enslaved Africans. They often stringently enforced those regimens which attempted to maintain a standard of health among enslaved Africans and which supported optimal labor production.

Slaveowners and overseers were concerned with whether or not Africans feigned illness. To an industrious and indebted slaveowner, a non-working, non-productive slave had the same value as a dead slave. A sick slave who was not cared for was useless. Slaveowners were on guard against false sickness among enslaved Africans. An absentee Louisiana sugar planter in Ascension and Terrebonne parishes noted, "People must be well taken care of when sick and must be punished always if they lay up when not sick. . ." (Sitterson 1967, 69). Enslaved Africans' oral histories have noted that feigning illness was used as a defiant response to the institution of enslavement. However, since prevailing stereotypes suggested that Africans were predisposed to lying and immoral behavior, the assumption among cautious overseers was that they were, more often than not, pretending to be sick, unless their illness was obvious. Solomon Northup related his experience in Louisiana after sustaining injuries from labor punishment:

> . . . when the busy season of cotton picking was at hand, I was unable to leave my cabin. Up

> to this time I had received no medicine, nor any attention from my master or mistress. The old cook visited me occasionally, preparing me corn-coffee, and sometimes boiling a bit of bacon, when I had grown too feeble to accomplish it myself.
>
> When it was said that I would die, Master Epps, unwilling to bear the loss, which the death of an animal worth a thousand dollars would bring upon him, concluded to incur the expense of sending to Holmesville for Dr. Wines (Eakin and Logsdon 1968, 134).

The extent of medical care was consistent with the slaveowners' desire to profit from his investment. It also created a precarious situation for the enslaved African, who might be accused of feigning illness or who may not have reported the illness at all. For a multitude of reasons a condition or illness may not be immediately attended to. Certainly, when a valuable slave was threatened with death, doctors were called in quickly and care was administered with some consistency.

CHAPTER 3

BRUTALITY/PUNISHMENT AND THE ISSUE OF MEDICAL HEALTH CARE

> My missis and boss both were cruel, for I know how dey had dem poor nigger[s] beat. I saw my grandma whipped until she had scars on her dat was dere when I got grown. My other grandma got branded with hot irons. When dey would be in de fields, the driver was always over dem with a bull whip; and he sho didn't mind using it.
>
> *Silas Spotfore*

Brutality/punishment is a signal feature of the system of enslavement in North America. Slaveowners speak of plantation punishments; necessary and accepted activities to teach and remind Africans of their bondage and to redress "slave crimes." However, more than the implication of "punishment," enslaved Africans recall slaveocracy brutality, arbitrary violence and physical retribution for their powerlessness. In retrospect, the enslaved African and the slaveowner probably agreed more on the factual nature of brutality/punishment than any other aspect of the institution of enslavement. While slaveowners described what they considered the necessary punishment to control and contain the African population; enslaved Africans, in their letters, narratives, and oral histories, describe physical violence and abuse.

Among Louisiana historians, there is contention as to who imported the most brutal system of enslavement, the French, Spanish or the Americans? Enslaved Africans of southeastern Louisiana do make some slight distinctions, e.g. "'my master didn't whip us much, but I know of others who whipped slaves all the time.'" It is interesting to note that French and Spanish participant/observers of the slaveocracy blame the Americans; and the Americans blame the "foreigners," the French and Spanish creoles. Among the former enslaved African interviewees of

Louisiana, Mary Harris provided her opinion:

> The plantation was owned by Mr. Gaudet, and I've heard-tell that Frenchmen were the hardest people and almost squeezed blood out of their slaves. With Americans it was different. So just set it down when you hear of brutal treatment, that it was foreigners (Clayton 1990, 95).

Other former enslaved Africans express the opposite opinion, citing that it was the Americans who were the most violent and brutal while the French and Spanish creoles were lenient on the Africans. The voice of the African however, regardless of their opinions, indicates that both groups provided significant examples of violence and brutality; and that both groups expressed, at times, some sense of concern for Africans who were brutalized. Regardless of which people perpetrated "the most" violence against African people in the slaveocracy, the system in its entirety promoted a continuous cycle of medical risk due to physical violence:

> Slaves faced one medical risk which their masters did not—the effects of punishment, most commonly whipping. Whipping caused unspeakable pain and often resulted in loss of blood, as well as shock and infection. Paddles did not lacerate the skin as whips did, but they raised large blisters. Which was more painful, whipping or paddling? We cannot say because the degree of suffering depended, in part, on the strength of the man wielding the instrument. Nor is it easy to assess the impact of punishment and deprivation on mental health; but it seems reasonable to infer that the systematic attempt to keep black people fearful and to impress upon them their inferiority and dependence was fertile breeding ground for personality disorders, psychoses, depression, aggression, and anxiety (Rosengarten 1986, 184–85).

Overseers are considered the primary source of brutality/punishment of enslaved Africans. Overseers were responsible for making sure labor was performed; ensuring that the labor was productive and efficient; reporting medical conditions immediately to the slaveowner; and providing security for the Whites. They often constituted a lower class of subsistence-oriented, property-less White males whose power rested in how well they managed their reputation as a professional overseer/slave labor manager. A no-nonsense, heavy-handed approach was often encouraged, noting that above all else, slaves would respond to punishment or the fear of punishment. Problems with enslaved Africans meant potential problems in establishing and maintaining a good reputation. Africans in Louisiana often expressed vehement anger toward and retaliatory sentiments against overseers (Porteus 1934, 48–63). Despite the tremendous role of the overseer in brutality/punishment, Africans could also expect such treatment from the slaveowners.

Whites and Africans recount numerous incidences of brutality/punishment. Englishman Benjamin Henry Boneval Latrobe, considered the founder of architecture in the United States, wrote in his diaries observations of various aspects of the lives of enslaved Africans. According to Latrobe, the Africans in New Orleans were generally kept well by their masters, except that the "Creoles are in all these respects comparatively cruel to these unfortunate people" (Latrobe 1951, 53). Latrobe recounted an incident in New Orleans involving a slaveowner named Mrs. Tremoulet:

> Mrs. Tremoulet had her [the enslaved African woman] stripped quite naked, tied to a bed post, & she herself, in presence of her daughter, Mrs. Turpin (the mother of three beautiful Children), whipped her with a Cowskin till she bled. . .William was called & made to whip her till she fainted. This scene made a noise in the house & the blood betrayed it (Latrobe 1951, 53–54).

Latrobe goes on to state that the wife of the president of the Bank of New Orleans "did actually whip a negress to death, and treated another so cruelly that she died a short time afterwards" (Latrobe 1951, 54). Frenchman Elisee Reclus' observations on enslavement in Louisiana (1863) include his asking a young Creole boy "'if he wanted to grow up?'" The boy affirmed that he did so that he could "'beat the slave woman'" (Dunbar 1982, 348).

Latrobe describes the arbitrary nature of slaveowner cruelty; however, in many documented incidences of brutality and punishment rationales were offered regarding the behavior of enslaved African people. In southeastern Louisiana, the 1811 slave uprising (the "Louisiana Revolt of 1811" or the Deslondes Slave Revolt), is recorded as the largest uprising of enslaved Africans in the United States (Wall 1990, 101–102). The event provides the example of the extreme punishment of and brutality against Africans who attempted to take their freedom by force:

> The slaveowners shot these leaders of the revolt and had their heads placed on poles along the River Road to frighten and intimidate the other slaves. One of those captured by the slave owners, a man called Daniel, was put on a ship and brought down the river to New Orleans. He was taken off the ship at the Vieux Carre (French Quarter) and taken to the front entrance of the St. Louis Cathedral. Here, with the approval of Church officials, Daniel was shot and his head was cut off (Thrasher 1994, 7).

One of the early chroniclers of Louisiana history, Francois-Xavier Martin describes the punishment of enslaved Africans involved in the Pointe Coupee conspiracy of Louisiana. Martin notes that "The slaves attempted a resistance and twenty-five of them were killed before those that had been selected for trial were arrested and confined. Fifty were found guilty; others were severely flogged. Sixteen of the first were hung in different parts of the parish; the nine remaining were put on board of a galley, which floated down to New Orleans. On her way one of them was landed near the church of each parish along the river, and left hanging on a tree" (Martin 1882, 266). In such cases, eyewitnesses such as Latrobe, Reclus and Martin provide details regarding the acts, but do not indicate whether or not medical care was sought or provided for those Africans who were jailed or otherwise survived the brutality/punishment. The obvious rationale is that these enslaved Africans were considered to have committed criminal acts. However, enslavement itself afforded Africans criminal status by virtue of their social rank. There are cases, however, where Africans in Louisiana, going to the gallows, were provided medical care so that they would be alive when executed. Further, in the New Orleans execution of an enslaved African woman named Pauline, she was granted a brief stay of execution so that doctors could determine if she was pregnant (Castellanos 1895, 173).

The case of Madame Delphine Lalaurie provides an example of individual slaveowner brutality/punishment against enslaved Africans. The Lalaurie case of 1834 in New Orleans has been described as an early case of newspaper sensationalism (Darkis 1982, 383–399). According to a local newspaper:

> These slaves were the property of the demon, in the shape of a woman, who we mentioned in the beginning of this article. They had been confined by her for several months in the situation from which they had thus providentially been rescued, and had been merely kept in existence to prolong their sufferings and to make them taste all that the most refined cruelty could inflict (New Orleans Bee 1834, April 11).

In the Lalaurie case, "refined cruelty" refers to the enslaved Africans having been kept generally malnourished, whipped with cowhides, a few said to have been murdered and buried on her property, kept in chains in an upper level prison on the Lalaurie residence, tortured and left (bound) in the house which caught on fire (Darkis 1982, 383–399; Castellanos 1978, 52–62; Saxon 1928, 202–217). When seven of the enslaved Africans were brought from the burning house they required medical attention (New Orleans Bee 1834, April 11).

While the Louisiana oral histories of enslaved Africans consistently point out how quickly slaveowners responded with medicines and physicians; they also state that the brutality/punishment meted out to African people was just as swift and efficient. Lydia Jefferson who was enslaved in Avoyelles parish, Louisiana stated that her mother died as a result of the beating she received from the "nigger driver." The "nigger driver" was a plantation position usually assigned to an enslaved African male who carried out the supervisory and punishment tasks of the overseer or slaveowner. Jefferson's mother was pregnant with her and her twin sister at the time. After the beating from the "nigger driver" Jefferson's mother died giving birth to the girls. Jefferson described the process of brutality/punishment as she observed it on her plantation:

> de overseer make men and women too, pull off de clothes what dey has on, and dey would find de largest ant bed dey could and make'em sit naked in it. Lord have mercy, it jes' make my flesh crawl to think 'bout it. And de overseer always strip de men, and women naked in de field and whip 'em. For a woman what is pregnant, dey dig a hole in de ground and lay her over de hole and whip her. Dat's de way dey did my mama (Cook and Poteet 1979, 285).

Numerous narratives of former slaves provide accounts such as the one above. However, very few accounts discuss the medical care provided to slaves after they were so severely punished (except for the argument that brine was used, not as further punishment, but was rubbed into the lacerations after whipping for medicinal purposes). This raises the issue of whether or not denial of medical care/treatment by slaveowners was also a form of punishment for Africans who broke slaves laws. If so, does the overwhelming acknowledgement of slaveowners' generosity in extending medical care for labor injuries, disease and pregnancy constitute their attempt to obfuscate the issue of brutality/punishment?

Because enslaved Africans acknowledge that they generally received prompt medical attention for acute conditions and labor related injuries, enslavement and medicine scholars have attempted to argue that enslavement was a benign and civilizing institution

(Phillips 1968, 82–92). They tend to support the theory that slaveowners were more victims of the slaveocracy than the slaves themselves (Dart 1924, 332–333). They also temper this view with the slave narratives and oral histories which often mention love and/or a filial relationship with the slaveowner and his family. Yet the slave narratives and oral histories which mention love sentiments toward the slaveowner often include the overwhelming reality of physical violence against African people. However, not all Africans who discussed the institution of enslavement after the Civil War expressed love for the slaveowner. Henrietta Butler who was born and enslaved in Lafourche Parish, Louisiana, noted that her Mistress, Emily Haidee "was mean as hell." She stated that the slave mistress forced her to breed, and that "She was always knockin' me around" (Clayton 1990, 38).

The son of a wealthy West Virginia slaveowner, B. M. Dietz, in the Louisiana testimonies, reiterated the treatment enslaved Africans describe in their narratives and oral accounts. According to Dietz "About three weeks before peace was declared my father bought thirty-three slaves, mostly for pity's sake. The man that owned them was so mean [that] he would beat them until they were bleeding, and then wash them off with salt water" (Clayton 1990, 50). A former enslaved African woman, Ceceil George related, "Down here dey strip you down naked, and two men hold you down and whip you till de blood come" (Clayton 1990, 84). As a child, Mary Harris worked in the main house fanning flies from the slaveowner's dinner table, tending the fire, gathering wood, and disposing of ashes. Harris stated: "I never got a whippin', either, because I was good and did my work and never talked back. My ma told me she was brutaly (sic) beaten. . ." (Clayton 1990, 94–95).

Elizabeth Ross Hite of Trinity Plantation, Louisiana described several instances of brutality against enslaved Africans. According to Hite the slave master owned over one hundred slaves and never whipped them because he was "too busy making money." However she noted that other slaveowners routinely engaged in punishment activities:

> Dey would put you in a stark [stocks]. Your hands and foots was buckled up and you stayed dere for months. . .De mean master would tie de

slaves to a tree and beat dem to death.

Old lady Oater ran away and built a home in de ground. She had six children. De driver caught her one day and whipped her to death. He beat her until her skin peel off and she died. Den he unloosened her from de tree and buried her in de ground in front of de quarters. De drivers used a platted rawhide whip (Clayton 1990, 102–103).

Hunton Love, born and enslaved in Bayou Lafourche, Louisiana discussed an aspect of the physical violence against enslaved African women.

Susan was bought and told to follow her new master. She was just about in childbirth and wouldn't move. When urged, [she] said, 'I won't go! I won't go! I won't!' For that she was given one hundred fifty lashes.

Another woman was throwed in a big bed of ants which they had caused to 'semble. She was tied down with heavy weights so she couldn't budge. She was tortured awfully (Clayton 1990, 162).

Enslaved Africans did not fail to acknowledge the special punishment meted out to pregnant enslaved African women. It demonstrates that punishment was a necessity of the slaveocracy and not just the personal proclivities of a select few slaveowners. It also helps us to understand the desire on the part of the slaveowner to protect his investment in unborn children. This special punishment, described in this research as, "the Whipping Hole" has consistent characteristics. In the oral history of Frances Doby of Opelousas, Louisiana:

France's mother, named Henrietta Alexander, was a slave of Lucius Dupre. Mr. Dupre was a good "mars", and sometimes he had to whip the slaves for disobedience. When a pregnant woman was to be punished, a hole was dug in the ground. Her abdomen [was] placed in the hole and her back [was] exposed. She was given twenty-five lashes (Clayton 1990, 61).

Rebecca Fletcher's oral testimony provided further detail:
> Some of the overseers were mean men: They wanted slaves to have babies 'cause they was valuable. So when a slave was about to produce a baby and he wanted her whipped, he had a hole dug in the ground and made her lay acrost it. And her hands and foots were tied, so she had to submit quiet-like to the beatin' with a strap (Clayton 1990, 66).

Fletcher associated "the Whipping Hole" experience with a comment on how close death came to enslaved African women:

> I heard tell that when a woman was a-bornin' a child, that death went 'round her bed seven times a-studyin' whether he'd take her or not. I got three children living and I don't know how many dead, so I reckon he had plenty [of] chances at me (Clayton 1990, 66).

Octavia Fontenette of New Iberia, Louisiana described "the Whipping Hole" experience during enslavement:

> . . . the slaves on the other plantations didn't have it so easy. I know 'cause I used to sneak off and play in the fields: They didn't make us children work. We used to see the white master on the other farms beatin' their poor slaves. One day we saw them dig a big hole and make a poor woman get in it face down with her clothes off, and they beat her till she bled. We snuck off home and told the others about it, what we had seen, but they fussed at us and told us we better not never go over there again. And you know, it was years after [later] I found out why they made those

women do that: They was pregnant (Clayton 1990, 72).

Robert St. Ann of Gueno Settlement, Plaquemine Parish Louisiana recalled another dimension to "the Whipping Hole":

> . . . I seen 'em take a woman what was prejudice (pregnant), and dey make a hole big enough for her to put her stomach in. Dey raise her clothes and beat her wid a strap till de blood come, den dey pour brine over her (Clayton 1990, 190).

Enslaved Africans were quick to point out the treatment they received from "good" masters. Albert Patterson of Laso Plantation, Plaquemines Parish Louisiana noted that the slaveowner was not cruel and that he refused to use the "nigger dogs" on Africans, however he stated:

> I seen de blood cut out of niggers dat deep, seen it wid my own eyes. But not Colonel White, he not cruel. He wouldn't whip, he'd punish. He had a iron band he'd rivet to go around the ankle, and he had a iron band to go around the neck and a piece of iron standin' up in de front, de back, and each side. You had to hold your head just so, and you couldn't lay down. You had to pad that iron band 'cause it was so heavy it would cut your neck (Clayton 1990, 179)

Gracie Stafford, born and enslaved on Myrtle Grove Plantation in St. James Parish, Louisiana stated: "The old folks used to say that the master was hard on slaves, and had em whipped until the blood sometimes stained the ground. My parents said they never was treated cruel like that 'cause they always was good, but my aunt said she was put in stocks 'cause she wouldn't give in" (Clayton 1990, 197).

Valsin Mermillion has been described as "The most cruel master in St. John [the] Baptist [Parish]" Louisiana. One of his former slaves Mrs. Webb said that "One of his cruelties was to place a disobedient slave, standing, in a box, in which there were nails placed in such a manner that the poor creature was unable to move. He was powerless even to chase the flies or sometimes, ants crawling on some parts of his body" (Clayton 1990, 209). Mrs. Webb also relates the story of how Mermillion graphically gave a young, enslaved African male an ultimatum—plow or dig his own grave. After his failure to comply, the African was shot and then buried in the hole he dug for himself (Clayton 1990, 209). Solomon Northup details at length the brutality/punishment that he suffered as an African kidnapped and sold into enslavement. At one point he described the physical results of a beating he received: ". . .I had become stiff and sore; my body was covered with blisters, and it was with great pain and difficulty that I could move. . .My wounds would not permit me to remain but a few minutes in any one position; so, sitting, or standing, or moving slowly round, I passed the days and nights" (Eakin & Logsdon 1968, 27). Other Africans enslaved in Louisiana suffered brutality of an inexplicable nature. An enslaved African named Gonzales was found "On Monday morning, his dead body was drawn from the Mississippi. The head was entirely severed from the body; the lower extremities had also suffered amputation. Several stabs, wounds and bruises, were discovered on various parts of the body" (Curry 1972, 221).

The prevalence of medical care provided to enslaved Africans, does not take into account the extent of punishment and brutality. While enslaved Africans' oral histories frequently acknowledge physical altercations with slaveowners and overseers, few cases document the resultant need for medical inquiry or care. In April, 1852 an enslaved African was stabbed in the ribs by his slaveowner, "the base of the left lung was found to have been slightly wounded. . . .the knife penetrating the diaphragm, its point wounded the omentum" (Ewing 1853, 764). This injury caused a puncture of the 'caul' or fold of the peritoneum which connects the stomach to other visceral organs. There are few, if any, extant records which indicate that Africans were rushed to the Louisiana hospitals with lacerations from whips, cut marks from chains and collars, knife or gunshot wounds.

The physical challenges of day-to-day labor took their toll on the majority of field hands. Illness, punishment and labor often intersected to compel the African to seek refuge in the next world.

Slavery and Medicine: Enslavement and Medical Practices in Antebellum Louisiana

Solomon Northup recalls his Avoyelles Parish, Louisiana experience with brutality/punishment and labor:

> It was now the season of hoeing. I was first sent into the corn-field, and afterwards set to scraping cotton. In this employment I remained until hoeing time was nearly passed, when I began to experience the symptoms of approaching illness. I was attacked with chills, which were succeeded by a burning fever. I became weak and emaciated, and frequently so dizzy it caused me to reel and stagger like a drunken man. Nevertheless, I was compelled to keep up my row. When in health I found little difficulty in keeping pace with my fellow-laborers, but now it seemed to be an utter impossibility. Often I fell behind, when the driver's lash was sure to greet my back, infusing into my sick and drooping body a little temporary energy. I continued to decline until at length the whip became entirely ineffectual. The sharpest sting of the rawhide could not arouse me (Eakin and Logsdon 1968, 133).

Northup indicated in his narratives, as do other oral histories from southeastern Louisiana, that enslaved Africans often labored ill and under the lash. In Northup's case the whip compounded the fever and impending illness, creating an increased risk/need for medical care. The antebellum scholarship which fails to address the physical violence against enslaved Africans serves to deny an important component of the totality of what medicine and enslavement meant to Africans in the United States.

CHAPTER 4

PROTECTION OF PROPERTY AND LEGISLATION

All masters had different laws.

Elizabeth Ross Hite

Antebellum observers were aware of the early slave codes of Louisiana, which stipulated the number of lashes administered to enslaved Africans. According to George Cable, "Even the requirement of law was only that he (the enslaved African) should not. . .get more than thirty lashes to the twenty-four hours" (Cable 1886, 6). Most interpretations of the Black Codes (or Slave Codes) of Louisiana suggest that Africans enjoyed notable privileges largely because their masters were, by law, granted the authority to permit them certain rights. An example of this privilege in Louisiana were the Sunday gatherings of enslaved Africans at Congo Square (Place Congo) in New Orleans. The medical care of enslaved Africans in Louisiana was loosely determined by the Black Codes and other official ordinances put forward by the French, Spanish and Americans. Louisiana, like other southern territories contained minor provisions regarding the medical care of Africans. For example, in the Code of Alabama of 1852 Title 5, Chapter IV states that "The master must. . .cause him (the slave) to be properly attended during sickness" (Code of Alabama 1852). In addition, certain Louisiana ordinances forbad ships carrying enslaved Africans from docking in order to "avoid contagion." By 1724 there existed a similar, more updated ordinance, which required a health officer to inspect slave ships before landing (Riddell 1925, 327–328).

While the Black Codes of Louisiana defined the rights and obligations of the slaveowner, it outlined some areas which impacted the enslaved Africans health status. These areas included

Slavery and Medicine: Enslavement and Medical Practices in Antebellum Louisiana

punishment for striking a white person, illicit intercourse (concubinage, etc.), stealing and congregation. In 1685 the Black Code was included in the "Regulations, Edicts, Declarations and Decrees Concerning the Commerce, Administration of Justice, and Policing of Louisiana and other French Colonies in America." The 1685 Article which spoke to the medical health issues of enslaved Africans stated:

> Slaves incapacitated by old age, illness, or otherwise, whether or not disease is incurable, shall be fed and maintained by their masters, and in case they have been abandoned, the said slave shall be sent to the alms-house to which the master shall be condemned to pay six sols (silver coins) per day for the food and care of each slave ("Regulations. . ." 1940, 378–379).

Later, the Black Code of 1724 included the provision which is remotely related to health care, that slaveowners should "Provide at length for the clothing of slaves and for their subsistence" (Gayarre' 1903, 533). Similar to the 1685 Article, the most specific provision which addressed medical/ health care in 1724 is found in Article 21:

> Slaves who are disabled from working, either by old age, disease, or otherwise, be the disease incurable or not, shall be fed and provided for by their masters; and in case they should have been abandoned by said masters, said slaves shall be adjudged to the nearest hospital, to which said masters shall be obliged to pay eight cents a day for the food and maintenance of each one of these slaves; and for the payment of this sum, said hospital shall have a lien on the plantations of the master (Gayarre' 1903, 534).

Slavery and Medicine: Enslavement and Medical Practices in Antebellum Louisiana

One hundred years later the Louisiana Slave Code (1824) was obscure and non-responsive to the issue of medical/health care of the enslaved African. Article 173 indirectly addressed this issue:

> The slave is entirely subject to the will of his master, who may correct and chastise him, though not with unusual rigor, nor so as to maim or mutilate him, or to expose him to the danger of loss of life, or to cause his death (Civil Code of the State of Louisiana 1825, 90–94).

While the Black Codes of Louisiana admonished the slaveowner for "unusual" punishment, they served largely to provide protection and security for the White slave owning population. Medical/health care issues of Africans were not a significant feature of the Black Codes. The Codes' rigid laws regarding acts of commission on the part of Africans put them in constant jeopardy, and did proscribe punishments in which the African would have required medical care. Section 3 of the Black Codes stated:

> Any slave who shall wilfully and maliciously strike his master, or his master's or mistress' child, or any white overseer appointed by his owner to superintend said owner's slaves, so as to cause a contusion or shedding of blood, shall be punished with death or imprisonment at hard labor for a term of not less than ten years (Civil Code of the State of Louisiana 1825, 90–94).

Aside from the Black Codes, most official documents of southeastern Louisiana do not specifically address the issue of health/medical care of enslaved Africans. They do, however, define the African as property, state their value, and imply the slaveowner's responsibility. The 1824 marriage contract of Elizabeth Arsenne and Cains Gracchus Fleurian de Belmare describe the property value of the future wife: "2. Indivisible half of a negress named Reinen aged about 45, domestic. which is estimated at the sum of $300. The future wife is owner, co-jointly with her sister. 3. A negress named Sophia, aged about 26, domestic, estimated at $1100. 4. a negress named Henrietta, daughter of the negress Sophia, aged 11, estimated at $600" (Heartman Collection 1824).

In a case involving the separation of property of a husband and wife in the Parish of West Feliciana, Louisiana in 1829, the wife was decreed approximately 640 acres "and that the slaves Ede, Esther, Sylla, Frank, Rose, Mary, Henry, Ann, Caroline, Bob, Comfort, Saul, Sarah, Bill, Charlotte, Adeline, and Harriet are also her separate property, and that she be put into immediate possession of the aforesaid property" (Webb 1983, 42 –43). The language used in the sales of enslaved Africans also protected property for slave owning Whites. Examples of bills of sale for enslaved Africans include the language which ensured that the African was not ill or diseased. In the Parish of East Feliciana, Louisiana in 1825, Eliza, described as "a certain negro girl" was twenty three years old. She was sold by Henry Smith to Zachariah Netty. In this sale for $460.00, Smith guaranteed "which girl I warrant of the maladies prescribed by law" (Heartman Collection 1820 –1825). Cordia, who was 12 years old, was sold in September of 1819 for $800.00, the language concerning Cordia stated: "sound serveable and healthy and a slave for life. I also warrant and defend the right and title of said negro from me" (Heartman Collection 1810–1819). Buyers and sellers had some measure of comfort regarding their purchases of enslaved Africans; part of the appeal of the sale was due to binding promises of compensation if necessary:

> Madam Lopez sells her slave, Vincent, against whom there are no general mortgages, resulting on her nomination as tutor of her children.
>
> Madam Lopez guarantees title to the buyer,

SLAVERY AND MEDICINE: ENSLAVEMENT AND MEDICAL PRACTICES IN ANTEBELLUM LOUISIANA

and can assure the buyer he will not be troubled in his possession of said slave, as she has sufficient means on the share of her children to compensate buyer of the slave
Land of the succession has not yet been sold.

(Signed) Tessier (Heartman Collection undated).

In another bill of sale, Thomas Purnell of West Feliciana, Louisiana sold to Samuel Clark several Africans. For the sum of $1,825.00 he sold, "the following negroes that is to say one negro man Edward aged about twenty years/ one negro woman Martha aged about twentyfive years/ one negro boy John aged about four years/ one girl Harriett aged about two years/ one negro woman Leah aged about fifteen years/ one negro woman Hannah aged about twentyfive years." They were sold "warranted and defended forever" and "sound in body and mind and slaves for life" (Heartman Collection undated). Another example from Assumption Parish, Louisiana, a 50 year old "negro man" was sold by Abraham Armstrong to Benjamin Winchester for $470.00. This transaction took place December 4, 1819 and includes the standard sales clause which guaranteed the African at the time of sale. In this record of a slave sale, Armstrong sold the African man "warranted free of all vices, defects and diseases" (Assumption Parish 1813–1844).

Slaveowners went to great length to protect their slave property. The enslaved African in antebellum Louisiana possessed few legal rights. Unlike other jurisdictions, he or she could appear in court as a plaintiff only to claim freedom and then only under guarded circumstances. However, enslaved Africans did appear often as defendants having been accused of a crime. Enslaved Africans could also testify against another slave, but never against a White person. However, these limitations did not prevent some enslaved Africans and free people of color in Louisiana from being involved

SLAVERY AND MEDICINE: ENSLAVEMENT AND MEDICAL PRACTICES IN ANTEBELLUM LOUISIANA

in numerous lawsuits at the parish or district level. An example is the case of Arsene, an enslaved African woman who filed suit for her freedom largely because her owner threatened to sell her for $650.00 in 1845. The case represented a dispute over international jurisdiction of an enslaved African (*Arsene v. Pigneguy* 1847).

Because enslaved Africans were commodities or "products," the laws that governed the buying and selling of slaves were similar to the laws that governed the buying and selling of property. Slaveowners considered their slaves significant financial investments. Legal historian Judith K. Schafer describes numerous court cases that were brought to the Supreme Court of Louisiana during the antebellum period, and many of these cases concerned the selling of "defective" slaves. Schafer asserts that approximately 1200 cases were heard during this time involving enslaved Africans (Schafer 1987, 306).

Louisiana borrowed over two-thirds of the French Code Napoleon to construct its first Civil Code. Within the French Code is a clause that issues a warranty against vices, meaning that an individual could be reimbursed for a purchase that had hidden defects. The Romans also had this law pertaining to slaves in their concept of "redhibitia." Redhibitia meant that a slave sale could be cancelled if it was purposely withheld that the slave was a habitual runaway or the slave had a hidden physical illness or other vices or defects (Schafer 1987, 308). Therefore, according to the Louisiana Civil Code, slaveowners had to keep what is referred to as a "slave log." In this log there was documentation of every whipping the slave had been given, every injury or illness experienced by the slave, every escape attempt and any other account of the African regarding disobedience.

Of all of the cases that were brought to the Supreme Court of Louisiana suits for sickness and disease were the most prevalent. Although the majority of enslaved Africans could not read or write, due to the laws prohibiting them from learning to do so, many were aware of the fact that the best and most efficient way not to be sold was to falsely exhibit some type of illness or disease. This practice among enslaved Africans was used as an attempt to keep families from being separated. There were 166 slave sale cancellation cases brought to court in the 1850's because enslaved Africans had diseases, and 19 percent of the Africans involved in these cases died shortly after sale (Schafer 1987, 311). Many times fraud came into play because some slaveowners were experiencing financial hardships and desperately tried to get the most money from slaves considered to have defects. In one case, a slave with scurvy was sold for top dollar and the condition went unnoticed because wooden teeth were put into his mouth to replace the ones that had fallen out. The African was returned to his original owner and he was required to reimburse the payment to the purchaser with interest (Schafer 1987, 312).

From the narratives and oral histories of former enslaved Africans there is no indication that the enslaved masses were aware of the legal structures which determined punishment and impacted health care. While Africans speak extensively of physical violence, medical care, labor, spirituality/religion, rape/breeding/concubinage and psychological abuse, they do not state that they knew of any specific information about the Black (Slave) Codes; or that the slaveowners verbally reminded them about the codes per se. This is consistent with the legal denial of education to the enslaved African population. Regarding official documents, enslaved Africans were aware that many sales transactions were in fact transfers of property to the surviving spouses and heirs of farms and plantations; or distributions of property to satisfy debts or marital separations..

CHAPTER 5

LABOR AND MEDICAL HEALTH CARE

> You see, what caused my ma to be sickly, I was de oldest child, and dey made her work too hard with de other children. One of my sisters was born right in de fields. Dey just dug two holes, one in de front and one in de back. She gets down in dat hole and gives birth to de baby; de baby just rolls out in de hole. Den de boss has someone to take de baby to de house, and makes my ma get up and keep right on hoeing. I never will forget.
>
> *Mary Ann John*

According to Dr. Samuel Cartwright, "A white man, like a blooded horse, can be worked to death. Not so the negro, whose ethnical elements, like the mule, restrict the limits of arbitrary power over him" (Cartwright 1857, 159). Cartwright believed that it was impossible that enslavement labor could have been harmful to Africans. However, enslaved Africans frequently spoke about the harmful aspects of enslavement labor and the arbitrary power of slaveowners. Yet few scholarly enterprises have discussed the connection between the labor of enslaved Africans and their need for medical health care. Much of the labor performed by enslaved Africans represented major risk factors. Africans who worked in the fields were often required to perform arduous and dangerous labors that White slaveowners and European immigrant laborers shunned. Extant records also indicate that Africans were frequently overworked by overseers. According to former enslaved Africans many aspects of agricultural labor were diverse and difficult. One of the most difficult labor activities performed by enslaved Africans was clearing the land. Few antebellum physicians acknowledged the environmental risks endured by enslaved Africans:

Slavery and Medicine: Enslavement and Medical Practices in Antebellum Louisiana

> The treatment of wounds and stings inflicted by venomous animals on the negroes, who from being generally employed in clearing and cultivating lands in the southern states, are necessarily more exposed to the risk of suffering from injuries of this nature. . .and it is really surprising, when we consider with what a variety of venomous animals our woods abound, that accidents do not more often occur to this race of people (Tidyman 1826, 334).

However, given the environmental risks involved it was still believed that "nature has armed the negro with a thicker cuticle than the white" (Tidyman 1826, 334). In addition to clearing the land, enslaved Africans labored as skilled tradesmen, built levees and drainage ditches; and served as soldiers and sailors, domestic servants, and of course in the intensive agricultural pursuits of cash crops including: indigo, sugar, cotton, rice and tobacco (Usner 1979, 25–48). According to C. Duncan Rice in The Rise and Fall of Black Slavery "Louisiana gained a reputation which made it the most terrifying of all the various hells of the deep south to which blacks from the older slave economies of the tidewater states could be sold" (Rice 1975, 287).

Former slaves like Sam Boykin of Morehouse Parish, Louisiana stated that enslaved Africans were subject to a number of challenges related to cotton labor:

> In the fall, we would go to the field early before the frost melted; our feet would get cold because we would not have on any shoes. To keep warm, we would wrap up in our sacks and hide under the cotton baskets but the overseer would find us and kick the baskets from over us and run us out to work in the frost. If you picked one or two hundred pounds of cotton one day, you had

that amount to pick every day or get punished (Cade 1935, 313).

In this example environmental factors, the lack of necessary resources, coupled with labor requirements created medical health risks including the potential for frostbite, lacerations from punishments, exhaustion and fatigue. Other former enslaved Africans of Morehouse Parish, Louisiana described labor conditions in which enslaved African children were required to work in the field; where disabled and elderly Africans performed child care duties for the field slaves; where mothers who labored in the fields often nursed their babies there; and where after the most significant amount of field work was performed for the season, Africans were forced to engage additional labor and tasks away from the fields (Cade 1935, 313).

Skeletal evidence and oral testimonies have indicated that enslaved Africans suffered physical trauma related to labor. Labor related conditions included hernias in both men and women from lifting heavy objects. Africans also experienced arthritis in the hands, elbows and shoulder joints indicative of their employment in intensive craft work. Arthritis also occurred in those involved in skilled labor and those who performed activities such as "pounding pig iron or digging out ore from the banks" (Kelley and Angel 1987, 207–209). According to formerly enslaved Edward De Biuew, born in 1861 in Lafourche Parish, Louisiana:

> My ma died 'bout three hours after I was born. Pa always said they made my ma work too hard. I was born in de fields. He said ma was hoein'. She told the driver she was sick; he told her to just hoe right-on. Soon, I was born, and my ma die[d] a few minutes after dey brung her to the house (Clayton 1990, 48).

Rebecca Fletcher, born in 1842 in Louisiana related that in

Slavery and Medicine: Enslavement and Medical Practices in Antebellum Louisiana

general, "Slaves had to go to field before daybreak and didn't come home till after dark. Then they cooked dinner and lunch to take with'em [the] next day" (Clayton 1990, 65).

Cecil George, born in 1846 in the Great Swamp Plantation, Charleston County, South Carolina, and enslaved in Louisiana, indicated that on the sugar plantations all of the enslaved Africans worked in the fields, including the youth and the elderly. She emphasized that "dey make every child on de plantation tote sugar cane just de same" (Clayton 1990, 84–85). Daffney Johnson born around 1850 on the Miller Don Plantation in Gretna, Louisiana confirmed that the "colored driver" (also known as the "nigger driver") of the plantation "sho did push us out in dem sugar cane fields" (Clayton 1990, 129). The majority of enslaved Africans of southeastern Louisiana, who worked in the sugar fields and plantations, confirm that much longer working hours (sixteen to eighteen hour days) were demanded of them (Rice 1975, 287; Olmsted 1861, 249–257).

Albert Patterson, born in 1850 in Lasco Plantation in Plaquemines Parish, Louisiana stated: "We raised sugarcane and made sugar—no refinery; we'd boil it in big kittles. There was a colored man from Mississippi that knew when the sugar grain [granulated]. We'd work in de fields in de day and make sugar at night" (Clayton 1990, 178). African women were often required to perform this difficult labor as well. Mandy Rollins' grandfather was a slaveowner in Louisiana and she recalled that the labor she performed was no different than enslaved African males:

> All dese houses stand now on de land where I used to work like a mule. I've plowed, hoed, stripped cane, pulled corn, and most everything dat a man ever did. 'Fore we worked dis land, I helped another woman cut down de trees right where dese cabins is now (Clayton 1990, 187).

SLAVERY AND MEDICINE: ENSLAVEMENT AND MEDICAL PRACTICES IN ANTEBELLUM LOUISIANA

Robert St. Ann of Gueno Settlement, Plaquemines Parish, Louisiana was born in 1844, like many former slaves he re-counted that he had a "good master," who never whipped his slaves. Yet "Cousin Bob," as he was known, provided specific details of rice labor among enslaved Africans:

> In de old slave days, we used to cut wid [a] sickle and cradle, [and] den tie it in bundles to dry. Dat was de best rice too. We'd cut like [on] Thursday and hull it [on] Saturday. You works den on a plantation. Dat's work dat has to be done right now! We starts cuttin' first of August. To thrash it we used to put a post in de ground about four feet deep, den we'd pack it and stomp it 'cause it had to be hard ground. Den we'd hitch de horses two abref (abreast) to de post. We puts de rice on de round, [and] de horses keep circlin' as fast as dey can. You put a fast one on de outside and de old one next to de post, and you keeps turnin' de rice, and de horse keeps trompin' on it. Den you cleans all de dirt out—keep fannin' de rice till it's clean—den you puts it in bags. We got fifty to seventy-five barrels in a day. You up before day-break, and you work hard wid de crop till you gets through 'cause de crop won't wait on you (Clayton 1990, 190).

While Robert St. Ann discussed the various aspects of rice labor, Shack Wilson, born before 1865 in Clinton, Louisiana expounded upon the connection between labor (specifically cotton) and punishment. Wilson's father had been a slave driver and died of labor-related injuries:

> They used to whip slaves if they didn't pick enough cotton. They put four pegs in the ground and tied one leg to one peg, the other to the other,

Slavery and Medicine: Enslavement and Medical Practices in Antebellum Louisiana

> and the arms were tied together. They were stripped of all clothing and whipped with a rawhide, [and said], 'Do pray master, do pray master, hi-yi hi-yi' until their cries almost died away. Then they'd [be] put to picking cotton with all that suffering. If a slave run away, they'd put a pack of 'nigger dogs' on their trail. Some people call them 'blood-hounds,' but they used to be called 'nigger dogs.' (Clayton 1990, 213)

It is not uncommon to find narratives and oral histories of former enslaved Africans attesting to the demanding labor; how labor impacted health and mortality; how the threat of harsh labor was used to control Africans; and how harsh labor served as an actual form of punishment.

In southeastern Louisiana the life of an enslaved African in domestic work was considered markedly different from the life of those who were required to work in the sugar, cotton, indigo and rice plantations. This difference was mainly due to the large numbers of agricultural slaves and the persistence of free Africans and free people of color (Black Creoles or gens de la coleur libre) in and around the city of New Orleans. Enslaved Africans possessed aspirations of a better socio-economic condition within the slaveocracy, often proud and many boasting of their status in the "big house." Physical evidence from a New Orleans cemetery "suggests that the slaves buried in this cemetery may have lived slightly better lives than those on rural plantations" (Owsley et al. 1987, 196). Despite the tentative nature of the research findings, enslaved Africans confirm that this phenomena was largely true for Africans required to work as domestic servants, especially in the well-to-do residential homes of White Creoles and Americans in New Orleans.

In East Feliciana Parish, Louisiana on the Weston Plantation, enslaved Africans were required to work as skilled laborers,

SLAVERY AND MEDICINE: ENSLAVEMENT AND MEDICAL PRACTICES IN ANTEBELLUM LOUISIANA

domestic servants and mostly as plantation hands in the cotton fields. According to the new plantation mistress, "The negroes have a large basket which they carry on the head when full. This is what they pick cotton in. I think it is as pretty a sight as I ever saw, the negroes (women and all) coming up to the gin, balancing these big baskets with the snowy cotton on their heads, contrasting so with their black faces" (Anderson 1960, 248). The new mistress of the Weston plantation also noted that enslaved Africans at the age of sixty years and beyond did not work in the cotton fields; but that a retired "Granny" in particular, had "worse then work" because she was required to take care of approximately 30 enslaved African babies while their parents worked in the cotton fields (Anderson 1960, 248).

Enslaved Africans who labored in the plantation fields were often described as "half" or "full" hands, "effective" or "non-effective" hands depending upon their ability to perform to an adult male's standard (Wall 1990, 164). Half or non-effective hands usually referred to pregnant women, small children, the elderly and disabled slaves. The profit potential of major southern planters depended upon the labor of full hands (Govan 1942, 513 –535). In addition to the requisite labor of enslaved Africans of southeastern Louisiana in sugar and cotton, most plantations and farms were self-sufficient units or shared community processing mills. According to the P. A. Champomier "Statement of the Sugar Crop made in Louisiana, 1854" there were a total of 1,457 sugar plantations in Louisiana in 1854. The "Estimated average no. working slaves per plantation" ranged from 11 to 108 enslaved Africans. The average number of enslaved Africans working in sugar on a given plantation was 56. There were 751 Creole (of Spanish and/or French ancestry) planters and 710 American planters working in sugar. Each enslaved African working in sugar was estimated as having produced six hogsheads, or between 6,000 to 6,750 pounds, of sugar each. A hogshead represented approximately one thousand pounds (Wall 1990, 142); however,

SLAVERY AND MEDICINE: ENSLAVEMENT AND MEDICAL PRACTICES IN
ANTEBELLUM LOUISIANA

Champomier estimated a hogshead at 1,125 pounds (Moody 1924, 201).

Sugar planting and harvesting (grinding) was a highly detailed, labor intensive occupation in Louisiana (Wall 1990, 139–142). By the 1850's the Tchoupitoulas plantation near the city of New Orleans contained more than one hundred enslaved Africans. These Africans labored at one time in sugarcane and then rice. Sugar production on the Tchoupitoulas Plantation is said to "have left much to be desired in the matter of sanitation and efficiency" (Soniat 1924, 311). The Africans' labor experience in sugar included carrying the "cane to the carrier, which in turn transported it to large iron rollers where it was crushed; the juice thus extracted would run into large wood tanks, and then it would be poured into huge iron kittles and boiled to the granulating point" (Soniat 1924, 311). The iron sugar caldrons (kettles) were as much as five feet in diameter, approximately three feet high and required large amounts of wood to keep a fire burning underneath them during the granulating period. With this simple open kettle process enslaved men and women spent large amounts of time cutting and hauling wood for sugar labor. The labor related medical risks of the sugar industry included accidents caused by machines: "...workers were caught in belts, caught in the rollers, struck by pieces of broken machinery, and worst of all, scalded or otherwise injured by steam explosions" (Wall 1990, 142).

In addition to the inherent dangers of agricultural labor, wet nursing, forced breeding, and concubinage were labors which created additional medical health risks for enslaved African women. African women who worked in the sugar or cotton fields often worked up to childbirth. Frequent births meant the risk of inadequate healing time between delivery, plantation labor, post-partum recovery and a new pregnancy. Many enslaved African women report numerous pregnancies and births within their life time. Wet nurses (sometimes called "nurse mammies") performed the breast feeding of infants while the mothers worked in the

SLAVERY AND MEDICINE: ENSLAVEMENT AND MEDICAL PRACTICES IN
ANTEBELLUM LOUISIANA

fields. Ellen Betts, born during enslavement on Bayou Teche in St. Mary's Parish, Louisiana noted the effects of nursing: "I don't do nothin' all my days but nuss, nuss, nuss. . .I nuss so many chillun it done went and stunted my growth, and dat's why I ain't got nothin' but bones to dis day. When de cullud women have to cut sugarcane all day till midnight and after, I has to nuss de babies for 'em and tend to de white chillun, too" (Mellon 1988, 381). Nursing the White children was an important occupation for many enslaved African women. While it appears a large portion of White women required this task, M. Le Page Du Pratz, who spent sixteen years in Louisiana and wrote extensively of his observations, warned against it:

> A French father and his wife are great enemies to their posterity when they give their children such nurses. For the milk being the purest blood of the woman, one must be a step-mother indeed to give her child to a negro nurse in such a country as Louisiana, where the mother has all conveniences of being served, of accommodating and carrying their children, who by that means may be always under their eyes (Du Pratz 1774, 362).

Despite the fact that Du Pratz reprimanded White women who allowed their children to be breast fed by enslaved African women, and felt that they were "sacrificing" their children, enslaved African women of southeastern Louisiana commented frequently on the practice.

Breeding and concubinage were enslavement labors, which are considered difficult to research. In their article, "The Slave-Breeding Hypothesis: A Demographic Comment on the 'Buying' and 'Selling' States," Richard Lowe and Randolph Campbell assert that "it must be remembered that demographic evidence cannot conclusively prove or disprove the existence of deliberate slave

SLAVERY AND MEDICINE: ENSLAVEMENT AND MEDICAL PRACTICES IN ANTEBELLUM LOUISIANA

breeding" (Lowe and Randolph 1976, 412). Breeding, like the extent of concubinage, cannot be quantified; however, when enslaved Africans speak and their voices are the center of the analysis, they confirm their perceptions of the frequency of the practices among slaveowners. It should be noted too that like women, enslaved African males were victims of breeding labor. They were victimized by the demand/expectation to perform in the role of "buck" on the plantations. Furthermore, they sustained the emotional hardships, like their female counterparts, of seeing the children sold away from whatever family unit the enslaved Africans managed to establish. Moreover, enslaved African males witnessed their mothers, sisters, daughters, etc. forced into various systems of sexual exploitation, unable to protect their womanhood.

Many scholars attempt to avoid the bondage aspect as it applied to "kept" African women. Harriet Jacobs described the helplessness and vulnerability of enslaved African females to the sexual advances of slaveowners in her work Incidents in the Life of a Slave Girl (1861). According to Jacobs her slaveowner, a physician by the name of Dr. Flint,

> began to whisper foul words in my ear. Young as I was, I could not remain ignorant of their import. . .He was a crafty man, and resorted to many means to accomplish his purposes. . . I was compelled to live under the same roof with him—where I saw a man forty years my senior daily violating the most sacred commandments of nature. He told me I was his property; that I must be subject to his will in all things. . .The mistress, who ought to protect the helpless victim, has no other feelings towards her but those of jealousy and rage. . . My master met me at every turn, reminding me that I belonged to him, and swearing by heaven and earth that he would compel me to submit to him . . .O, what days and

nights of fear and sorrow that man caused me! Reader, it is not to awaken sympathy for myself that I am telling you truthfully what I suffered in slavery. I do it to kindle a flame of compassion in your hearts for my sisters who are still in bondage, suffering as I once suffered (Gates 1987, 360–363).

In addition to the agricultural and domestic labor tasks, enslaved African women were required to work as concubines in the New Orleans slave market. This market was well known for providing wealthy male consumers with "fancy" and "yellow" girls whose African heritage and admixture with Europeans produced for them the desirable features and hues they called mulatto, octoroon and quadroon. Sometimes these terms are used interchangeably, primarily because some antebellum Africans with European admixture were indistinguishable in skin tone and color from one another (Bankole 1995, 122, 137, 148). Louisiana is characterized as the primary place in the South to acquire "yellow" girls. According to Mary Reynolds, her slaveowner, on a trip to Baton Rouge, Louisiana, brought back a "yaller gal" who served as a seamstress and a concubine. Reynolds recalled that the slaveowner built this woman a house a distance from the slave quarters, and she bore him several children who resembled their father (Mellon 1988, 20–21).

Concubinage was not limited to cities like Baton Rouge and New Orleans, there was also concubinage on the remote farms and plantations of Louisiana. Rachel O'Connor, the antebellum mistress of Evergreen plantation in Feliciana, Louisiana, commented frequently on the subject in her letters written between 1823 and 1845. In a letter to her sister, O'Connor remarked:

> I'm glad to hear of your house girls behaving so well. I have no doubt of your judging mean low white men being the chief cause of their

> disobedience. It is always the case where they are. They cause more punishment to be inflicted amongst the poor ignorant slaves than all else they commit. Otherwise any white man that encourages the likes are next to the old evil one in badness (Webb 1983, 150).

Very often the scholarship focuses on data and documentation such as the above to assert that the incidence of forced concubinage reflected an agreed upon arrangement, between slave and master (or overseer); particularly where the slave woman was eventually freed by will and the Supreme Court (Schafer 1987, 165–182). This concubinage involving enslaved African women should not be confused with the "keeping" of free women of color, often cited in the New Orleans literature referencing the Quadroon Balls and system of placage. Closer to Louisiana enslavement reality, Solomon Northup related the story of Eliza and her daughter Emily. Eliza was an enslaved woman who was "kept" by her wealthy slaveowner, Emily was their daughter. Eventually they were sold and mother and daughter were separated. Yet, according to Northup, the child Emily, would follow the fate of her mother, and would not be resold by the slave trader until she grew up:

> He would not sell her then on any account whatever. There were heaps and piles of money to be made of her, he said, when she was a few years older. There were men enough in New Orleans who would give five thousand dollars for such an extra, handsome, fancy piece as Emily would be, rather than not get her. No, no, he would not sell her then. She was a beauty—picture—a doll—one of the regular bloods—none of your thick-lipped, bullet-headed, cotton picking niggers if she was might he be d—d (Eakin and Logsdon 1968, 58).

SLAVERY AND MEDICINE: ENSLAVEMENT AND MEDICAL PRACTICES IN
ANTEBELLUM LOUISIANA

Furthermore, the case of Pauline of New Orleans in 1846, is another example of the risks of concubine labor. Pauline, an enslaved African woman deemed a quadroon, was found guilty of brutalizing and torturing her mistress. Pauline was the bound concubine of a master, a Peter Rabbaneck, who is said to have told his wife of the situation; the mistress in turn reacted with hostility toward Pauline. In the absence of the master Pauline whipped and confined the mistress (and her children) until another enslaved African woman reported the incident. The mistress recovered from her injuries; she and her children were eventually abandoned and left destitute by Rabbaneck (Saxon 1929, 213–217; Castellanos 1895, 52–62). Pauline was kept in the Orleans parish prison until her execution (by hanging) on March 28, 1846. This example of concubine labor is important because, it is consistent with the historical record regarding the outcome of such situations. The victim of the sexual labor relationship, the enslaved African woman, is punished; the White characters to the drama are not held responsible by the church or state.

The historical record regarding breeding and concubinage indicates that the rape of African women was common and not considered a criminal activity. Forced and coerced concubinage is considered to have been a frequent practice in southern Louisiana history. Generations of White males "broke" the miscegenation laws and initiated what has been called a "common degeneracy." John Hope Franklin noted in his work that the rape of enslaved African women generally reflected trespassing under the Slave Codes; while concubinage was "socially acceptable" in several southern cities (Franklin 1994, 124 and 139). Victoria Bynum in her work, Unruly Women "The Politics of Social and Sexual Control in the Old South," provides numerous examples showing that "men considered lower class women, particularly African Americans, a sexual proving ground. . ." (Bynum 1992, 109). Slaveowners could not admit forced or coerced sexual relations with bond African women to their wives; and it would appear more of them refused to claim their progeny from these situations than some

Slavery and Medicine: Enslavement and Medical Practices in Antebellum Louisiana

contemporary scholars advance. Generally, enslaved African women could not legally hold White males accountable in the courts and since enslavement followed the condition of the mother, the slaveowners benefitted from the exploitation of African women because the results (live births) often represented a monetary or labor profit.

Overseers were notorious sexual predators and used their position of power to exploit enslaved African females. Rachel O'Connor of Evergreen Plantation in Louisiana, often commented on the "wicked" nature of the overseers she hired. However, the enslaved females caught in these forced and coerced liaisons were punished (Webb 1983, 120, 134, 140–141, 176). Lid, enslaved by Rachel O'Connor, was "caught" with the overseer Mulkey. The overseer was reprimanded, retained his position, and Lid had an iron collar placed around her neck. O'Connor expressed in an 1834 post script of a letter, "I begin to feel sorry for Lid. The iron is rather tight on her neck" (Webb 1983, 134). In a later letter to her brother regarding the concubinage incident involving Lid, O'Connor remarked:

> I should be glad if you let the iron be taken off Lid's neck. I begin to feel sorry for her. She was a good girl before that villain came here, and I scarcely think there is one negro woman in existence that is not guilty of the same wickedness. They are poor ignorant beings, born to serve out their days, and are led astray by such vile wretches as Mulkey, who will, no doubt, have to account ere long for the sin they commit and are the cause of being committed (Webb 1983, 140).

O'Connor made the assumption that despite being "born to serve out their days," enslaved African women like Lid had a choice. With all of her contempt for the overseer, Mulkey, the punishment for his sin would occur "ere long." Lid's punishment,

SLAVERY AND MEDICINE: ENSLAVEMENT AND MEDICAL PRACTICES IN ANTEBELLUM LOUISIANA

as with the paradigm for concubine labor, was swift. In an earlier letter O'Connor remarked that enslaved African women on her plantation had given birth to three mulatto babies that particular month. Yet she made no comment on the White fathers of these babies. Julia Woodrich, formerly enslaved in Lafourche Crossing, Louisiana related a circumstance of concubine labor and her sister:

> I 'member how my master used to would come and get my sister, make her take a bath and comb her hair, and take her down in the quarter all night, den have de nerve to come around de next day and ask her how she feel. He used to wear a big straw hat, cottoneyed pants, and red shoes. Dat's de reason dere is so many mulatto nigger children now (Clayton 1990, 218).

In antebellum culture White women were generally idealized and therefore had their sexuality guarded and preserved; African women were afforded no dignity to their physical persons or their sexuality. They were stripped naked and whipped in front of others; or undressed and probed during slave sales. White women of the time, especially among the wealthy, engaged in such social customs as separate sitting and drawing rooms for males and females. Further, instead of initially undressing for a physician's examination, White women of means would point to an anatomically correct doll to indicate to the physician where the problem area was located. Many antebellum social customs developed for White women by men, placed a higher value on their femininity, sexual preservation and modesty; while African women were made available for a variety of sexual abuses due to the lust of White males in positions of power (Wall 1990, 129). However, poor White women and those who defied masculine societal convention and authority also had their sexual dignity challenged. According to Bynum "poverty defeminized white women much as race defeminized black women" (Bynum 1992, 7).

SLAVERY AND MEDICINE: ENSLAVEMENT AND MEDICAL PRACTICES IN ANTEBELLUM LOUISIANA

Breeding labor, like the institution of enslavement, included the system of reward and punishment. Good breeders were given such "gifts" as calico dresses and less harsh labor; childless women or bad breeders were consigned to arduous field labor. Since breeding labor included the exploitation of men and women, "bucks" and "breeders" were put together and both were ordered and/or encouraged to breed. In 1835 Rachel O'Connor rewarded enslaved African women in this manner:

> I must request the favor of you to add twenty-eight yards of cheap calico in your memorandum for me. Please let it be gay. I have always given a dress of such to every woman after having a young child I am now in debt to four that has young babes, and fine ones too. They do much better by being encouraged a little and I have ever thought they deserved it (Webb 1983, 167).

Enslaved Africans of southeastern Louisiana speak with great consistency of breeding labor. For example, Frances Doby, born in 1838 and enslaved in Louisiana, recalled:

> Her ma had plenty [of] children—Oh, maybe twenty or twenty-five children—so dey don't make her work in de field. No, she work in de house 'cause she always either was nursin' a niggah baby or carryin one.
>
> De master, he had two kind of niggahs: one for de breedin, and de other for de workin' in de fields. Well, Francis' ma was de kind dey keeps for makin' children, and [she] used to stay and do housework or something easy in de house wid de white folks (Clayton 1990, 52).

Manda Cooper, like Francis Doby recalled the breeding labor of

SLAVERY AND MEDICINE: ENSLAVEMENT AND MEDICAL PRACTICES IN ANTEBELLUM LOUISIANA

her mother, and how much this type of labor was worth to the slaveowner:

> My ma never worked in the fields: She had a baby every year. She had twins one time, so the old master taken care of her. She brought him more money having children than she could working in the field. None of us had the same father. They would pick out the biggest nigger and tell her they wanted a kid by him. She had to stay with him until she did get one. When I got old enough to breed, [I] never could have no children. I stayed in the field (Clayton 1990, 44).

Mary Harris was quite cooperative with the Works Progress Administration interviewers, however; her son's statement regarding breeding and enslavement caused the interviewer, Zoe Posey, to record, "It was our first experience with a madman!" Harris' son told Posey:

> '. . .My mother tells me about the brutality of those days, how they whipped unmercifully their slaves.
>
> 'But every slaveholder was not like that,' we ventured.
>
> 'Yes'm, I'm bitter. And the more I think about it, the madder I get. Look at me. They say I could pass for white. My mother is bright, too. And why? Because the man who owned and sold my mother was her father. But that's not all. That man I hate with every fiber of my body. And why? A brute like that, who could sell his own child into unprincipled hands, is a beast. The power—just because he had the power and thirst for money'

SLAVERY AND MEDICINE: ENSLAVEMENT AND MEDICAL PRACTICES IN
ANTEBELLUM LOUISIANA

(Clayton 1990, 95).

Mary Ann John, born in Opelousas, Louisiana in 1855, escaped breeding labor:

> . . .my ma always told me if we had not of been set free when us was, in about two years they would of made me have a baby. They had a big old husky man on de place dey would send all de gals to. If dey didn't want to go, dey given dem a lashin' and make dem go. If dey did not get pregnant de first time, dey was forced to go back. You see, dat nigger didn't do a thing but get babies. You see, dey always sold dem. I was sure glad I was never forced to do anything like that (Clayton 1990, 129).

For enslaved African women the results of breeding labor were significant. African women suffered the high mortality rate of pregnant women in the 19th century and they also suffered from a myriad of conditions such as: general menstrual problems, prolapses of the uterus, abortions, difficult pregnancies and births, vesico-vaginal fistulas, and uterine diseases (see Table 1. Touro Infirmary Pregnancy, Abortion and Uterine/Vaginal Conditions 1855–1860). Related to the mortality rate of enslaved African women is the mortality of enslaved babies. Enslaved African babies experienced a higher mortality rate than White babies due to numerous factors (Kiple and Kiple 1977, 284–306; Steckel 1986, 721–741). When frequent births and mortality were not immediate issues, menstrual disorders were frequently cited. Menstrual disorders included amenorrhea, dysmenorrhea and menorrhea. African women suffered from the painful cramps of dysmenorrhea, which could have been caused by such conditions as endometriosis and pelvic inflammation. In the Touro Infirmary records, African women suffered significantly from amenorrhea, the absence of menstrual bleeding, which was likely a signal of physical exertion, pregnancy or the onset of menopause. The discharge of excessive menstrual blood, menorrhea (menorrhagia), was also a problem related to pelvic inflammation and infections, but might have also been linked to hormonal imbalances and tumors of the uterus.

Prolapses of the uterus or vagina, also known as "falling of the womb," was a frequent medical condition among enslaved African women. This condition occurred when the uterus became displaced from its normal position and pushed toward the vagina. Falling of the womb occurred among women who had numerous/frequent pregnancies/births; and it is suggested that it also occurred among those who labored in the fields during pregnancy. The stretching of the ligaments of the uterus, due to frequent pregnancies and childbirth, not only occurred in African women who labored in the fields, but was also linked to other slave labors and the poor general health of enslaved Africans. On the Destrehan plantation in Jefferson Parish, Louisiana, Nicholas N. Destrehan prepared a list of slaves valued at $35,275.00 at the time of his death in 1848. Laura and Mary Ann were enslaved by Destrehan and both were listed with falling of the womb. Generally, this did not seem to affect their monetary value. Laura, who was 35 years old, was valued at only $300.00; while Maryann, age 30, was valued at $700.00 ("Destrehan's Slave Roll" 1924, 302–303). The Touro Infirmary Admission Record Book (New Orleans, Louisiana) for 1855 to 1860 cites five cases of prolapses of the uterus among enslaved African women. The five women were Maria (patient number 37), Hannah, Maria (patient number 89), Margaret and Ellen. They were all between the ages of 19 and 24 (except for Maria (89) whose age was not listed). Three of the women were listed as married, the other two were listed as single. Three of the women were born in Louisiana, one in Maryland and the birth place of one was not listed (Margaret). The admission record does not detail the number of previous births to the onset of prolapses of the uterus. However, we know that Ellen had one child listed with her, and Maria (89) was pregnant and suffered from the condition at the same time.

Slavery and Medicine: Enslavement and Medical Practices in Antebellum Louisiana

Enslaved African women had spontaneous (miscarriages) and elected abortions. Eight of the 25 conditions in Table 1 refer to abortions performed at the Touro Infirmary of New Orleans from 1855 to 1860. Difficult pregnancies include those resulting in cesarian sections, some performed by African midwives and others in the hospitals. General uterine conditions included diseases, ovarian dropsy, and vaginal fistulas. Alice, a 35 year old enslaved African woman, was brought to the Touro Infirmary in New Orleans in 1858. She was diagnosed with uterine disease and spent 34 days in the hospital. Regarding post-partum conditions, there is little discussion or documentation regarding the after pain that occurred after child birth among enslaved African women. There is significant documentation among former enslaved Africans that women were required to labor in the fields immediately after delivery. Other records indicate that prolific breeders where "pampered" before and after delivery of the babies.

TABLE 1. TOURO INFIRMARY. PREGNANCY, ABORTION AND UTERINE CONDITIONS OF ENSLAVED AFRICAN WOMEN 1855–1860

Patient No.	Name	Condition	Marital Status	Cost
37	Maria	Prolapses Uterus	Married	$30.00
40	Rosetta	Dysmenorrhea	Married	$14.00
59	Hannah	Prolapses Uterus	Single	$36.00/$15.00
89	Maria	Pregnancy and Prolapses of Uterus	Married	$25.00
103	Martha	Pregnancy	Married	$ 2.00
114	Margaret	Prolapses Uterus	Single	$10.00
165	Martha	Abortion	Married	$33.00
213	Ellen &Child	Prolapses Vagina	Married	$48.00/$10.00
223	Emma	Abortion	Single	$17.00
235	Lavinia	Abortion	Married	$16.00
343	Ann Maria	Amenorrhea	Married	$10.00
356	Eliza	Amenorrhea	Married	$10.00
362	Rachael	Pregnancy	Married	$78.00/$25.00
428	Martha	Abortion	Married	$17.00
488	Fanny	Abortion	Married	$32.00
491	Mary	Abortion	Married	$14.00
503	Mary	Amenorrhea	Married	$28.00
590	Julice	Pregnancy	Married	$36.00
670	Eliza	Abortion	Single	$ 5.00
700	Mary Anne	Ovarian Dropsy	Married	$72.00

SLAVERY AND MEDICINE: ENSLAVEMENT AND MEDICAL PRACTICES IN ANTEBELLUM LOUISIANA

780	Harriet	Pregnant	Married	$43.00
782	Louisa	Abortion	Married	$19.00
797	Marie	Pregnant	Not Indicated	$48.00
799	Eliza	Pregnant	Not Indicated	$49.00
895	Alice	Uterine Disease	Married	$34.00
			Total Cost:	$776.00
			Total Number:	25 (3.75%) out of 680

PART TWO

AFRICANS, MEDICAL THEORIES AND PRACTICES

The medical care of enslaved Africans was dependent upon four issues. First, it was dependent upon the human/subhuman controversy. Enslaved Africans early on in the slaveocracy had their humanity questioned, to the extent that the lower South, particularly Louisiana, led the United States in advancing the theories which questioned the physical and psychological nature of the African. Second, the medical management of enslaved Africans comprised a body of knowledge which provides insight into the thinking of the slaveowner. Slaveowners practiced medicine upon the African with some consistency, based upon preserving their chattel property investment. Further, licensed medical doctors and hospitals generally welcomed slaveowner business. They made special provisions for slaveowners to bring in slaves through advertising and offering of low fees. Third, medical experimentation, treatments, surgical procedures and post-mortem examinations are important to understanding the African presence in the development of medical knowledge in the old South and the extent of medical exploitation of the African. Enslaved Africans were regularly used in medical procedures, but, they are rarely acknowledged for having "participated" in the advancement of early medicine. Finally, few enslavement and medicine scholars have considered the Africans' perception of medicine and the medical care they received as slaves.

CHAPTER 6

HUMAN/SUBHUMAN ISSUE: PHYSIOLOGICAL AND PSEUDO-SCIENTIFIC THEORIES

> The slaves are put in stalls like the pens they use for cattle—a man and his wife with a child on each arm. And there's a curtain, sometimes just a sheet over the front of the stall, so the bidders can't see the "stock" too soon. . . .They have white gloves there, and one of the bidders takes a pair of gloves and rubs his fingers over a man's teeth, and he says to the overseer," You call this buck twenty years old? Why there's cup worms in his teeth. He's forty years old, if he's a day." So they knock this buck down for a thousand dollars. . .he makes 'em hop, he makes 'm trot, he makes 'em jump. . .Then, the bidders makes offers accordin' to size and build.
>
> *James Martin*

> We had a good master: He never beat any of us. He say, 'My slave's human like me.'
>
> *Robert St. Ann*

Europeans had specific ideas about the physicality and personality traits of African people, particularly enslaved Africans. Berquin-Duvallon traveled to Louisiana in 1802 and made several observations about the behavioral qualities of Africans:

SLAVERY AND MEDICINE: ENSLAVEMENT AND MEDICAL PRACTICES IN ANTEBELLUM LOUISIANA

> The negro creoles of the country, or born in some other European colony, and sent hither, are the most active, the most intelligent, and the least subject to chronic distempers; but they are the most indolent, vicious and debauched. Those who come from Guinea are less expert in domestic service, and the mechanical arts, less intelligent, and oftener victims of violent sickness or of grief (particularly in the early days of their transportation), but more robust, more laborious, more adapted to the labors of the field, less deceitful and libertine than others (Berquin-Duvallon 1806, 81).

As noted previously, M. Le Page Du Pratz in the 18th century authored a major work on the history of Louisiana. Du Pratz held definite opinions about the behavioral and attitudinal qualities of Africans, specifically those from Senegal. Du Pratz felt that "The Negroes must be governed differently from the Europeans; not because they are black, nor because they are slaves; but because they think differently from the white men" (Du Pratz 1774, 357). Based on his sixteen years in Louisiana, Du Pratz felt that the Louisiana Africans "imbibe a prejudice from their infancy, that the white men buy them for no other purpose but to drink their blood" (Du Pratz 1774, 357). In addition to the European's attribution of a "different disposition" to African people, racial ideology was central to the slaveocracy, particularly as the system was manifested in the lower South. Even the medical theories of the English colonists included supremacist notions (Puckrein 1979, 179–193). Slaveowners, whether educated or not, were privy to the racial doctrines of the times. Certainly White racial supremacy was appealing to their separate and collective ethnocentricities. The idea of a superior White race was also useful in justifying the institution of enslavement, the treatment of African people (enslaved and free), and the attempted enslavement and subsequent removal of Native Americans. Racial ideology of the 1800s rejected the notion

SLAVERY AND MEDICINE: ENSLAVEMENT AND MEDICAL PRACTICES IN ANTEBELLUM LOUISIANA

that the condition of slavery was a dominant factor in the intellectual and physical condition of African people. Rather, it accepted, more often vigorously and sometimes passively, the notion that Africans were simply not human beings:

> In order to decide what is our duty concerning the Africans and their descendants, we must first clearly make up our minds whether they are, or are not, human beings—whether they have, or have not, the same capacities for improvement as other men (Child 1836, 148).

Thomas Jefferson, questioned the humanity of Africans as did many of the prominent White statesmen and founding fathers. However, in their philosophical ideas some felt that should it be ultimately proven that Africans were—White supremacy would continue to prevail. Notable commentary regarding racial ideologies comes from personalities such as Samuel Stanhope Smith (1787), George Fitzhugh (1854), Theodore Parker (1846) and Louis Agassiz (1863). Even those who did believe in the humanity of Africans, often expressed the idea that they were of a different "human" species. Among those who expressed uncertainty, the question still left Whites' suspicious of the Africans' existence. Samuel Cartwright reiterated the feeling of many of the time, "Our Declaration of Independence, which was drawn up at a time when negroes were scarcely considered as human beings, 'That all men are by nature free and equal,' and only intended to apply to white men. . ." (Cartwright 1859, 336)

Whites addressed the question of the humanity of African people by developing laws and an economic institution which oppressed the African; and at the same time heralded the equality and democracy of Whites. White supremacy and the enslavement of Africans often included a religious basis in support of the management of enslaved African people. For example, in his 1754

SLAVERY AND MEDICINE: ENSLAVEMENT AND MEDICAL PRACTICES IN
ANTEBELLUM LOUISIANA

essay entitled "Some Considerations on the Keeping of Negroes," John Woolman stated:

> We allow them to be of the same Species with ourselves, the Odds is, we are in a higher Station, and enjoy greater Favours than they: And when it is thus, that our heavenly Father endoweth some of his Children with distinguished Gifts, they are intended for good Ends: but if those thus gifted are thereby lifted up above their Brethren, not considering themselves as Debtors to the Weak, nor behaving themselves as faithful Stewards, none who judge impartially can suppose them free from Ingratitude (Ducas 1970, 7).

The human/subhuman issue operated in two arenas: first, in the psychological arena Africans were perceived as intellectually inferior and possibly incapable of intellectual improvement (except in the case of interbreeding with Whites). Miscegenation, which was illegal, but frequent in social practice, especially in southeastern Louisiana, was thought to improve the intellectual abilities of Africans; while at the same time debilitate the genetic stock of Whites. The intellectual and psychological state of Africans was considered so precarious that pro-slavery advocates offered arguments that Africans had a higher insanity rate than Whites—especially free Africans (Deutsch 1944, 469–82). Second, the human/subhuman issue addressed the physical nature of African people. There is conflict among antebellum racial ideologists as to whether Africans were physically inferior to Whites. According to author and essayist George W. Cable: "The negro of colonial Louisiana was a most grotesque figure. He was nearly naked. Often his neck and arms, thighs, shanks, and splay feet were shrunken, tough, sinewy, like a monkey's" (Cable 1886, 6). Many people believed that Africans were physically inferior to Whites; and that this inferiority made them better suited to the intensive agricultural labor demanded by the slaveocracy. This contradiction was

SLAVERY AND MEDICINE: ENSLAVEMENT AND MEDICAL PRACTICES IN
ANTEBELLUM LOUISIANA

explained through the logical composition that: a) Africans were physically inferior to Whites because they were not human; b) some (non-human) animals possess a unique ability to perform hard labor (e.g. mules, horses, etc.); therefore c) the African is an animal. The African presented such a different physical presence to White society that explaining certain attributes became a passion for many. Antebellum racial theorists made commentary on Africoid features: heavily melanated skin, broad noses, full lips, and curly course hair. According to Dr. P. Tidyman:

> The colour of the skin in the negro gives him a decided advantage over the white, by enabling him to endure the scorching heat of the sun with less suffering; whilst he is protected by the very nature of his constitution from the unhealthiness of hot climates, which are so inimical to the whites, especially among those who may be necessitated to labour in low swampy situations, and inhale a deleterious atmosphere. . .negroes are seen working with cheerfulness and alacrity, when the white labourer would become languid and sink from the effects of a torrid sun (Tidyman 1826, 306).

Tidyman saw certain advantages among Africans over Whites. Dr. Samuel Cartwright, however, expressed a marked difference between the physical natures of the "the two races" with a confirmed supremacist analysis:

> . . .the Anglo-Saxon and the negro, have antipodal constitutions. The former abounds with red blood, even penetrating the capillaries and the veins, flushing the face and illuminating the countenance; the skin white; lips thin; nose high; hair auburn, flaxen, red or black; beard thick and heavy; eyes brilliant; will strong and

unconquerable; mind and muscles full of energy and activity. The latter, with molasses blood sluggishly circulating and scarcely penetrating the capillaries; skin ebony, and the mucous membranes and muscles partaking of the darker hue pervading the blood and the cutis; lips thick and protuberant; nose broad and flat; scalp covered with a coarse, crispy wool in thick naps; beard wanting or consisting of a few scattering woolly naps, in the "bucks," provincially so called; mind and body dull and slothful; will weak, wanting or subdued (Cartwright 1852, 208).

The human/subhuman issue had a tremendous impact upon medicine and enslavement. Nowhere in the United States did enslavement and medicine link to racial supremacist notions more completely than the lower South. Southern doctors theorized about the African intellect and physical body; and they offered medical ideas tailored to the African. Doctors also conducted studies, performed procedures and surgeries geared toward categorizing the differences between Whites and Africans and wrote extensively on the course of endemic and epidemic diseases with reference to enslaved African people. Leading the discourse on the differences between Africans and Whites, and the effects of certain diseases on the African constitution, was Louisiana physician Samuel Cartwright. Cartwright is considered to have made a significant contribution to the development of medical understanding in the old South. Cartwright was well respected and relentless in his pro-slavery arguments. He defended the anti-abolitionist arguments using medical, scientific and biblical sources. Medical scholar James Guillory notes that Cartwright "apparently felt it his duty to prove that slavery was the only condition proper for the Negro race. Working toward this end, he published many articles during the 1850's and even during the Civil War" (Guillory 1968, 212). Cartwright and his colleagues, through their writings and lectures, addressed an audience of physicians, researchers, members of scientific societies and medical students (Stephens 1989, 55–78).

CHAPTER 7

MEDICAL MANAGEMENT, PRACTICES AND THE HOSPITAL EXPERIENCE

> . . .the niggers in slavery used to get sick. There was jaundice in the bottoms. First off, they would give a sick nigger some castor oil, and if that didn't cure him, they gave him blue moss. Then, if he was still sick, they had a doctor, which they paid to look after the slaves, to come out to see him.
>
> *Cato Carter*

> Dere wont no horspitals. De only "horspitals" "niggers" had in dem days wuz when dey took dem out o' de house tuh de graveyard yasser dat wuz de next place dey took em.
>
> *Henry Baker*

> De slaves was well-treated when dey got sick. My marster had a standin' doctor what he paid y de year. Dey was a horspital building near de quarters an' a good old granny woman to nuss de sick. Dey was five or six beds in a room. One room was for de mens an' one for de wimmins. Us docor was name Richardson, an' he tended us long after de War.
>
> *Isaac Stier*

The medical management of enslaved Africans was important business to the individual slaveowners and to the slaveocracy itself. From the very beginning, slaveowners took a serious interest in the medical management of enslaved Africans. Le Page Du Pratz offered slaveowners this advice:

> The first thing you ought to do when you

> purchase negroes, is to cause them to be examined by a skilful surgeon and an honest man, to discover if they have the Venereal or any other distempter. When they are viewed, both men and women are stripped naked as the hand, and are carefully examined from the crown of the head to the sole of the feet, then between the toes and between the fingers, in the mouth, in the ears, not excepting even the parts naturally concealed, though then exposed to view. . .observe carefully over all the body of the negro, whether you can discover any parts of the skin, which though black like the rest, are however as smooth as a looking-glass, without any tumor or rising. . .There are always experienced surgeons at the sale of new negroes. . .(Du Pratz 1774, 358–359).

After the purchases made at the slave market, slaveowners often, from that time forward, served as "doctors" to increase the physical health of enslaved Africans. Part of the overseers' job was to report illnesses as quickly as possible to the slaveowner. Further, mistresses often attempted to "doctor" slaves back to adequate health. When the folk medicine of the slaveowners failed, they turned to licensed medical practitioners. Professional physicians in Louisiana advertised extensively in such dailies as *The Picayune* (Vol. 1, Vol. 2, 1837, 1838). Medical historian John Duffy describes New Orleans, Louisiana as "one of the leading medical centers in the United States" by 1855 (Duffy 1957, 306). New Orleans contained one of five medical institutions available in the lower South (Mitchell 1944, 441). Therefore, many Louisiana physicians kept residential practices on the plantations of the largest slaveowners. Others eked out an existence as physicians on-call for emergencies. Insurance companies, medical doctors, infirmaries and hospitals all benefitted from the institution of enslavement. But on the main, slaveowners took direct action regarding the medical care of Africans:

SLAVERY AND MEDICINE: ENSLAVEMENT AND MEDICAL PRACTICES IN
ANTEBELLUM LOUISIANA

Many planters, of course, seldom consulted the physician on the diseases of the blacks. Indeed, except for the large plantations, and in those instances where an epidemic might strike a particular region, the planter relied upon his own judgement and prognosis of sickness. For this reason, planters generally kept a book of medicine, and for all practical purposes, the planter, his wife, or the overseer, became the plantation physician (Haller 1972, 246).

Enslaved Africans participated in their medical management. They tell us in their narratives and oral histories that they served as nurses and distributed medicines. They also relate the experiences of those responsible for their medical care—slaveowner, mistress or doctor. With or without the assistance of licensed medical doctors, slaveowners were armed with their own materia medica, which was often a compilation of their own or their neighbors' tried and true remedies.

Part of the medical management of enslaved Africans included making decisions that affected the entire slave population. There was always the threat of purchasing sick Africans. Andrew Durnford of Louisiana is listed as a free man of color who was also a slaveowner and managed his own sugar plantation. He bought his property from one of the largest Louisiana slaveowners, John McDonogh. According to the Durnford letters ". . .I find more difficulty respecting my purchases. . .If a few getts sick on the way I will have to stay up and expend what few dollars I may have left" (Whitten 1970, 237). Durnford experienced a typical slaveowners difficulty with high prices for slaves, problems in transporting slaves after purchase, and especially the issue of illness before, during or after the sale of Africans. For example:

I have been advised not to buy and leave them

in these houses of detention on A/C of diseases of all sorts. I could have bought today a family of eight for 2500. The father a likely black man the mother a mulatto woman, two girls of 7 & 6, two twins of 3 to 4, one of one year or more, one of 2 months, but I decline, for reasons of being put in the house of detention and getting sick (Whitten 1970, 239).

From the frequency with which slaveowners and enslaved Africans mention and discuss sickness, injury and disease, we know that concern for medical conditions was a signal feature of the slaveocracy. Slaveowners worried about the expense that could result from sickness and mortality; enslaved Africans described their care, or lack of care, as a matter of routine. There was always an aspect of sickness to be concerned about in the antebellum South. Children often suffered debilitating illnesses and often mortality from worms. Enslaved African women were at double risk during pregnancy; and at times the ravages of contagious diseases seemed unstoppable among large African populations.

When Rachel O'Connor became the "Mistress of Evergreen" plantation, she was not aware that one day she would be running the plantation almost single-handedly. Her tasks included the supervision of slaves, hiring overseers, estimating and acquiring adequate supplies and accounting for the crops. Her letters to her family, particularly her sister and brother, detail southeastern Louisiana's constant battle with sickness and disease. O'Connor wrote extensively about the illnesses she suffered, those of enslaved Africans, and the sickness, which pervaded the Feliciana area. According to O'Connor in 1829, her doctor-in-residence was "very attentive to the sick ones and soon has them able to work again. Mr. Bowman has lost several slaves this fall and winter past; one fine young man died last night. Mrs. Pirrie and Dr. Ira Smith has some dangerously ill at this time" (Webb 1983, 44). Cholera was a significant threat to the Louisiana territory and O'Connor wrote extensively about the disease:

> I have written often and enclosed many receipts to cure cholera . . . There has several died of cholera at the landing, but they were landed from steamboats either from N. Orleans or from above, and died in a few hours and were buried instantly. Some market Negroes from Point Coupe that were sent on board the boats with their marketing caught the disease and died, but no others has taken it yet. St. Francis Ville is perfectly healthy at this time, but I do not let the Negroes go there or any other place. I am very afraid of it. The boats are all stopped running. They cannot get men to work on board. They have refused six dollars per day, owing to their dying so fast (Webb 1983, 84).

Evergreen Plantation suffered cycles of enslaved Africans out from field labor due to sickness. During times of sickness or other extreme labor need, slaveowners like O'Connor would "borrow" or "lend" enslaved Africans from/to neighboring plantations. O'Connor did not leave the "doctoring" to her physician-in-residence, Dr. William L. Denny. In 1840 she wrote to her sister "I have not laid up one day for 8 or 9 months past and am constantly nursing sick Negroes. There has not been one day past for several months that there has not been more or less very sick. Two are sick now. On the 26th of last month little Sam died. He was seven years old on the 13th. O, my dear sister, no pen can convey to you my distresses" (Webb 1983, 228). On several occasions O'Connor shared her home medicine remedies with family and neighbors.

Enslaved Africans commented on the medical management of the slaveowner; and also their role in alleviating illnesses. Ellen Broomfield of Louisiana recalled less sickness than other enslaved Africans and noted:

Slavery and Medicine: Enslavement and Medical Practices in Antebellum Louisiana

> In [the] Spring they give us sulphur and molasses to purify our blood. And candy was made out Jimson weed and sugar, and that was good for worms.
>
> When folks had too much blood, they cupped them. Well, it was like this: You take a cup of water and put in it a piece of cotton. Put [it] to [the] temple and set [the] cotton on fire; that draws blood. [I] saw my ma do it many a-time (Clayton 1990, 32).

Henrietta Butler of Lafourche Parish, Louisiana served as a nurse on the plantation. She recalled that the mistress' older brother served as a doctor to the enslaved Africans and that the mistress herself served in that capacity also:

> He would give us pills when we got sick. I rember one day one of the mens had lockjaw. That old woman made a fly blister and put on dat poor nigger and let it stay until it blistered. Then [she] took a stiff brush and roughed over dat sore place. When she did, dat nigger hollered and his jaws come unlocked (Clayton 1990, 38).

With the various types of injuries and illnesses that Africans suffered it was inevitable that they should spend time in either a plantation or city hospital or infirmary. New Orleans possessed a number of hospitals and infirmaries including: Charity Hospital, Franklin Infirmary, The Circus Street Infirmary and the Orleans Infirmary among others. Many of these hospitals in New Orleans offered and advertised their services to slaveowners inviting enslaved Africans as patients, and providing slaveowners with attractive rates. One such medical facility was Touro Infirmary. Touro Infirmary was founded by Judah Touro (1775–1854) as a non-sectarian, charitable hospital to help the indigent sick of New

SLAVERY AND MEDICINE: ENSLAVEMENT AND MEDICAL PRACTICES IN
ANTEBELLUM LOUISIANA

Orleans. It opened in 1852 in the old plantation house known as "Paulding Mansion." Touro, a businessman of Jewish descent, was a major philanthropist and bequeathed thousands of dollars to Hebrew and other interests in New Orleans and other parts of the United States. In his last will and testament Touro established the Hebrew Hospital of New Orleans:

> I give and bequeath to found the Hebrew Hospital of New Orleans the entire property purchased for me, at the succession sale of the late C. Paulding, upon which property the building now known as the "Touro Infirmary" is situated; the said contemplated Hospital to be organized according to law, as a charitable institution for the relief of the indigent sick, by my executors and such other persons as they may associate with them conformably with the laws of Louisiana (Huhner 1946, 131).

When the infirmary opened, it contained 24 beds and accepted all people regardless of creed or race. It collected fees from patients on a sliding scale from $1.00 to $5.00 per day; surgical procedures were performed for an additional charge. From approximately 1862 to 1869 the hospital closed to keep the Union army from appropriating it during and after the Civil War; the hospital reopened after the Civil War. From 1854 to 1859, which marked the formative years of Touro Infirmary, medical care was administered through the contract with Dr. Joseph Bensadon who served as the Resident Surgeon of the infirmary. It is suggested that a number of patients during this time were from Dr. Bensadon's private practice, along with the walk-in patients (Burnett 1979, 1–4; Kahn 1991, 4–5).

Touro Infirmary, like many antebellum hospitals in New Orleans, regularly admitted slaves. While some medical facilities were strictly for the use of slaves, Touro admitted enslaved

SLAVERY AND MEDICINE: ENSLAVEMENT AND MEDICAL PRACTICES IN
ANTEBELLUM LOUISIANA

Africans, White Americans, French and Spanish Creoles, and of course White European immigrants. The Admission Book of the Touro Infirmary (See Appendix B) gives a wealth of information regarding the patient. However, this basic account of the patient's admission does not list such information as causes, symptoms and cures of specific conditions; nor does it provide any data on previous health conditions of the patients listed. The admission book does however contain twenty-one categories that provide information regarding enslaved Africans. The categories are: (1) No. (Patient Number), (2) Name of Patient, (3) Place of Birth, (4) Occupation, (5) Last Place From, (6) Residence in New Orleans, (7) Date of Admission, (8) Hour of Admission, (9) Date of Discharge, (10) Date of Death, (11) Age, (12) Whose Account, (13) Deposit, (14) Rate Per Day, (15) Malady, (16) How Long Sick, (17) Married or Single, (18) No. of Ward, (19) Total No. of Days, (20) Amount, and (21) Remarks.

Each patient in the Admission Book of the Touro Infirmary is numbered. Between 1855 and 1860 1,584 patients were admitted to the Touro Infirmary. Of this number, 43% or 680 (two sequential numbers are missed in the admission record during this period) were enslaved Africans. The next category of the admission record is "Name of Patient." This is important because enslaved Africans are most often identified by one name (forename), and few are listed with a forename and a surname. Individuals who were not slaves, and those which the record indicates were born abroad, are usually listed with a first and last name. Masculine and feminine identity of enslaved Africans was determined by forename. "Place of Birth" is the next category. In this section we discover where enslaved Africans were born. Most of them have an immediate connection to the South (See Table 2. Touro Infirmary Place of Birth of Enslaved Africans 1855–1860). In the Admission Book of the Touro Infirmary enslaved Africans are also identified by occupation, which was consistently listed as "slave." "Occupation" is the primary indicator of the African's status. Each person is assigned an occupation. For example, European immigrants are listed as engaging in such occupations as "seaman," "clerk," "peddler," "cobbler," and "servant." Enslaved Africans are listed as "slave." As the nation got closer to the Civil War, Touro Infirmary (about 1859) began listing many of their first-name-no-last-name patients as "servants" or used another word descriptive of the work they did, e.g. "field hand," "levee hand." This was an attempt to move away from the use of the word "slave." In addition, first-name-no-last-name patients who were not born abroad, and who were most likely enslaved Africans, are also listed under occupation as: "plantation," "laborer," "cook," "nurse," "drayman," "canal hand," "press hand," "steve-dore," "servant (girl/boy)," "levee hand," etc. The data presented includes only those 680 individuals specifically listed as "slaves."

TABLE 2. TOURO INFIRMARY PLACE OF BIRTH OF ENSLAVED
AFRICANS 1855–1860

State (Place) of Birth	Number	Total
Alabama	29	29
Arkansas	5	5
Maryland	54	↓
Baltimore	7 (61)	61
Carolina	4	4
Connecticut	1	1
Florida	8	8
Georgia	28	28
Kentucky	40	↓
Louisville	5 (45)	45
Louisiana	59	59
New Orleans	33	33
Opelousas	2	2
Bayou Sara	1	1
Shreveport	1 (96)	1
Mississippi	9	9
North Carolina	43	43
South Carolina	38	↓
Charleston	3	↓
Alexandria	2 (43)	43
Tennessee	17	↓
Nashville	1	↓
Memphis	1 (19)	19
Texas	5	5
Virginia	221	221

Washington	2	2
"Not Known"	1	1
Not Indicated	23	23
Total	680	680

"Last Place From" is the category which indicates where the person came from before entering New Orleans. Many of the enslaved Africans listed in Touro's records during this time, came from places other than New Orleans and other than their place of birth, which would indicate their movement through slave sales or the movement of their slaveowners. This is consistent with New Orleans holding the position as the most significant slave trading market in the lower South and the United States in general (Wall 1990, 148).

The next category, "Residence in New Orleans," gives specific information as to how long the patient was in the city of New Orleans. The record ranges from "2 days," to several years; or a "—" (dash) indicating that the enslaved African is "from" New Orleans. "Date of Admission" gives the month and date, sometimes the year (the year is listed at the top with the first listed patient and is always listed in the upper right hand corner of the admission book). "Hour of Admission" is listed in whole time and either in the A.M. or P.M. (7 A.M., 5 P.M.). "Date of Discharge" is listed as month and date, except in the case of death when it is not listed at all.

The "Date of Death" is the next category and is listed by the month and date the person died in the infirmary. There were 48 recorded deaths of enslaved Africans at the Touro Infirmary between 1855 to 1860 (See Table 3 Touro. Infirmary Recorded Deaths of Enslaved Africans 1855–1860).

Slavery and Medicine: Enslavement and Medical Practices in Antebellum Louisiana

Table 3. Touro Infirmary Recorded Deaths of Enslaved Africans 1855–1860

Patient No.	Name	Date of Death	Age	Condition	Remarks
32	Jerry	Feb. 19, 1855	19	Typhoid Fever	
139	Jimbo	Aug. 15, 1855	24	Gas. Enteritis	
239	Sophia	Dec. 4, 1855	21	Anasarca	
247	Ben	Dec. 31, 1855	34	Athesma	
275	Malinda	Feb. 26, 1856	35	Typhoid Fever	
320	Mary Ann	May 29, 1856	27	Phethisis	$10/Burial
349	George	June 7, 1856	32	Injury	
352	Alley	June 20, 1856	15	Phethisis	
354	Nelson	June 18, 1856	48	Injury	
400	Lafayette	Aug. 25, 1856	28	Typhoid Fever	$12/Burial
418	Jack William	Sept. 4, 1856	36	Typhoid Fever	
479	Adam	Nov. 18, 1856	52	Pneumonia	$10/Burial
495	Rachael	Apr. 3, 1857	24	Dropsy	
524	Judy	Feb. 16, 1857	36	Not Determined	
533	Loomus	Apr. 10, 1857	?	Scrofula	
559	Ann	Mar. 20, 1857	38	Pleurisy	
580	Isham	Apr. 3, 1857	12	Tetanus	
626	Allen	May 13, 1857	21	Dysentery	
640	Sarah	May 16, 1857	24	Int. Fever	
653	Esther	June 2, 1857	23	Typhoid Fever	
684	Jack	June 18, 1857	33	Pneumonia	
697	David	Aug. 21, 1857	50	Apoplexy	$12/Burial
756	Jim Butler	Nov. 7, 1857	50	?	
790	Louisa Hester	Nov. 29, 1857	19	Peritonitis	
820	Bob	Feb. 2, 1858	30	Consumption	
848	Lucinda	Mar. 17, 1858	13	Pleuropneumonia	$12/Burial
865	Abraham	Mar. 19, 1858	25	Congestion of Brain	$10/Burial
900	Nancy Ann	July 25, 1858	17	Gonorrhea	
908	Thomas	June 6, 1858	48	Dropsy	
916	Henry	June 17, 1858	22	Typhoid Fever	
919	Dock	June 23, 1858	—	Dropsy	
929	Harriet	Aug. 29, 1858	17	Sec. Syphilis	
932	Jim	July 24, 1858	35	Chron. Dysentery	
944	Patty Mussina	Aug. 2, 1858	65	Schirrus of Glands	
976	Phil	Aug. 21, 1858	35	—	
981	Colter	Sept. 11, 1858	30	Ulceration of Rectum	
993	Tom	Aug. 24, 1858	24	—	
997	Joseph	Aug. 30, 1858	27	—	
1008	Jane	Sept. 17, 1858	40	Yellow Fever	
1215	Ben	Nov. 11, 1858	—	Consumption	
1268	Frederick	Jan. 22, 1859	65	Dropsy	
1309	Jack	Jan. 14, 1859	40	Pneumonia	
1313	Jim	Feb. 4, 1859	38	Not Listed	

1317	Polly/Child	Mar. 19, 1859	20	Not Listed
1321	Jim	Mar. 25, 1859	40	Not Listed
1366	Zachariah	June 23, 1859	60	Typh. Pneumonia
1398	Amy	Sept. 27, 1859	25	Anemia

Total Number: 48 (7%) out of 680

Sixteen of the deaths were female and thirty-one were male. A total of $66.00 was recorded in burial fees for enslaved Africans. Six deaths were recorded from September 1859 through April, 1860, but they were not listed as slaves, due to the pre-Civil War practice of listing Africans actual slave occupation as noted above. A total of thirty Africans who died were single; thirteen were married; and the marital status of four of the enslaved Africans was not indicated in the record. Finally, the average age at death was thirty years old.

The Admission Book of the Touro Infirmary lists an "Age" for each patient. This category gives us an idea of how old the enslaved African was at the time of admittance to the Infirmary. For example, on February 15, 1855 at 5 P.M. an enslaved girl from Virginia named Henrietta was 15 years old and admitted for Gonorrhea. During this time a few African women were admitted with their children and are listed by the first name of the woman followed by "and child." It would appear that very small children were admitted in this manner; or perhaps children under the age of 14. The admission record itself does not indicate the frequency of admittance of children from 3 to 14 years of age. However, 28 children between the ages of 3 to 14 years were admitted between 1855 and 1860 (see Table 4. Touro Infirmary Enslaved Africans Age Distribution at Time of Admission 1855–1860).

"Whose Account," is the category which indicates who was responsible or paying the hospital bill. In the case of enslaved Africans this person was usually the slaveowner, a secondary slaveowner (such as individuals and businesses who rented the African's labor), an overseer, or a family member. It also appears that several prominent or frequent account holders admitted groups of Africans on the same day, sometimes indicated by the ditto sign (") sometimes written as (do). The account holders entries varied, we usually get the first and last name, or often the first initials and the last name and then sometimes just the last name. There were 680 accounts for enslaved Africans between 1855 and 1860. During this period there were 223 Account Holders. The majority of Account Holders represented only had one account. There are multiple account holders in the record including: D. Donovan (10), T. Foster (63), Dominique Madden (19), J. L. Moore (13), T. J. Pipkin (62), H. J. Ranney (64), A. O. Sibley (33), Col. R. A. Stewart (18) and New Orleans slave trader Bernard Kendig (24). Several companies in New Orleans held accounts for slaves, and the City of New Orleans held an account for one enslaved African. During this period there were six female account holders identified as such by "Mrs." in front of the surname (See Table 5. Touro Infirmary Account Holders Named for Enslaved Africans 1855–1860).

TABLE 4. TOURO INFIRMARY ENSLAVED AFRICANS AGE DISTRIBUTION AT TIME OF ADMISSION 1855–1860

Age	Number of People
3	2
4	1
5	4
6	1
8	1
9	2
10	3
12	7
13	2
14	5
15	17
16	9
17	11
18	14
19	19
20	18
21	23
34	8
35	31
36	11
37	13
38	10
39	1
40	25
41	2
42	5
43	4
44	9
45	11
46	1
47	1
48	8
50	8
51	1

Slavery and Medicine: Enslavement and Medical Practices in Antebellum Louisiana

22	33	52	2
23	19	53	3
24	41	55	3
25	44	56	1
26	44	57	5
27	26	58	2
28	30	60	4
29	14	62	2
30	46	64	1
31	5	65	2
32	14	67	1
33	6	68	1
		69	1

Age not listed. 42

Total............680

TABLE 5. TOURO INFIRMARY ACCOUNT HOLDERS NAMED FOR ENSLAVED AFRICANS 1855–1860

A. Brown and Co. —1
Abrams, J.P. — 2
Allen, N.W. — 1
Andrews and Co. — 2
Andrews, G. — 1
Andrews, J.S. —2
Armstrong, J. —1

Bates, George —1
Batson, Will —6
Bayley, G.M. — 1
Bein, J.D. — 3
Bell, J.M. — 3
Bell and Boyd — 1
Belleville Iron Wks—2
Bernard — 1
Bidwell, D. —1
Blass, G. Anjele — 1
Blocks, Daniel — 3
Blenderman, John — 1
Bogart, G.C. —1
Boulware, E. —1
Bowdich, Capt. — 1
Bradford, G.M. — 2
Bradford, Judge —4
Breeden, Mark —1
Brenan, R. —1
Bridwell, David —1
Brown — 1

Hagan, A. —1
Hall and Street —1
Hall, Rodd & Putman—2
Hansell, H.H. —1
Hardenbrook —1
Harrell, Mr. — 1
Harrison, R.M. —1
Horrell Gayle & Co.— 3
Harvey — 1
Haskell — 1
Hasman, T. (?) — 1
Hatcher, C.F. —1
Hays, H.M. —2
Henderson, Geo. —1
Henderson, Terry — 1
Hoffman, H. — 1
Hogan, Mr. — 1
Holmes, Dr. —1
Holmes, Luther — 1
Huggins, Capt. —1
Huntington, B.W. —2

Intosh, Mr. — 1
Israel, Mrs. E.M. — 2

J.A. Beard and Co.—3
Jamison, S. — 2
Johnson, L. —3
Johnstone, T. —3

Parker, G.P. —1
Patterson, G. —1
Patton, Thos. F. —1
Paxton, William H. –1
Payne, G.E. —1
Pendegrast, Richard—2
Philips, Adler —1
Philips, H.B. —4
Pierce —1
Pinkhard, G.M. — 5
Pillsbury, Edward —1
Pipkin — 1
Pipkin, T.J. — 62
Poitevent, Capt. —4
Poitevent, W.J. —12
Porter, George —1
Post – L Mel — 1
Post, R.B. —1
Purvis, George — 1
Putman, J.M. —1

Quick, M.C. — 1

Ramsey, H.J. —8
Ranney, H.J.(Maj.)–64
Rehan, J.C. —1
Ricardo, D.J. —1
Rice, N.F. —1
Ricketts — 1

102

SLAVERY AND MEDICINE: ENSLAVEMENT AND MEDICAL PRACTICES IN ANTEBELLUM LOUISIANA

Brown, Henry — 7
Brown, J.D. —2
Brown, Wm. —1
Bustamente, Mrs. — 1
Boyd, S. —2

Calder, J. —1
Calder, James —5
Calder, John — 1
Caldwell & Sisk — 1
Campbell, W.L. —1
Carre', W.W. —4
Carter, E.H. —1
Casey, T.J. — 4
City of New Orleans—1
Clark, Dr. — 2
Clark, T.L. —1
Cohen, J. —1
Collings, Mrs. —1
Cotter, W. —2
Condon, R. — 5
Cooks, Mr. B. — 1
Cook, G.W. — 1
Cousin, Capt. —1
Cromwell, O.G. —1
Crookes, H.M. —1
Cuddy Brown & Co.—3
Cummings, R.C. —1
C.W.Rutherford&Co.–1

Davis, C.H. —1
Davis, George — 1
Davis, J. —1
Davis, R.W. —2
Delk, P.A.B. —1
Denegre, W.O. —1
Donnella, O.G. —3
Donnovan, D. —10
DuBois & Mish —1

Eaton &Henderson —1
Edgar, Mr. —1
Edwards, D. —1
Elmore, W.A. —2

Fassman, H.A. —2
Felger, Mrs. —1
Finch, M. —1
Finney, Thomas —2
Forsyth, Mr. —1

Jonas, George — 1

Kendig, B. — 24
Key, Mr. — 2
Key, W.J. — 4
Kilpatrick, W.W. —1
King, Geo. R. —2
Knapp — 1
Knapp, Dr. —1

Labat, D.C. — 1
Lane, L.W. —1
Leathers, Capt. T. —2
Leeds Co. —4
Levy, A. — 1
Levy, J.S. —2

Levy, L.C. —1
Levy, Lionell — 3
Levy, W. —1
Lisk, O.M. — 1
Longsfield, J.H. —1
Lousdale, H.J. — 1
Lyons, G.H. — 1
Lytle, C.W. —1

Madden, Dominique–19
Macgee, Mr. — 1
Macgee, Mrs. —1
Macon, William C. —1
Magee — 1
Marks, A. — 1
Matthews, Mr. —1
Matthews, T.E. —1
Matthews, T.J. —1
McCann & Patterson–5
McCelland, Jerry —1
McGinnies —1
McGuire, Nimrod —1
McIntosh, J. — 3
McKelvery Agent — 1
McKnight, Thos. —9
McLanathan, J. —1
McQueen —2
Miot, G.R. —1
Mitchell, J. —5
Moise, Columbus —1
Moore, J.L. —13
Morgan, T.H. —1
Murphy, Mrs. —1

Robertson, J.B. —1
Rock, Mr. —1
Rodd, E.W. —2
Rutherford, C.M. —1
Rutherford and Long–1

Shaw and Gunts —1
Sheilds, Thos. —1
Sibley, A.O. —33
Sidle, D. — 6
Simpson, M.M. — 1
Smith and Harris —1
Stadeker — 1
Stevens, W.G. — 3
Stevenson & Co. — 2
Stewart, Col. R.A. —8
Stinson, Jos. —2
Stockton, Jas. —2
Sullivan, D.O. —4

Tisdale, N.O.J. — 1
Tisdale, R. — 1
Tompkins —1
Turner, T.S. —1
Turpin, John —1

Ure, Capt. — 2
Ure, T.M. — 2

Van Benthayzen, W. –1
Van Horn, J.D. —1

Walker, A.W. —2
Walton, Col. —1
Weiners, Mr. — 1
Wheeler, Paul (?) —1
Wilbur, Thos. —1
Williams, Scott —1
Wilson, P.H. —1
Wooten, G.J. —1

Yancy —4

Not Determined — 7
Not Listed —1

Total:
Account Holders: 223
Number of Accounts: 680

SLAVERY AND MEDICINE: ENSLAVEMENT AND MEDICAL PRACTICES IN ANTEBELLUM LOUISIANA

Foster, John —1
Foster, T. —63
Fortier, T. —1
Frisby, T. J. —1

Gale, John —1
Glass, Thomas A. —2
Graham, D.S. —4
Graham, Mr. —2
Grant, Capt. —2

Morton, Mr. —4
Mussina, J. —1

Oakey and Hawkins —1
O'Rourk, S. —1

"Deposit" is a category which is not often used in the Admission Book during this period of time; and is rarely used with enslaved Africans. When used deposits could range rather high for non-African patients and was related to their ability to pay the account—either through a third party or because they had the financial means to pay more than other non-African patients. "Rate Per Day" is an interesting category, which for enslaved Africans was fixed at $1.00. The Rate Per Day was a little higher for some non-Africans and even higher for those who possessed the means to pay. The non-African patients were charged from $1.50 per day to as much as $5.00 per day.

"Malady" is the category which indicates the reason or the diagnoses for the patient's admittance to the Touro Infirmary. This category too yields an abundance of information regarding the various conditions, diseases and illnesses suffered by enslaved Africans. The first eleven African patients for the year 1855 were listed with a variety of "maladies" including: dysentery, syphilis, typhoid pneumonia, secondary syphilis, intermittent fever, gonorrhea, bronchitis, prolapses (of the) uterus and dysmenorrhea. The most common maladies were Catarrh (16), Diarrhea (80), Dysentery (39), Intermittent (32+) and other fevers, Pneumonia (24+) and other pneumonias, Rheumatism (14), Syphilis (17+) and other related syphilitic disorders, Typhoid fever (18) and Yellow Fever (18). 75 maladies were not listed in the admission record (See Table 6. Touro Infirmary Maladies Attributed to Enslaved Africans 1855–1860).

The "How Long Sick" category tells us that the patient was known to possess the malady for a specific period of time. For Example, David, a 26 year old enslaved African born in South Carolina, and having lived in New Orleans for 2 years, suffered from typhoid pneumonia for "8 days." Choice, a Georgia-born African suffered from the same ailment for "3 weeks" before being brought to Touro Infirmary. Enslaved Africans suffered days, weeks and months from various conditions, ostensively before being brought into the hospital for treatment.

The marital status of enslaved Africans is contained in the category "Married or Single." It should be noted that many enslaved Africans diagnosed with sexually transmitted diseases such as syphilis and gonorrhea were also listed as "single." Sometimes an African was listed as married and we are told for how long, "2 weeks", "1 month" etc. We don't know however, if husband and wives were admitted to the infirmary together. This was possible since groups of Africans were admitted at the same time by a single account holder. We should be cautioned that more than one admission of an enslaved person, over the five year period was also possible, but not determined with accuracy. According to the Touro Admission record for 1855 to 1860, 24.5% of the enslaved Africans were married, while 67.5% were listed as single (see Table 7 Touro Infirmary Enslaved Africans Gender 1855–1860).

TABLE 6. TOURO INFIRMARY MALADIES ATTRIBUTED TO ENSLAVED AFRICANS 1855–1860

Abortion–8
Abscess–3
Amenorrhea–3
Amputation–2
Anasarca–1
Anemia–6
Apoplexy–1
Arthritis–1
Ascites–2
Asthma–1

Blenorrhagia–2
Bronchitis–7
Burn–1
Bubo–2

Cataract–1
Catarrh–16
Cholera–5
Cholera Morbus–1
Cholic–3
Congestion Brain–1
Constipation–7
Consumption–2
Convulsions–2
Cuts–2
Cystitis–1

Debility–6
Delirium Tremens–2
Diarrhea–80
Dirt–Eating–1
Dislocation of Humorous–1
Dislocation Thumb–1
Dislocation Toe –1
Dropsy–5
Dropsy(Ovarian)–1
Dysentery–39
Dysmenorrhea–2

Eczema–1

Fistula–1
Fistula on Arm–2
Fistulous Abscess—1
Flatulence–1
Fractures–5
Frostbitten–1

Gangrene–1
Gastritis–3
Gastro Enteratis–2
Gastrodynia–1
Gonorrhea–6

Hemiplegia–2
Hemorrhoids–4
Hernia(Femoral) –1
Hernia(Inguinal)–1
Hernia(Umbilical)–1
Hydrocele–1
Hydro–Pericarditis–1
Hysteria–8

Indigestion–1
Indisposition–12
Indurated Gland–1
Indurated Testicle–1
Injury–45
Intermit Fever–32
Itch–1

Measles–10

Node on Tibia–1
Nostalgia–1
Necrosis–1
Neuralgia–3
Neuro Pheneumonia–1
Not Listed–75

Orchitis–3

Paraplegia–1
Pericarditis–1
Peritonitis–1
Phthisis–5
Pleuritis–1

Pleuro–Pneumonia–4
Pneumonia–24
Poisoned by Oak Vine–1
Pregnancy–6
Pregnancy/Prolapses–1
Prolapses Uterine–3
Prolapses Vagina–1
Puncture Wound–1

Renal Hemorrhage–1
Retention of Urine–1
Rheumatism–14
Rubeola–8

Scalp Wound–1
Schirrhus of Gland–1
Scrofula—2
Scrofulous Tumor–1
Scrotal Hernia–1
Sprain–1
Syphilis–17
Syphilis Secondary–6
Syphilis Tertiary–2
Syphilitic Erupt.–1
Syphilitic Pneum.–1

Tetanus–1
Tonsillitis–6
Tumour–3
Typhoid Fever–18
Typhoid Pneum.–8

Ulcer–2
Ulcer of Rectum –4
Ulcer on leg–5
Undetermined–18
Uterine Disease –1

Variola–3
Varicosella–1

Worms–1

Yellow Fever–18

SLAVERY AND MEDICINE: ENSLAVEMENT AND MEDICAL PRACTICES IN ANTEBELLUM LOUISIANA

Enteritis–1   Pleurisy–8
Epilepsy–7
Erithema–1
Eruption Disease–1

Fever–10
 (B.R.) Fever–1
 Continued   Total: 680
 Fever–2

In addition, in the Admission Book of the Touro Infirmary, 75.2% of the enslaved Africans were male and 24.6% were female (See Table 8. Touro Infirmary Enslaved Africans Gender 1855–1860). "No. of Ward" is a category that was not used in the Touro Infirmary Admission record during this period. There is a notation of "£" that, when it is used, is used for African and non-African patients.

TABLE 7. TOURO INFIRMARY MARITAL STATUS OF ENSLAVED AFRICANS 1855–1860

	Married	Single	Not Indicated	Total
Number of Enslaved Africans	166*	460**	54	680
Percentage	24.5%	67.5%	8%	100%

*One enslaved African woman was designated as a widow.
**This table an estimate; it includes 45 children who were under the age of 16; 25 of the 45 are children under the age of 12.

TABLE 8. TOURO INFIRMARY ENSLAVED AFRICANS GENDER 1855–1860***

African Males	African Females	Not Listed	Total
512	167	1	680
75.2%	24.6%	.02%	100%

***Gender was determined by the traditional European male-specific and female-specific names given to Africans. For example, John, Bill were considered male; Ann, Mary were considered female.

Therefore, we don't know if Africans were housed in the same areas as non-Africans; yet the preference of the time was to segregate the two groups of people. "Total No. of Days," is the category indicating the number of days the patient spent in the Infirmary before being discharged from the infirmary or perhaps dying. For example, a Florida-born African, Jerry, was admitted February 10th to the Infirmary with Typhoid Fever; he spent 9 days in the hospital and died February 19, 1855.

The "Amount" category was multiplied by the rate times the number of days. Therefore, Jerry's account holder, Mr. Harrell paid $9.00 on his account. The last category for the Admission Book is "Remarks." Information in this section varied, but usually listed whether or not the account was paid, marked as "PD" or "Paid." This section also indicated other situations, such as if the patient was discharged with the malady, whether or not surgery was performed, if the patient died, or whether extra charges (usually in conjunction with surgery or burial) were assessed. Surgical procedures involving Africans were performed at the Touro Infirmary between 1855 and 1860 and are frequently mentioned in the remarks section. Surgeries were relatively expensive. In the Touro Infirmary record surgical costs ranged from $10.00 to $100.00 (See Table 9. Touro Infirmary Surgical Procedures Performed Upon Enslaved Africans 1855–1860).

TABLE 9. TOURO INFIRMARY SURGICAL PROCEDURES PERFORMED UPON ENSLAVED AFRICANS 1855–1860

Number	Surgical Remarks	Amount	Medical Condition
59	Surgical Extra	$ 15.00	Prolapses Uterus
89	Delivery	$ 25.00	Pregnancy & Prolapses
102	Operation	$ 50.00	Hernia
122	Operation	$ 10.00	Psychosis
180	Operation	$ 50.00	Injury
213	Extra	$ 10.00	Prolapses Vagina
256	Pleurisy from Injury	$ 10.00	Pleurisy
266	Operation	$ 50.00	Fracture Cranium
288	Extra for Surgery	$ 20.00	Injury
312	Extra for Surgery	$ 35.00	Not Listed
313	Extra for Surgery	$ 52.50	Scrofulous Tumor
362	Extra	$ 20.00	Pregnancy
367	Extra	$ 12.00	Phethesis
375	Extra	$ 25.00	Injury
380	Extra	$ 10.00	Injury
383	Extra	$ 21.00	Injury

Slavery and Medicine: Enslavement and Medical Practices in Antebellum Louisiana

392	—	$ 25.00	Dislocation of Thumb*
407	Extra	$100.00	Injury
411	Extra	$ 50.00	Fracture Patella
456	Extra	$ 15.00	Scalp Wound
462	Extra	$ 20.00	Hemorrhoids
469	Extra	$ 25.00	Hemorrhoids
497	Extra	$ 50.00	Undetermined
641	Extra	$ 20.00	Tumour
671	—	$ —	Amputation of Arm**
1273	—	$ —	Hand Amputation
		Total:	$720.50

27 (4%) surgical procedures listed out of 680
*This was not indicated as an extra cost amount.
**No remarks or extra amount was listed for this amputation of the arm.

CHAPTER 8

MEDICAL EXPERIMENTATION, TREATMENTS, SURGICAL PROCEDURES AND POST-MORTEM EXAMINATIONS

> Oh, de blood done sign my name, oh, de blood.
> Oh, de blood done sign my name, name.
> Oh, de blood done sign my name.
>
> *Enslavement Hymn*

Enslaved Africans were subject to medical experiments and procedures, surgeries and post-mortem examinations. Medical doctors left various detailed records regarding these areas of enslavement and medicine. While much has been written on medical experimentation, few scholars have acknowledged the powerlessness of enslaved Africans. Few records indicate that enslaved Africans were ever asked permission to have experiments, treatments or procedures performed upon them. No extant records reveal that enslaved Africans ever refused treatment. Records indicate that slaveowners permitted the use of slaves, particularly for experiments which could result in the African being able to return to labor.

The narratives and oral histories of enslaved Africans do not significantly discuss the incidence of medical experimentation. Africans confirm "doctoring," or the failure to provide medical care by the slaveowner, but do not provide any information outside of the realms of such procedures as births and amputations. This is probably due in part to the masses of enslaved Africans understanding of medical experimentation as another form of "doctoring" or "nursing." Medical experimentation was not widespread, but when it did occur, and where there was a nearby enslaved African population, they were regularly used and this added to the medical risk factors inherent in the system of

SLAVERY AND MEDICINE: ENSLAVEMENT AND MEDICAL PRACTICES IN
ANTEBELLUM LOUISIANA

enslavement.

New Orleans led the way in medical experimentation in the old South. Medical historian James Morris notes that even radical procedures such as blood transfusions were first performed in the United States in New Orleans at Charity Hospital (Morris 1975, 354). Many of these experiments were reported in the *New Orleans Medical and Surgical Journal* and they detail the use of Africans as subjects. For example, Dr. William M. Boling of Montgomery Alabama carried out an experiment with phosphorus ("Phosphoric ether") based on a previous experiment conducted by Dr. Ames who used phosphorus as a cure for pneumonia.

The subjects in this experiment were a healthy "mulatto" boy named Sam who was seven years old; and a healthy "Negro" man who was twenty-five years old. While both subjects were recorded as being in good health, the man had a "small ulcer on the foot" (Boling 1853–54, 729). No conclusive results were obtained from either subject. According to Dr. Ames, certain amounts of phosphorus acted as a sedative and reduced the pulse, while excessive amounts of phosphorus acted as a stimulant, and caused the pulse to speed up. In the course of the experiment, Dr. Boling observed Sam behaving a little "giddy" from the ounce and a half of alcohol administered with the phosphorus. According to Boling:

> The two hours immediately succeeding each of the last two doses, Sam spent riding in my buggy with me, and attending to my horse at the different stopping places; and though I noticed him carefully, no appreciable effect was manifested—the variation in the pulse alone excepted—otherwise than that he seemed a little merry, which was fairly, I think it will be admitted, attributable to the alcoholic part of the dose— about half an ounce in one instance, and an ounce in the other. It would scarcely seem necessary, while the large quantity of alcohol would render it

improper, to repeat, or to carry the—joke any further with Sam (Boling 1853–54, 729).

Boling cited that both subjects remained in good condition throughout the experiment, even though they could have experienced "nausea, vomiting, a burning sensation or feeling of oppression at the epigastrium, local inflammation of stomach and bowels" (Boling 1953-54, 731). In addition, Dr. Ames said his subjects experienced a reduced pulse with "2 drops of the saturated tincture." Dr. Boling stated that his patients (especially the man) should have been depressed to "an extreme state of sedation" with 272 drops in nine and one half hours (Boling 1853–1854, 726–738).

In another case published in the *New Orleans Medical and Surgical Journal* a doctor was called to a twenty-eight year old African woman who suffered from "sanguine nervous temperament." She was pregnant, but had begun to menstruate on June 1, 1846. She also had pain in the "back and region of the womb." She was said to be in good condition at this time, and the doctor administered medication. On June 2, 1846, the doctor was called again because the woman was dying. Her condition had deteriorated and she seemed bleak and unresponsive. She had been hemorrhaging heavily. The doctor administered urtica urains and the hemorrhaging ceased. When the menstrual flow began again, she was given urtica urains and opium. The next morning, she had regained some strength, and was given urtica urains, acetate lead and opium. Despite this the woman was exhausted and "she was not able to return to labor, until the 13th of July, although kept on tonics the whole time" (Johnson 1849–50, 452). The lead acetate was used as an astringent which is considered poisonous, but was used therapeutically in the past. Opium was used to assist in subsiding the pain. Both of these medicines could have been harmful to the patient and especially the developing fetus.

On February 17, 1849 in another case involving the use of

urtica urains on menorrhagia, an African woman named Eliza, who was thirty years old suffered from excessive menstrual flow and "complains of giddiness and blindness when attempting to rise, with ringing in her ears" (Johnson 1849–50, 453). Eliza was administered castor oil and urtica urains. This case also indicates that Eliza was "operated twice." Apparently the menorrhagia had subsided and the doctor decided that it was unnecessary to return until March 1.

Post mortem examinations were necessary to gain the depth of understanding required by medical practitioners of the antebellum period. However, "dissection was frowned upon as immoral, irreligious, and a posthumous disgrace and was seriously impeded by state laws prohibiting the legal acquisition of cadavers, forcing teachers of anatomy to resort to the heinous practice of grave robbing to secure bodies" (Breeden 1975, 321). The availability of cadavers was an inducement to acquiring good numbers of medical school students. Medical historian James O. Breeden found that grave robbing, while condemned by antebellum society, was a thriving business in some areas of New England and in Virginia. Africans played an important role because of their social status as enslaved persons. Among Americans of African descent there is mythology, a preponderance, which still persists from antebellum times—tales of "night doctors," and "gown men" who sought the bodies of Africans for "unnatural acts" (Fry 1975, 170–211). In New Orleans, Louisiana the medical mythology among Africans surrounding scientific horrors included the stories about "Needle Men"—Charity hospital medical school students, eager to procure cadavers for their studies. Also the "Black Bottle Men" of Charity Hospital were said to have given patients cascara and magnesia thought to hasten death and also provide the necessary corpses for post-mortem examinations (Saxon, Dreyer and Tallant 1945, 75–78).

In 1795, an example of a post-mortem examination, was a 30 year old African woman named Phillis who required medical attention for a hypogastric tumor. In addition she was pregnant, yet continued to menstruate. She apparently lost the baby in 1795, but continued to suffer from painful menstrual hemorrhaging and increased weight. By 1808 she was considered to be of "enormous size" and "could (to the astonishment of all about her), still walk about her house, and would even visit some of her relations, who lived at the distance of half a mile" (Callaway 1808, 139). While the menstrual hemorrhaging ceased she died of other "symptoms." Then, according to Dr. Callaway:

> Having obtained permission, her body was opened in the presence of several gentlemen, and the following appearances were marked: the omentum covering the abdominal viscera, to appearance healthy, but increased (to speak within the bounds of moderation) to fifty times its natural size. Its blood-vessels, which composed the principal part of its bulk, measured one-fourth of an inch and upwards in diameter. It was attached to a tumor, presently to be described, into which its blood-vessels evidently penetrated (Callaway 1808, 140).

We are not told who gave permission, however as the post-mortem examination proceeded, the doctor(s) examined the intestines, abdomen, spleen, stomach, liver and removed the tumor. The doctor(s) continued on to examine the "ligamenta lata et rotunda, the ovaria, the tubae fallopianae, and vagina" which were found to be normal (Callaway 1808, 141). The uterus was found to contain various tumors. The uterus was removed and according to Callaway, "the whole weight of the uterus, with its connections, was thirty-six pounds" (Callaway 1808, 142). Phillis' case represents one of the early explorations into the problems of the uterine cavity, she would be a precursor to African women like Anarcha and others who were (while living) subjected to and survived numerous gynecological surgeries and experiments.

SLAVERY AND MEDICINE: ENSLAVEMENT AND MEDICAL PRACTICES IN ANTEBELLUM LOUISIANA

Anarcha and other enslaved African women under the care of Dr. J. Marion Sims have come to symbolize, probably more than any other case of medical experimentation, the faceless, nameless, voiceless African of the slaveocracy. Her dilemma existed as a woman in need of medical care; but she also served as a "guinea pig" until the procedure could be repeated with success. As an enslaved African woman, Anarcha was seventeen, pregnant and had to undergo a difficult birth. The birth of her child left her with the condition known as "vesico-vaginal fistula." Numerous enslaved African women suffered from this condition which included symptoms of urinary and rectal incontinence. While operating on a White woman, Sims stumbled upon a technique which he felt would address vesico-vaginal fistula. This procedure involved the patient being placed in a knee-elbow position. Air pressure was used to dilate the vagina and a forerunner to the speculum was used. Anarcha suffered through thirty procedures before closure of the fistula. Other enslaved African women underwent this painful operation as well. In the end, Sims had perfected the technique and developed the Sims speculum. According to medical historian John Duffy:

> . . . had Sims not lived in the South where slaves were available, his "experiments" would not have been possible. These repeated operations were performed for the large part without anesthesia and must have caused considerable suffering. It is highly unlikely that any surgeon, northern or southern, would have experimented on white women in such a way, nor that the patients themselves would have submitted to such a lengthy ordeal—one covering several years (Duffy 1976, 139).

There are many surgical cases of vesico-vaginal fistulas involving African women listed in the *New Orleans Medical and*

SLAVERY AND MEDICINE: ENSLAVEMENT AND MEDICAL PRACTICES IN ANTEBELLUM LOUISIANA

Surgical Journal. In 1855 and 1858 Dr. Nathan Bozeman operated on "a colored girl" sent to him by another doctor in Selma, Alabama. She was twenty-eight years old and described as "spare built, and rather delicate-looking." Her last pregnancy involved the difficult birth of a twin which left her with urinal retention and leakage difficulties. Bozeman operated experimenting with zinc sutures when the norm had been to use silver. According to Bozeman the woman was discharged "entirely well, having complete control over her urine" (Bozeman 1860, 190–191). Unlike other enslaved African women, this patient was subjected to only one surgical procedure for vesico-vaginal fistula.

The next case discussed involved another "colored girl" called Mary who was thirty years old and had six children. Mary, who was from St. James Parish, Louisiana was brought to Bozeman by Samuel Cartwright. The account indicates that Mary had suffered from vesico-vaginal fistula, recto-vaginal fistula and a retroversion of the uterus since she was twenty-three years old. Bozeman described Mary as "somewhat reduced in flesh, and has the appearance of one who has endured great suffering" (Bozeman 1860, 191). There were two vesico-vaginal fistulas to close, and regarding the retroversion of the uterus, Bozeman noted "There was the most complete retroversion of the uterus I have ever seen" (Bozeman 1860, 192). Mary was operated upon three times to close the fistulas, Bozeman stated his feeling about the surgeries:

> Our failure, at subsequent operations to close these small openings, as well as the one in the bowel, is such that every surgeon may expect now and then to meet with. One who is constantly operating is liable to become careless in attending to small matters, which frequently leads to unfavorable results when it might not otherwise have happened. I am not exempt from this fault myself, and I think if I had taken a little more pains with my operations in this case, I would not

now be under the necessity of recording my two failures (Bozeman 1860, 194).

If Bozeman expressed concerns about the failure of the procedures, it would be important to know how Mary felt about the persistence of the doctors in attempting to perfect the suture. Regarding the third patient Bozeman cites a case involving an enslaved African woman named Matilda, described as a "colored girl, property of Col. M. Stamper, of Early County, Ga." (Bozeman 1860, 195). Matilda, who was twenty-one years old in 1855, suffered from urethra-vaginal fistula, vesico-vaginal fistula, contraction of the vagina, amenorrhea, and poor general health. Like many physicians, Bozeman followed the surgical techniques offered by J. Marion Sims for vesico-vaginal fistulas. Matilda was operated upon ten times over a period of more than three years. Despite the physician's persistent efforts, he noted: "Instead now of advanciug (sic) our patient towards a cure, the reverse was observed. . .our patient was placed where we started with her" (Bozeman 1860, 198). Matilda was discharged "uncured" with Bozeman lamenting about the failure of his procedures. However, we are not given any insight into the perspective, feeling, attitude or health condition from any of these three women involving the painful and time-consuming surgical procedures for vesico-vaginal fistulas.

In addition to being an important part of the development of an effective treatment for vesico-vaginal fistulas, enslaved African women also were in the forefront in the development of cesarean section procedures in the United States. Louisiana figured significantly in the numbers of cesarian sections performed in the antebellum South. According to Duffy's research,

> . . .all of the cesarean sections in Louisiana were performed on slave women. The usual practice in cases where the pelvis was deformed or too small was to resort to craniotomy, cutting up

the head of the fetus in order to facilitate delivery. The fear of abdominal incisions was so great that it was generally considered much safer to destroy the child than sacrifice the life of the mother. The high risk which was involved in any abdominal surgery makes it more than a coincidence that so many of these early patients were slaves, and clearly indicates that southern surgeons and physicians were far more willing to try new procedures upon slaves than upon other women (Duffy 1976, 141–142).

The failure of many traditional scholars to assay the gross victimization of enslaved African women (and men) is an oversight which must be addressed. It would include asking the primary questions which would logically provide a more detailed analysis and observation than we currently possess. We believe we can answer simple questions like: why were enslaved African women utilized more than White women of the time regarding procedures such as vesico-vaginal fistula and cesarian sections? Why were so many enslaved African women patients not addressed by name? In the physicians' records, the responses and feelings of enslaved African women patients were not recorded. How will we assess the validity of the physicians' records regarding the frequency of their surgical procedures and outcomes (successes and failures) involving enslaved African men and women? And finally, what does this research area tell us about the issue of medical ethics and enslaved Africans in the antebellum period? These questions and others would yield added understanding to the discourse on enslavement and medicine and the historical development of cures for such conditions as vesico-vaginal fistula.

Analysis of other types of surgical procedures (involving enslaved Africans) which were numerous in the antebellum period may shed more light upon these questions since Africans were significant "patients" for these procedures for a variety of reasons.

SLAVERY AND MEDICINE: ENSLAVEMENT AND MEDICAL PRACTICES IN ANTEBELLUM LOUISIANA

In April 1854, a slaveowner called in a Dr. Brooks of Wheelock, Texas to examine her "negro man, Caleb, aged about forty years" (Brooks 1854–55, 457). For approximately one year, Caleb suffered from a "large tumor growing on the left side of his neck" (Brooks 1854 –55, 457). The growth of the tumor was said to be very rapid and caused respiratory problems. Brooks attempted to remove the tumor enlisting the assistance of two other physicians and allowing other individuals to view the surgery.

Four other cases from South Carolina represented the types of illnesses and injuries enslaved Africans suffered. The first involved an African woman named Betty, twenty years old, who suffered from "inflammation of the fibula." The second case was Robert, a "mulatto" thought to have been between thirty and forty years old who suffered from gonorrhea. The third case was Hector, who suffered a leg injury from mill work, began experiencing the effects of gangrene—and faced a second amputation. Finally, Simon, forty years old, suffered from a labor related dislocation of the hip (Bailey 1859, 740–745).

Betty, according to Dr. Bailey, "has for several years past suffered from pain and inflammation of the fibula" (Bailey 1859, 740). Her leg was swollen, prone to secretions and generally interfered with her labor responsibilities:

> She is at times totally incapacitated for work, the irritation being so great as to cause fever and painful swelling of the lympathic glands of the groin (Bailey 1859, 740).

Betty was operated on, prescribed an opiate for the pain and given anodyne and potassium. To the extent that the surgery was successful, Betty was "able to resume her accustomed duties" (Bailey 1859, 741).

On two or three previous occasions Robert had suffered from

gonorrhea. He had swelling of the "right scrotum and testis." The surgery performed on Robert consisted of two separate punctures of his scrotum. The doctor removed eight ounces of "clear serum," then he "injected about 3 oz diluted tinc. iodine" (Bailey 1959, 741). Robert was given anodyne and sulphur of magnesia. Bailey concluded that Robert "has since suffered no inconvenience" since the procedure (Bailey 1859, 741).

Hector labored as a miller and, when his shirt was caught in the wheel, he injured his right foot, crushed his leg, broke a rib and suffered bruises and other severe lacerations and punctures. Bailey commented on his decision to amputate Hector's leg:

> I examined carefully the crushed leg and the rest of the calf, and saw no reason why I should not attempt to save the knee joint as the limb appeared perfectly healthy at point, of election, and the negro was very valuable to his owners. I accordingly resolved to amputate at the point above, named (Bailey 1859, 742).

Hector was given sulphuric morphine, morphine and brandy. On the ninth day Bailey remarked: "I am surprised to find my patient so comfortable this morning—he is cheerful and hopeful" (Bailey 1859, 743). Hector's stump began to be consumed by gangrene and, with the aid of one of Bailey's friends and the slaveowner, Bailey began to amputate the stump further. Having concluded that Hector had "entirely recovered" Bailey made this observation of Hector's demeanor throughout the ordeal:

> This case is remarkable as showing the influence exerted by the mental over the physical organization. At the time of the accident, and ever after, the patient exhibited a presence of mind and strength of will that was wonderful. He remarked, that during the rapid revolutions of the wheel, 'he

dodged his head to prevent his brains being knocked out,' and accommodated himself to his unnatural position, which no doubt prevented his being mangled and killed on the spot. He was always hopeful, and exhibited a patience and cheerfulness under suffering that was worthy of all admiration (Bailey 1859, 744).

Simon was struck in a labor accident in the hip joint. Bailey attempted to correct the dislocation by "reduction by manipulation." Bailey noted that, "The head of the bone was felt distinctly to change its position downwards and forwards with a slight rubbing sound. Two more trials were made in like manner, and I began to despair of reduction by this method, when a distinct snapping sound was heard, and the head of the bone slipped into the acetabulum. I directed the patient to be kept quiet. . ." (Bailey 1859, 745). At this point, Bailey gave Simon sulphuric morphine. Despite continued pain and some swelling Bailey concluded that Simon "seems to be doing well in all other respects" (Bailey 1859, 745).

Another case of amputation involved an enslaved African woman named Rachel who was 20 years old. Rachel's slaveowner was Miss Martha Bullock of Arkansas. In January, 1857 Rachel suffered from frostbite of the legs and feet from a snowstorm. When she came across an open fire she put her legs and feet too close and unknowingly burned herself. After various remedies were tried the gangrene continued to advance and the doctor made the decision to amputate both of her lower legs. After amputation, Rachel seemed to recover slowly but steadily (McElrath 1859, 195–197). Dr. McElrath, in detailing the case of Rachel, spends time justifying the radical procedure, noting that she would have been in pain for a significant duration and that amputation would have eventually been necessary.

CHAPTER 9

"NEGRO/SLAVE DISEASES" AND OTHER ILLNESSES ATTRIBUTED TO OR AFFECTING ENSLAVED AFRICANS

No more sickness,
No more sorrow,
When I lay my burden down.

Enslavement Hymn

In the available research in the field of enslavement and medicine no other area is as intriguing as the material available on "Negro/Slave Diseases." The identification of "Negro/Slave Diseases" was a direct manifestation of the human/subhuman issue. Extending from that basic premise, people of African descent would logically contract and manifest diseases and illnesses that were race-specific, and more importantly, different from those contracted by Whites. The "Negro/Slave Diseases" that extended from a racial supremacist orientation include: Negro Consumption, Cachexia Africana, Drapetomania, and Dysaesthesia Aethiopica. Other illnesses that significantly affected Whites, and yet caused them to observe closely their course in the African, include: Dysentery, Yellow Fever, Cholera and Diarrhea. However, all of these illnesses share some specific racial components when applied to enslaved Africans in the antebellum South.

Negro Consumption (also called Struma Africana and "Negro Poison") was thought to be a race-specific condition among people of African descent, specifically, enslaved Africans. Some scholars have linked the condition to pulmonary disorders or other lung-based problems. According to *De Bow's Review*:

SLAVERY AND MEDICINE: ENSLAVEMENT AND MEDICAL PRACTICES IN ANTEBELLUM LOUISIANA

Some physicians, looking upon negro consumption through Northern books, suppose it to be a variety of phthisis pulmonalis—but it has no form or resemblance to the phthisis of the white race, except in the emaciation, or when it is complicated with the relics of pneumonia or a badly-cured pleurisy. Others regard it as a dyspepsia or some disease of the liver or stomach; the French call it mal d'estomac. But dyspepsia is not a disease of the negro; it is, par excellence, a disease of the Anglo-Saxon race. I have never seen a well-marked case of dyspepsia among the blacks. It is a disease that selects its victims from the most intellectual of mankind, passing by the ignorant and unreflecting (*De Bow's Review* 1851, 212).

Negro Consumption could not, therefore, have been contracted by Whites. According to the above observation, it could not be confused with other, perhaps similar disorders, not on the basis of physical diagnosis, but on the basis of racist assumption. However, Negro Consumption symptoms included mucous on the gums, an accelerated pulse, ashy skin, and thin blood. Africans afflicted with Negro Consumption were given to dirt-eating, displaying a "sulky" disposition and/or paranoia. The major cause of Negro Consumption, however, was "generally mismanagement or bad government on the part of the master, and superstition or dissatisfaction on the part of the negro" (*De Bow's Review* 1851, 213). Negro Consumption was also said to be compounded by the prevalence of conjurers among enslaved Africans; and their belief that "fellow-servants are against them." Negro Consumption also manifested itself because Africans believed that their "master or overseer cares nothing for them or is prejudiced against them" (*De Bow's Review* 1851, 213).

Samuel Cartwright emphasized that Negro Consumption was

not related to the consumption of the White race, except when it results in "emaciation," and when it is "complicated with relics of pneumonia or badly cured pleurisy." Cartwright suggested that the cause of Negro Consumption was superstition, largely because the African feels that he has been poisoned. This state leads to a condition of depression and possibly dirt eating. Cartwright suggested that the patient should be rubbed down with an oil. In addition, he should be given "tartar emetic-half grain, capsicum-five grains, and teaspoonful of charcoal, and a tablespoonful of gum gusiacusm -3 times a day" (*De Bow's Review* 1851, 213).

Cachexia Africana gets its name from its chief symptom, dirt-eating. Its other symptoms include a host of physical and psychological ailments, among those are: emaciation, no desire to eat, melancholia, heart palpitations, sleepiness and an appetite for dirt or chalk. According to W. M. Harvey and John Lindesay in 1799, Cachexia Africana "occurs in those who have, generally speaking been badly cloathed, ill fed and lodged, and whose constitutions have been worn out by hard labour" (Harvey and Lindesay 1799, 282). These authors placed an emphasis on environmental factors in addition to racial factors. However, they noted that the Africans condition could improve better than Whites when moved to different areas:

> It is remarkable that negroes, subject to this disease, have been much benefited by living in a low situation, near to marshes, which quickly prove fatal to whites; and I have long ago observed this, before I had formed any theory upon the subject (Harvey and Lindesay 1799, 284).

Similar to Negro Consumption, Cachexia Africana also contained a major psychological component. The African's condition in enslavement, being so profoundly challenging, produced a host of debilitating symptoms. Harvey and Lindesay noted that, "The mind, partaking of the sufferings of the body, is affected with nostalgia, brooding over their ill treatment, separated forever from their friends and relations, and doomed to suffer without daring to complain" (Harvey and Lindesay 1799, 282).

Cachexia Africana was thought at times to be an epidemic which killed Africans in large numbers. Cachexia Africana was also attributed to the poor diet of enslaved Africans. Enslaved Africans usually only ate twice a day, and usually the meal was a mixture of cornmeal and salt. Their diet generally lacked meat and vegetables. Another aspect of Cachexia Africana was attributed to the living conditions of enslaved Africans. Traditionally, the living conditions of enslaved Africans consisted of crowded, drafty quarters with a rudimentary wood or dirt floor. Proper ventilation was often difficult, especially with the necessary use of cooking/warming hearths. According to one antebellum report regarding slave housing, "one of the most prolific sources of disease among negroes, is the condition of their houses and the manner in which they live. Small, low, tight and filthy, their houses can be but laboratories of disease" ("Department of Agriculture. . ." 1846, 325). The close contact Africans had with the soil put them at risk for various parasitic conditions. Cachexia Africana was similar to hookworm disease, named after a parasitic intestinal worm. Like Cachexia Africana, dirt-eating was a symptom of hookworm disease. According to V. Alton Moody, hookworm disease was acquired:

> . . .either directly through the mouth or through skin infection. Water, or food that had been contaminated with infected mud or water, might become the source of infection. Penetration through the skin, however, was practically the only source of the disease. The habit of going barefooted gave ample opportunity for infection through the skin of the feet. Within a few weeks the little worms had found their way into the

blood, thence to the heart, to the lungs, into the throat and then through the stomach to become lodged on the walls of the intestines (Moody 1924, 271–272).

There were no cases of Negro Consumption, Cachexia Africana or hookworm disease in the Touro Infirmary Admission Record for 1855 to 1860. There was, however, in this record one case of worms and two cases of an unspecified consumption disorder contracted by enslaved Africans.

Drapetomania is a condition best described in the "Diseases and Peculiarities of the Negro Race" by Samuel Cartwright. Cartwright simply defined it as the "disease causing negroes to run away" (Cartwright 1859, 331). In addition to being a "disease of the mind," Drapetomania was treatable and preventable. The most important aspect of Drapetomania was that it was an issue of slave management, based largely on the treatment of enslaved Africans. Drapetomania was not only a race-specific illness, but was also—according to Cartwright's theories—grounded in pro-slavery religious doctrine (Wall 1990, 128–129). Cartwright asserted that Drapetomania was linked to the concept of Pentateuch. The Pentateuch refers to the first five books of the Bible viewed collectively. According to Cartwright the Pentateuch:

> . . .declares the Creator's will in regard to the negro; it declares him to be the submissive knee-bender. In the anatomical conformation of his knees, we see "genu flexit" written in his physical structure, being more flexed or bent, than any other kind of man (Cartwright 1859, 332).

Therefore, if Whites were to treat Africans with some semblance of equality it would be an abuse of God's will because of the position of the African. Cartwright noted, "those who made themselves too familiar with them, treating them as equals, and making little or no distinction in regard to color" do a disservice to Africans and were just as bad as those who were cruel and abusive to Africans (Cartwright 1859, 332). There were several cures for Drapetomania including: whipping the negative attitudes out of Africans, treating Africans kindly, feeding Africans well and providing adequate clothes and warmth. In addition, it was suggested that one family per slave house should be implemented and Africans should not be allowed to visit other farms or plantations. Furthermore, no liquor was to be given to slaves; and they were not to be "overworked" or exposed to inclement weather. Drapetomania could also be cured by punishing the African to submission and treating them like children (Cartwright 1859, 332–333). There were no cases of Drapetomania reported in the Touro Infirmary Admission Records from 1855 to 1860. There were however, twelve cases of "indisposition" and eight cases of hysteria reported in the Touro Infirmary Admission records.

Cartwright described Dysaesthesia Aethiopica as the "hebetude of mind and obtuse sensibility of body." Dysaesthesia Aethiopica was thought to be a mental disease which affected both the body and mind. In this state the African is said to be in a condition not unlike anesthesia. As a general deterioration of the blood, Dysaesthesia Aethiopica was said to produce sleepiness, dry skin, lesions on the body and a preponderance for mischievous behavior. This mischievous behavior prompted overseers to call the disease "rascality" because Africans were said to have broken equipment, destroyed crops and animals; and "they raise disturbances with their overseers and fellow servants without cause or motive" (Cartwright 1859, 333). Dysaesthesia Aethiopica would affect those slaveowners:

> who made themselves too familiar with them [enslaved Africans], treating them as equals, and making little or no distinction in regard to color; and, on the other hand, those who treated them cruelly, denied them the common necessaries of

life, neglected to protect them against the abuses of others, or frightened them by a blustering manner of approach, when about to punish them for misdemeanors (Cartwright 1859, 332).

Another important aspect of Dysaesthesia Aethiopica is that it was said to be more common among free Africans than those who were enslaved. Those enslaved Africans who contracted Dysaesthesia Aethiopica did so through contact with free Africans. According to Cartwright, Dysaesthesia Aethiopica:

> . . . attacks only such slaves as live like free negroes in regard to diet, drinks, exercise, etc. It is not my purpose to treat of the complaint as it prevails among free negroes, nearly all of whom are more or less afflicted with it, that have not got some white person to direct and to take care of them. . .I propose only to describe its symptoms among slaves (Cartwright 1859, 333).

In addition to the above, Dysaesthesia Aethiopica was not just caused by bad management among slaveowners and their overseers; but also by "idleness" among enslaved Africans. Cures for Dysaesthesia Aethiopica included stimulating the liver and kidneys of the enslaved African; giving him/her hard labor outdoors, good food and a warm environment. These remedies, given a chance, should have produced the following affects:

> His intelligence restored and his sensations awakened, he is no longer the bipedum nequissimus, or arrant rascal, he was supposed to be, but a good negro that can hoe or plow, and handles things with as much care as his fellow servants (Cartwright 1859, 335).

Like Drapetomania, there were no cases of Dysaesthesia

Aethiopica reported in the Touro Infirmary Admission Record from 1855 to 1860. The closest diseases in epidemiological analysis would be the previously mentioned hysteria and indisposition.

A major problem with the assertion of "Negro/Slave Diseases" is the lack of adequate information regarding their epidemiology. While we are provided several causes of Negro Consumption, Cachexia Africana, Drapetomania, and Dysaesthesia Aethiopica, we are not critically informed as to what type of African is likely to acquire the disease. Furthermore, we do not know scientifically how the diseases were spread, where they most frequently appeared; or where any significant numbers of the infected population lived. A general retro-epidemiological analysis of the four primary "Negro/Slave Diseases" reveals their chief commonality was largely a psychological dysfunction attributed to Africans. Another commonality of the diseases is, in order to exist, they "need" to vilify the African and elevate White society.

Outside of the realm of "Negro/Slave Diseases," enslaved Africans suffered from the same diseases and illnesses as Whites. However, Africans were thought to add a different quality to the ailments. These conditions were numerous and Africans in the United States experienced significant mortality (See Table 7). Antebellum disorders prevalent among enslaved Africans include, but were not limited to, dysentery, yellow fever, cholera and diarrhea. Antebellum society constantly battled conditions such as these. In doing so, some doctors believed that the African physical-immunological response to these ailments was indicative of a pathology different from Whites.

Dysentery (also called the flux and the bloody flux) was a significant condition which represented a severe intestinal infection. It's symptoms included chills, fevers, inflammation, diarrhea, and a characteristic bloody-water discharge. Dysentery among enslaved Africans of the antebellum period is described as:

Slavery and Medicine: Enslavement and Medical Practices in Antebellum Louisiana

> A low, grave form of typhoid fever, with frequent discharges of serosanguinous fluid from the bowels, sometimes attended with pain at stool, more or less severe, but not during the intervals. In short, a grave typhoid fever, with its diarrheal discharges changed from a "cider" to a sanguinolent character (Wooten 1854–55, 452).

In addition, a 1853 treatise on "The Negro and his Diseases," stated that "Dysentery is sometimes seen to take on a peculiar form among negroes. We know not how extensively this form of disease may have been noticed among them, or whether it should not be considered a modification of the disease induced by hot climate" (Grier 1853, 760). Dysentery was said to affect Africans primarily in the fall and winter seasons. It was frequently fatal due to the severe loss of bodily fluids. Some antebellum physicians found some success in treating dysentery with blue mass and opium in Africans and Whites who contracted the illness. Dysentery ranked among the most frequent medical cases reported in the Touro Infirmary Admission Record. Thirty-nine cases of dysentery were reported for enslaved Africans during the period 1855 to 1860.

Much like dysentery, cholera was an intestinal infection which affected enslaved Africans in significant numbers. One of the causes of cholera among Africans was thought to be bad food. Cholera caused dehydration like dysentery due to the diarrhea and vomiting that accompanied the illness. Cartwright proffered the idea of "cholera of the mind" as a condition affecting enslaved Africans. When this condition affected enslaved Africans they:

> die when their mind has a splinter of superstition run into it from the appearance of cholera, or some frightful disease among their comrades. . .This peculiar psychological condition, so fatal among negroes, might properly be termed a tetanus of the mind; a dream, a prophecy, or any

idle thing, when cholera or any malignant disease is about, acting the part of a splinter to excite it. To call it fear or panic, conveys a wrong idea of it (Cartwright 1854, 156).

Despite its purported frequency before 1855, enslaved Africans represented only six cases of cholera in the Touro Infirmary Admission Records from 1855 to 1860.

The scholarly literature on yellow fever in New Orleans, and other parts of Louisiana, is considerable due to several epidemics which produced high mortality rates in the antebellum South, especially among Whites. The most devastating of the yellow fever epidemics in Louisiana occurred in 1853 and was considered a monumental plague (Wall 1990, 131). In New Orleans, it is believed that yellow fever was brought to the territory by enslaved Africans around 1769. That idea, coupled with the extreme mortality rate among Whites in 1853, caused many to suggest that Africans had a significant resistance to yellow fever. This opinion was expressed in 1826:

> During the prevalence of the yellow fever in New Orleans or Charleston, and in other towns where the disease is strictly endemic, it is but seldom that we hear of negroes being attacked, whether they are strangers to the city or permanent inhabitants; occasionally a few cases may be discovered among them, but I believe where one patient is carried off by the disease, that three under skillful treatment recover; the fever with them yields more readily to medicine, and the symptoms are rarely so severe or inflammatory as to require bleeding (Tidyman 1826, 327).

The "black vomit" as yellow fever was sometimes called (also "Yellow Jack," and the "Saffron Scourge"), was sometimes thought to be noncontagious; and exposure to yellow fever once fostered the idea that a future immunity to the disease would follow. In southeastern Louisiana yellow fever was considered a "seasonal disease" that came with the extreme summer heat and humidity ("Yellow Fever at New Orleans" 1843, 288).

Yellow fever displayed a host a symptoms and stages or degrees of severity. Yellow fever symptoms included: vertigo, headaches, back pain, muscular soreness, sleepiness, rapid or weak pulse, respiratory difficulties, a coated tongue, nausea, vomiting and diarrhea. Sometimes yellow fever sufferers would experience remissions of one to two days before advancing to seriously debilitating stages that included: cavity bleeding (including bloody stools), yellow/green or black/bloody vomiting, loss of memory, high fever, yellow skin tone (jaundiced) and coma. In the Touro Infirmary Admission Records for 1855 to 1860, eighteen cases of yellow fever were reported for enslaved Africans. In addition, only one of these yellow fever cases, in 1858, resulted in death.

From 1855 to 1860 diarrhea was the most frequently cited condition affecting enslaved Africans at the Touro Infirmary in New Orleans. During this period of time eighty cases of diarrhea were reported. Diarrhea, a major endemic disease of antebellum society, normally represents a symptom of other disorders. The major symptom of diarrhea is liquid bowel activity. Its cause is usually contaminated food and/or water supplies. There are two types of diarrhea—acute and chronic. Chronic diarrhea most often required hospitalization since, of the two types, acute diarrhea had a span of a few hours to seventy-two hours. Chronic diarrhea may have been an indication of more serious intestinal disorders; and like dysentery, blood may accompany the condition. Cholera, dysentery and diarrhea were all endemic conditions, related to the geography and the available clean water supply:

> . . .the land was low and surrounded by marshes made the problem the more difficult.

> Without modern processes of filtration the use of water from the Mississippi, from bayous or from stagnant lagoons was fraught with fearful consequences. Cistern water was found to be the purest and best (Moody 1924, 267).

Cistern water was not readily available to enslaved Africans living in the slave quarters. Since these holding tanks had to be clean, well-constructed and able to hold large amounts of rain water they were normally situated for use near the slaveowner's main house. Many Africans had to rely on stagnant water near the quarters and fields. Historic archeology and oral histories of Africans and planters who made observations of southeastern Louisiana plantations do not illustrate that cisterns were provided to enslaved Africans on a regular basis. However, it appears that when endemic diseases such as cholera, dysentery and diarrhea produced high mortality rates and loss of investment, cistern water became a medical health necessity (Postell 1951, 94).

PART THREE

AFRICAN MATERIA MEDICA AND ENSLAVEMENT

There is general consensus that enslaved Africans contributed nothing significant to the field of medicine or to the medical care they received as slaves during the antebellum period. In addition, a type of "pure victim" theory is offered and supported, denoting that the African, so oppressed in the institution of enslavement, could not manifest any proactive human behaviors. A pervasive historical theme is that the slaves abject powerlessness is the defining feature of African American history and culture. Africans are not acknowledged for their role in the medical development of the antebellum South and other parts of the United States. This is due in part to the assumption that enslaved Africans were transformed and "immediately" forgot their identity and heritage during the Middle Passage. It is also suggested that a resultant process of self-denial and self-hatred took place with urgency. Because White society believed in this tabulae rasa theory, and in turn promoted it, it was assumed that no attention would be necessary or provided regarding the cultural antecedents of people of African descent. As C. Tsehloane Keto noted:

> . . .another very disturbing consequence of the hegemonic Europe centered perspective, is the way the trade in enslaved Africans is described in most American history textbooks. American history books tend to celebrate a miraculous social transformation of Africans in the middle of the Atlantic ocean. In an ocean that was once known as the Ethiopian Sea by the map makers of southern Europe in the sixteenth century, the Africans commit physical and cultural genocide by disappearing without a trace. They either complete a process that reformulates them into 'Negroes' on the coasts of West and West Central Africa or

> undergo the rapid social metamorphosis at sea. Once the Africans had transformed themselves into slaves, negroes, Negroes and Blacks, they were now ready to play their ascribed peripheral roles as social adjuncts to the Europe centered enterprise...(Keto 1989, 27).

Eurocentric scholars largely subscribe to Ron Bodin's idea of a "synthetic culture for blacks." Using John Blassingame's *The Slave Community* to make the assertion, Bodin states, "The opportunities provided to slaves (in Louisiana) by such an array of factors permitted much intraslave contact and helps explain the development of a new synthetic culture for blacks—one needed by second and third generation slaves (a race now without a country or an identity) and with little remaining formal knowledge of their African heritage" (Bodin 1990, 15). This was at a time when Anglo-Americans, the ancient (French descendant) population (and to a certain extent the descendants of the Spanish), often fought overtly for supremacy of their own separate ethnic and cultural identities in Louisiana (Wall 1990, 107). However, the scholarly emphasis has always been on finding and supporting evidence which would demonstrate a less than authentic African experience in America; rather than examining a priori evidence which speaks to an organic, though transplanted, African culture.

Therefore, the idea of African medicine could be broached because the concept of African ancestry is a problematic in the scholarship regarding African American history and culture. Yet the precedent for their interpretations was set by Whites who viewed African heritage as a subject of scorn during antebellum times. They responded by actively and/or passively attempting to inculcate the idea, not only of an innate African inferiority, but a past not worth remembering; or simply to the old world European mind-set, an African pas that was non-existent. Therefore, some Africans of the antebellum period articulated negative ideas about their identity. Marie Brown, who described to the Works Progress

Slavery and Medicine: Enslavement and Medical Practices in Antebellum Louisiana

Administration interviewer what life was like as a "free woman of color" during the institution of enslavement in Louisiana, simply stated: "The negro is a fallen race. . ." (Clayton 1990, 36). Yet some Louisiana interviewees, like others from the South, mention their African antecedents. For example, Frances Doby, born in Opelousas, Louisiana in 1845, indicated that her parents were from the Congo. The interviewer stated, "Like [the] people of Guinea, she is very tiny, the reason for her being known as 'Guinea'" (Clayton 1990, 60). Thomas Steptoe told the Works Progress Administration interviewer:

> My Mother's name was Jane Geambo, and father's surname was Johnson Jean Pierre Geambo, a Guinea Nigger. They brought my granpa from Africa. He was an African nigger: They stole him from there (Clayton 1990, 206).

Contrary to long-held beliefs, the narratives, oral histories, slaveowner records, medical records and case studies of the antebellum period indicate that Africans played an important role in the development of medicine during the period of enslavement. These documents also reveal that the African materia medica during the slaveocracy is much more complex than a catalogue of herbal/botanical cures and remedies. First, however, there must be some discussion of how African medicine was characterized by Whites. Second, enslaved Africans recalled definite perceptions of medicine that were often shaped by the behavior of the slaveowner; and, which shaped the Africans' attitude about the slaveowner. Third, the traditional African worldview of medicine figures intrinsically in the study of African American culture because it indicates largely what people of African descent thought culturally about what constituted medicine. Forth, evidence of a "religious" formulation is central to the medical corpus of Africans during their enslavement. Finally, enslaved Africans proactively participated in the care and treatment of illness/disease during the Holocaust of Enslavement.

CHAPTER 10

CHARACTERIZATIONS OF AFRICAN MEDICINE

> I was born in Africa, several hundred miles up the Gambia river. Fine country dat; but we are called heathen in dis Christian—no, I don't know what to call it—in dis enlightened heathen country. But the villagers in that country are very kind. When you go into house, first question is, have you had anything to eat? Bring water, you wash, and den eat much you want; and all you got do is tank them for it—not one fip you pay. If you are sick, nurse you, and make you well—not one fip you pay.
>
> *[excerpt from Mr. Johnson's speech given at the fifth annual meeting of the Massachusetts Anti-Slavery Society in Boston, January 26, 1837.]*

Among Samuel Cartwright's work is a body of knowledge which seeks to analyze disease and illnesses attributed to African people. In Cartwright's theory on race, it would not have been possible to discuss the medical understanding of African people—it would not have existed. Cartwright, his colleagues, and contemporaries believed that African people were not capable of conceptualizing or utilizing a medical universe. Notwithstanding Cartwright's racial theories, he conceded that the African psyche could indeed outwit the most adept physician of the time. Cartwright believed that:

> The African mind is so constituted that superstition and panic immediately begin to dig the negro's grave, on the occurrence of a few fatal

cases, from any unusual or malignant complaint among them and will speedily kill him, unless counteracted—kill him in defiance of any medicine in the materia medica and in defiance of the best directed efforts of the most skillful physician . . . (Cartwright 1854, 155).

Cartwright unknowingly saw only a glimpse into what comprised traditional African medicine. His assertion was that superstitious thoughts and ideas among enslaved Africans also caused a notable mortality rate. It is interesting to note that he used the term "defiance", thus acknowledging the Africans' power in a seemingly powerless institution. Cartwright's limited understanding of African culture did not dissuade him from attempting to manipulate an aspect of it. Cartwright attempted to reduce Africans fears of cholera by ritually destroying their faith in plantation medicine men:

I took about three hundred negroes, sick and well, a mile or two back into a dry, open place in the swamp, where there was no house to be seen, or any preparation begun for building any. . .The ashy-colored, dry skin conjurers, or prophets, who had alarmed their fellow-servants with the prophecies that the cholera was to kill them all, and who had gained, by various tricks and artifices, much influence over their superstitious minds, were by my orders, at twilight, called up, stripped, and greased with fat bacon, in presence of the whole camp—a camp without tents or covering of any kind, except some bushes and boards over the sick from the carts that conveyed them to the camp. After being greased, the grease was well slapped in with broad leather straps, marking time with the tam tam, a wild African dance that was going on in the center of the camp among all those, who had the physical strength to participate in it. This procedure drove the cholera out of the heads of all who had been conjured into the belief that they were to die with the disease; because it broke the charm of the conjurers by converting them, under the greasing and slapping process, into subjects for ridicule and laughter, instead of fear and veneration (Cartwright 1854, 149).

Cartwright believed that it was the African mind which fostered the problems of well-being. The goal of this event was to get the African back to productive labor for the slaveowner. Cartwright considered his attempt at simulating an African ritual a success and presented the outcome:

The next morning, by times, all who had been able to join in the dance the overnight, were ordered into the cane-field to work. There were no more cases of cholera, or deaths from that disease after the removal, except one man who had strayed away from the camp, and except also among some half dozen who had been left to take care of the houses, about half of whom died. The removal included not only the negroes, but the horses, mules and dogs, that there might be no excuse for revisiting the houses and haunts of civilized life. They remained in the camp at night, and labored in the fields by day for some six weeks before they were brought back to the houses, and during all that time they enjoyed good health (Cartwright 1854, 149).

Much later "Negro Folklorists" would support Cartwright's theory expressing it this way, "Let a negro once be convinced that he has been bewitched, and he will sink into deep despondency, his face will become clouded and sad, and his health rapidly decline. On the other hand, when he believes the baleful influence to have been counteracted the progress of his recovery is equally phenomenal" (Pendleton 1890, 204).

Many post-bellum folklorists on the Africana experience expressed a keen cultural and intellectual chauvinism in relating information about African beliefs, attitudes, customs, rituals and traditions. Their corpus contains rudimentary glimpses into the African world experience. They speak of the significance and diversity of the Uncle Remus/Br'er Rabbit (in Louisiana sometimes called Compair Lapin) tales. They also speak of the incredulous "Negro mind" regarding information about loup garous, Jack o' Lanterns, ghosts, and Raw Head and Bloody Bones. Therefore, the idea of African medicine was placed in the realm of superstition, witchcraft, conjuring, gris-gris, root doctors, charms, Voodoo, Hoodoo, Ju-Ju, trick-doctors, etc. (Pendleton 1890, 201–207). Some of the folklorists speculated on what they thought represented African medicine:

> It requires no belief in the supernatural whatever to make one afraid of persons whose business it is to devise poisons to place in the food of their victims, and if the evidence of our collection of compositions is to be trusted, there was on the plantations in the old days a vast amount of just that short of thing (Herron and Bacon 1896, 143).

Folklorists and observers like Julien A. Hall were unable to see beyond their own biases. Hall lived on a large Virginia plantation, where he once wrote "five or six negro families have their cabins near the big house, numbering in all, including pickaninnies, about thirty-five people." He went on to describe the enslaved Africans belief in conjuring as "a relic of barbarism and the dark ages" (Hall 1897, 242–243).

Slavery and Medicine: Enslavement and Medical Practices in Antebellum Louisiana

The activities that might be engaged by significant groups of Africans meeting in seclusion were an important concern of large slaveowners. The gathering of enslaved Africans was strictly forbidden by law and by the governing practices of individual farms and plantations. The slaveowners feared conspiracies and insurrections would result from such behavior. However, they also had to "guard their negroes against the imposition of those pretending to possess powers as conjurers or as 'voudous'" (Moody 1924, 278). Part of the duties of the patrollers (also called pattyrollers) was to make sure that these gatherings did not take place, especially at night. However, the southeastern Louisiana history of enslaved Africans indicates that secret meetings did occur (Thrasher 1994, 1–7). Antebellum society did not acknowledge African medicine. They reinforced the idea of African "superstitions" as being the main foundation of the African belief system.

CHAPTER 11

AFRICAN PERCEPTIONS OF SLAVEOCRACY MEDICINE

> Let me tell you right here, when you done been conjured, medical doctors can't do you no good. You got ter get anudder conjure doctor ter get it off you.
>
> *Rosa Milegan*

In the narratives and oral histories of African peoples of the old South, the narrators state matter-of-factly that they received medical care from the slaveowner. Often, the African commented upon the status and good intentions of the slaveowner by his or her action in providing medical care. Furthermore, some of the oral histories say that the slaveowner often refused to spend the money to provide care when folk medicine was the norm. Enslaved Africans often note that they were reminded that feigning illness would court punishment. Finally, the narratives and oral histories of enslaved Africans are significant because they overwhelmingly discuss brutality/punishment, labor, social relationships between the master and slave; and the issues of rape, forced concubinage and breeding. However, more often than not, these narratives and oral histories do not state whether or not Africans thought that the medicine that Whites provided was "good," "bad," or effective. Dr. Samuel Cartwright related a personal story regarding enslaved Africans stricken with dysentery and demanding a hardier diet, which the slaveowner refused to supply. When Cartwright asked the Africans about their condition, which had become "greatly debilited and emaciated," they stated, "'nothing at all, only young master don't know us people, and keeps us on white people's soup, that makes us weak'" (Cartwright 1854, 150–151). Post enslavement documents, mythology and folklore of Americans of

SLAVERY AND MEDICINE: ENSLAVEMENT AND MEDICAL PRACTICES IN
ANTEBELLUM LOUISIANA

African descent does suggest that at some point in the institution of enslavement in North America, enslaved Africans were suspicious of at least some of the medical practices of Whites.

Enslaved Africans in Louisiana gave insight and made critical comments about enslavement and medicine. Mary Reynolds, who was born in Black River, Louisiana and enslaved there remembers illness and responses to illness:

> I wasn't sick much, though. Some the niggers had chills and fever a lot, but they had'nt discovered so many diseases then as now. Massa give sick niggers ipecac and asafetida and oil and turpentine and black fever pills (Botkin 1973, 122).

Enslaved Africans in other parts of the slaveocracy also speak to enslavement and medicine, confirming the use of folk medicine such as asafetida and the motivation of slaveowners in acquiring medical doctors for slaves. Jenny Proctor, enslaved in Alabama stated:

> We didn't have much looking after when we git sick. We had to take the worst stuff in the world for medicine, just so it was cheap. That old blue mass and bitter apple would keep us out all night. Sometimes he have the doctor when he thinks we going to die, 'cause he say he ain't got anyone to lose, then that calomel what that doctor would give us would pretty nigh kill us. Then they keeps all kinds of lead bullets and asafetida balls round our necks, and some carried a rabbit foot with them all the time to keep off evil of any kind (Botkin 1973, 92–93).

Proctor gave insight on the African worldview and she remembered that the slaveowner in her experience provided a medical doctor when the threat of losing the slave investment and labor was imminent. Cato, also enslaved in Alabama recalled illness:

> Take me, I was never one for sickness. But the slaves used to get sick. There was jaundice in them bottoms. First off they'd give some castor oil, and if that didn't cure, they'd give blue mass. Then if he was still sick they'd get a doctor (Botkin 1973, 86).

Tines Kendricks, enslaved in Georgia, provided an example of how the accusation of feigning illness figured in medical care. Kendricks also related an experience which included the medical role of the mistress of the farm or plantation:

> Old Miss, she generally looked after the niggers when they sick and give them the medicine. And, too she would get the doctor iffen she think they real bad off 'cause like I said, old Miss, she mighty stingy, and she never want to lose no nigger by them dying. Howsomever, it was hard sometime to get her to believe you sick when you tell her that you was, and she would think you just playing off from work. I have seen niggers what would be mighty near dead before old Miss would believe them sick at all (Botkin 1973, 71–72).

Ellen Betts, born in Bayou Parish, Louisiana provided an example of how enslaved Africans, particularly women, provided care to other enslaved Africans. In addition, Mandy Rollins, on her plantation in Louisiana had access to a "colored doctor" (Clayton 1990, 187). Africans often served as doctors, nurses, assistants to doctors and worked in the sick-houses on the farms and plantations. According to Betts:

Slavery and Medicine: Enslavement and Medical Practices in Antebellum Louisiana

> I nussed de sick folk too—white and black. Sometime I dose with blue mass pills, and den sometime Doc fatchit {Fawcett} come along and leave rhubarb and epicac and calomel and castor oil and sech (Mellon 1988, 383).

Adam Hall from the Flowerton Plantation in Louisiana recalled: "I had my hip broke, my ankle broke, and my wrist broke. I couldn't move—couldn't get up—and them boys runned off and left me, yes, sir. One girl wouldn't leave me and got an old feller from over de bayou to come to me." Hall remembers that four White doctors came to provide care during this time (Clayton 1990, 92–93).

Enslaved Africans recognized that medical care was linked to the slaveowners' profit potential and labor needs. They also frequently mentioned that care was provided. Africans participated in their own medical care by dispensing medicines and performing some procedures such as bleeding (bloodletting, cupping or leeching) and delivering babies. The slaveowner also provided medical care through dispensing home remedies; and his wife played an important role in providing medical care. The overseer had the responsibility of reporting any illness or injury immediately to the slaveowner. This was essential in judging his effectiveness as a manager. His failure to do so could cost him his job and future employment as a plantation overseer.

CHAPTER 12

THE TRADITIONAL AFRICAN WORLDVIEW AND MEDICINE

> Dis man what I'm goin' to tell you about is one of the best kind of two-headed persons I ever knowed...even when we was coming up, [he] was very different from de rest of us children, and always said dat he could see things of de other world and talk to dem just as dat he could talk to us. He got so dat he could tell us things about ourselves dat happened at us homes at night when he was nowhere around. When we was about de age of twelve years, he explained to us dat dis was brought to him by de spirit.
>
> *Mrs. Equella Wheeler*

> ...the spirits has been after me all my life.
>
> *Wilkinson Jones*

Slaveowners, medical doctors and observers of Africans in the slaveocracy, often preoccupied with racial assumptions and supremacist privilege, failed to understand the African worldview. In Louisiana, by way of New Orleans, several major African ethnic groups were represented including, but not limited to Bambara, Wolof, Yoruba, Congo, Igbo, Fon, Coromanti (Midlo-Hall 1993, 403–405). The mixtures of various African ethnicities brought a blending of African cultures and cosmology, all reflecting certain basic (and often similar) principals and ideas referred to by Africalogists and other scholars as "traditional" African. The traditional African worldview permeates indigenous African cultures throughout the continent; and reflect the ancient Kemetic medical practices (Finch 1990, 121–140; Garrett 1978, 876–877).

SLAVERY AND MEDICINE: ENSLAVEMENT AND MEDICAL PRACTICES IN ANTEBELLUM LOUISIANA

The people of ancient Kemet left a substantial and influential body of medical knowledge. Physician and historian, Charles S. Finch notes that:

> A study of other African systems of medicine is more problematical, however, because of the absence of surviving written records. Thus, most of what we know comes from the testimony of European missionaries whose contemptuous view of traditional culture was most pointed when writing about traditional medical practices. Nonetheless, it can be shown that the best of the traditional healers in various parts of Africa acquired a startling level of proficiency and, contrary to contemporary opinion, were not without a medical science (Finch 1990, 129).

The European generally saw this Kemetic legacy and the blending and reflecting of other African cultures as more evidence of "a belief in witchcraft as these savages of the African bush who file their teeth and perforate the cartilage of their noses" (Pendleton 1890, 204). Identifying people of African descent as the perennial "savage," "heathen," "pagan," "primitive," denied Europeans the dispassionate voice necessary to explore the deep structure and diversity of Africanity in the "new world."

Philosophical thought focused on the differences between Africans and Europeans, consigning to the African gross negative connotations of being. The African, even under the oppressive nature of the slaveocracy, expressed and redefined an African philosophy, much like John Mbiti's analysis, which "refers to the understanding, attitude of mind, logic and perception behind the manner in which African peoples think, act or speak in different situations of life" (Mbiti 1970, 2). Very early on the African presence became an academic "problem" for researchers and analysts (Asante 1990, 152). Instead of seeking to understand the function and motive of, for example, the phenomena called Voodoo (Vodu, Hoodoo, Vodun, Vaudou), antebellum witnesses and their descendant chroniclers ridiculed and reinterpreted an important aspect of the African world experience. This misunderstanding of Voodoo is at the core of many of the interpretations of African medico-religious phenomena.

Many scholars agree that the antebellum seat of Voodoo in the United States was New Orleans, Louisiana (Tallant 1946, 3–40; Saxon 1929, 309–322; Raboteau 1978, 75–80; Mulira 1990, 34–68; Bodin 1990, 1–42, etc.). Jessie Gaston Mulira states that "New Orleans was the birthplace of Voodoo in North America" (Mulira 1990, 35) and provides scholarship which attempts a serious discussion of the subject before the Civil War. From antebellum times Voodoo has been assigned to the status of religious "sect" or "cult." The plethora of information on the African "religious" experience in the United States addresses a wide range of topics. The term "religion" does not adequately identify the African phenomenon being addressed. It is often used for expediency in discussing the spiritual histories of Africa, Asia and South America. Therefore it is necessary to move away from the vague concept of African "religions" and move toward a concept that this research designates as an *African Living Belief System*. There is a limited amount of information, however, which addresses the African American "religious" experience that seeks to provide an analysis of *what* constitutes the African component of African American religion. There are numerous contemporary studies which address "Blacks and Religion," "Black American Religion and Politics," and "Religion, Blacks and Mental Health." These scholarly studies discuss "Black Religion," or the "Black Church" with finality, offering scant or no attention to the African history, nature, quality, relevance and frequency of the African experience rooted in the continental African and enslavement experience of African Americans. The research interest has been away from exploring the possibility of transcendent Africanisms in American culture toward emphasizing "creolization" and "syncretism" (the fusion of two or more originally different phenomena which creates a new entity) in African American religion. The major problem with the European cultural conception of African "religion" is primarily the Europeans' historic inability to comprehend and respect an African spiritual complex because of the rootedness of racist practices and beliefs which persistently dehumanized Africans. Numerous texts offer us premises such as this: "From a religious perspective, Africa is a mixture of indigenous sub-Saharan cults, Christianity, and Islam" (Smart 1984, 59). It is necessary, therefore, to examine the term "religion" as it relates to the African and African American experience with attention to the concept of an African Living Belief System. Second, it is important to generally survey the scholarship which focuses upon African "religion" within the Afrocentric paradigm.

John Mbiti in *African Religions and Philosophy* notes, that of the approximately one thousand African languages and dialects, there has not been found a definitive equivalent to the European term "religion." The continued use of the term with reference to Africa perpetuates the connotation that those items which characterized European religious systems also characterize African "religious" systems. Mbiti states that African "religion" "permeate(s) all the departments of life, there is no formal distinction between the sacred and the secular, between the religious and non-religious, between the spiritual and the material areas of life...it nevertheless accompanies the individual from long before his birth to long after his physical death" (Mbiti 1970, 2–3). Jordan Ngubane notes in his *Conflict of Mind* that the African god-spirit-force that westerners try to identify, can for Africans, be a force which has ultimate value known as "UQOBO." Uqobo is infinite, self-perpetuating and is the manifestation of men, not an external force. As Ngubane expresses the quality of Uqobo, he states, "I am the value UQOBO ...I am a Universal Constant; I am a Cosmic Constant;/I am All-in-One; I am One-in-All./I am the circle which encompasses infinity;/I am the point that is the beginning of the circle;/I am the value behind the circle" (Ngubane 1979, 97 and 99). The concept of Uqobo is similar to the concept of Modimo as presented in *African Theology* by Gabriel Molehe Setiloane. According to Setiloane, Modimo is a vital force, which is the source of all life and exists within everything. It is a dynamic force like Uqobo in that it is perpetually evolving (Setiloane 1986, 1–48).

Mbiti, Ngubane and Setiloane introduce us to a worldview, a perspective of a god-force which gives way to conceptualizing an African Living Belief System. The African Living Belief System posited here is a composite of traditional African philosophy before the conquest of Africa and the intrusion of European Christianity, Arabic Islam, and the European trade in enslaved Africans. The African Living Belief System is a way of life. In this life all of the senses are engaged in a celebration of existence and the promulgation of the ancient Kemetic concept of Ma'at. Ma'at refers to the ancient Kemetic concept encompassing the ideas of truth, justice, balance, righteousness, harmony and reciprocity (Karenga and Carruthers 1986, 83–99) (See Table 10. General Conceptual Components of the African Living Belief System for some categorical ideas that relate to the concept of an African spiritual and value system).

TABLE 10. GENERAL CONCEPTUAL COMPONENTS OF THE
AFRICAN LIVING BELIEF SYSTEM

Concepts	Components
Consciousness:	Supreme being, deities, genius, infinity, empowerment, creativity, emotions, complementarity
Sound:	Song, word, instruments, incantation, drum, music, oral history, prayer
Sight:	Nature, symbols, alters, shrines
Feeling:	Community, oneness, harmony, purpose
Movement:	Dance, rhythm, space, continuity
Form:	Ritual, communalism, spirit manifestation, ceremony, dress, societies, sites, naming, divination
Tools:	Fire, water, earth, herbs, implements, food, colors, vegetation
Philosophy:	Non-hegemonic, non-proselytizing, order, union, reciprocity, ancestors, truth, justice, sacrifice, reincarnation, cyclical, healing, transformation, continuity, fertility, diversity

Slavery and Medicine: Enslavement and Medical Practices in Antebellum Louisiana

In the case of traditional African "religion," the concepts of sacred and profane are a holistic part of "religion" never perceived as separate. Traditional African people tend to focus on the task of the ritual which makes use of sacred objects and tools. The African Living Belief System offers a moral code sanctioned by the people, and influenced by God, the deities and the ancestors. Thus, the African Living Belief System encapsulates a holistic quality whose emphasis equally relates community, man/woman, deity, forms and the natural implements for living out the system of belief. Therefore, in the African Living Belief System, Africa relates to the traditional indigenous culture of the various ethnic groups on the continent of Africa. Living refers to the African emphasis on life as a dynamic, perpetually evolving condition which includes the way in which the ancestors "live" on long after their death. Belief is the thought/rationale behind the African's worldview, customs and behaviors. Finally, System is the totality of a complex, highly organized structure of ideas and behaviors which is passed on (actively and passively) from generation to generation.

The vast folklore on Africans in the Americas demonstrates the transmission, over time, of an African worldview in which Africanisms changed the Christian church into an entity which is distinct from the European form (Bradley 1975, 413–421; Raboteau 1978, 1–150). Africans, in their forced migration to the Americas, transported with them the worldview of the African Living Belief System which laid the basis for African inspired "religious" structures such as Voodoo, Santeria, Shango, Spiritualism, etc. Operating within the European Christian framework, post-bellum sects of Christianity were created (Black Theology, Black Baptists) and transformed by the African Living Belief System where we have, for example, a continuation of the traditional African concepts of ritual death and resurrection, call-response, nommo and other forms of oral expression redefining the Christian perspective.

SLAVERY AND MEDICINE: ENSLAVEMENT AND MEDICAL PRACTICES IN
ANTEBELLUM LOUISIANA

Scholarship on African "religion" is filled with terminology which separates the African "religious" tradition from the European and makes extensive use of negative Christian missionary ideas about Africa. Therefore, African "religion" (whatever the ethnicity, culture or linguistic structure) is termed as "animistic," "primitive," "savage," "barbaric," "heathen," "pagan," etc. These terms are classic examples of the European hegemonic perspective (Asante 1987, 4; Keto 1989, 14–15) and speaks to the time-worn strategy in European scholarship of studying and writing about Africans as objects in research, rather than the subjects of research (Asante 1980, 6–7; Asante 1987, 6; Asante 1990, 6). In addition, the phenomena of spirit manifestation (sometimes called spirit possession) among Africans was a fascinating display of African savagery to the antebellum European/American observer. To the initiated of the African Living Belief System, it was a natural part of human existence.

Well-established European historical analysts prefer to view Africans as beings who are constantly acted upon, as non-participants in their cosmology, rather than to view them, once again, as people who act and enhance their own cosmological destinies. What many scholars did not recognize was the fact that the *diverse* expression of African American religious behavior post-bellum (Mt. Sinai Holy Church of America, Inc., United House of Prayer for All People, Church of God—Black Jews, Moorish Science Temple of America, Father Divine Peace Mission Movement, Shrine of the Black Madonna, etc.) was in itself more characteristically African (Yoruba, Ifa, Shango, Ogun, etc.) than European (Christianity). Unfortunately, most of the literature favors objectifying people and terms with negative connotations; and reinforcing the mythological beliefs about the cultural superiority, in this case religion, of Europeans.

The Afrocentric interpretations of African "religion" emerged strongly in the 1980s sought to place Africa (Africans, African thought, activity, scholarship, etc.) at the center of any analysis involving African phenomena (Asante 1980, 6–7; Keto 1989, 1–4). This way of viewing Africa and Africans existed long before a term or conceptual framework was identified and utilized. Maulana Karenga echoed Cheikh Anta Diop and called it the "rescue and reconstruction." C. Tsehloane Keto and others termed it "Africa centered," and Molefi Kete Asante progressively posited "Afrocentricity." Therefore, works can be classified as Afrocentric if Africa (African people, phenomena, etc.) is subject, not object and if the research and reporting attempt is not inherently anti-African regardless of the research outcome or the race/ancestry of the researcher. This approach, attempted to reconstruct the negative effects, and invalidity of the prior schools of thought, and provided an enhanced, and some researchers suggest, an authentic focus to the study of the African experience.

An example of Afrocentric interpretations of African American religion is Sheila Walker's "African Gods in the Americas: The Black Religious Continuum." In her exploration of Africanisms in the African American religious tradition and spirit manifestation, Walker argues that spirit manifestation is a "common unifying feature," (Walker 1980, 26) of the African Living Belief System and exists, in some form, among Africans in the diaspora. Walker notes the "tangible relationship between humans and deities. In the United States former enslaved Africans and their descendants will say matter-of-factly, 'I was talking with Jesus,' as if he were a familiar neighbor" (Walker 1980, 31). While Walker acknowledges that one of the difficulties African Americans experienced in maintaining their African orishas was due to the fact that they were geographically the farthest from the African cultural continuum (Walker 1980, 33). This explains the strong manifestations of Africanisms in Haiti, Brazil and the Caribbean Islands (Holloway 1990, 1–18). In Walker's analysis enslaved Africans in America:

. . . had to leave their African gods behind,
they did not leave behind their sense of religion,

SLAVERY AND MEDICINE: ENSLAVEMENT AND MEDICAL PRACTICES IN ANTEBELLUM LOUISIANA

of what should be the nature of interaction between human and deity, and how a deity should be properly worshipped. They understood the new religion within the framework of the old, and it is this framework that has set the pattern for the black religions (sic) experience in the United States...(Walker 1980, 34).

Understanding and having identified many of the numerous of components inherent in the African Living Belief System, Walker is able to approach the study of African spiritual retentions in the United States with convincing explanations. In addition, Walker shares the same research findings as Michael Bradley who asserts:

> Slaves had ample opportunities to keep old ways alive. Most Africans lived in small groups on isolated frontier farms. They had minimal contact with white culture. Masters or overseers might swiftly crush visible African culture considered dangerous or economically nonproductive, but religion is primarily a non-material aspect of life. Thus, unobtrusive African religious concepts and practices had a good chance of survival. One seldom reads of attempts to destroy African traits (Bradley 1975, 414).

Many contemporary scholars and Afrocentricists have recognized the basic characteristics of the African worldview as related to the African's medical universe. In doing so they have been able to relate the various factors which have allowed traditional continental African culture to transmigrate time and space. Yet none of these scholars have argued the existence of a static, all encompassing, unaltered transfer of culture from Africa. According to Robert Ferris Thompson, Americans of African descent possess aspects of a descent language whereby in the:

Slavery and Medicine: Enslavement and Medical Practices in Antebellum Louisiana

> Metaphysical traditions of conjuring and healing with herbs and roots, there are words and phrases that cannot readily be traced to European origins. One of the most important words in black United States conjure-work, "goofer," refers to grave dirt, often inserted in a charm. In Kongo territory, earth from a grave is considered at one with the spirit of the buried person. "Goofer dust" harks back to the Ki-Kongo verb Kufwa ("to die"). Another important word in the lexicon of the charm makers is toby. A toby is a good-luck charm. In form and function it almost certainly derives from the tobe charms of Kongo (Thompson 1984, 105).

Janheinz Jahn recognized the European religious problem with African medical phenomena, particularly that of the medicine man:

> The fundamental objectives to the therapy of the 'medicine man' came from the circles of pragmatic European medicine—arguments which were appropriated also by the missionaries. In ignorance of African philosophy, its body of knowledge and its principles, Europeans asserted that the cures offered by the 'sorcer' had in most cases no connection with the illness that was being treated (Jahn 1989, 127).

Jahn asserts that the European/American attention to medicine is defined by three criteria:

> ... firstly, the remedy is effective only for a strictly defined malady; secondly, the effect of it is so reliable that its success can be predicted with great certainty; a failure leads to doubt of the

diagnosis. In the third place, given the same malady, the result is reproducible. . .(Jahn 1989, 128).

Any other aspect of the illness and disease that was not readily discernable was ignored. The clash of medical cultures occurred because people of African descent did not perceive a dichotomy between the remedy for the clear physical ailment and any attendant conditions or causal factors not as easily perceived. African American scholar and folk culturalist Beverly J. Robinson has reiterated that the African art of healing was a religious act, emanating from the traditional African worldview:

> The more common healers in the United States are known as spiritual healers or advisers, folk doctors, grannies, and midwives. Some practitioners are more fearsome, are known as root workers, hoodoo, juju, and voodoo doctors, hainsters, and conjurers. In traditional African culture preventive medicine was practiced by the traditional root doctors. . .African-American healing is rooted in belief and thus is a religion which places folk practitioners and their art in the world of the spiritual. . .the priest and medicine man, a major support system enslaved Africans transported to the West. . .The priest, medicine man, or preacher-type figure because an important catalyst in reinforcing this world view (Robinson 1990, 219).

This view is different from the attempt to grasp the holistic and circular African conceptual models utilizing Eurocentric linear patterns of analysis. In his chapter on "Folk Religion in the Slave Narratives" Olli Alho makes a distinction between the use of charms and folk medicine among enslaved Africans. According to Alho, "Charms seem to be directed against more or less

SLAVERY AND MEDICINE: ENSLAVEMENT AND MEDICAL PRACTICES IN
ANTEBELLUM LOUISIANA

anonymous powers that cause illness and disease, but folk medicines are directed against the specific illness" (Alho 1976, 202). This harkens back to Jahn's criteria of European and American medicine which fails to comprehend and/or acknowledge a broader view of medical health.

Traditional African culture, The African Living Belief System, with its cosmo-cultural focus on the attempt at maintaining harmony and balance, produced African diasporan descendants who could not forget their primary cultural orientation. The embeddedness of certain African cultural traits speaks to the latent behaviors of people of African descent manifested throughout the antebellum and postbellum periods. Therefore, Voodoo in antebellum America was, in addition to its spiritual construction, a *medical system* of "beliefs about health and illness that facilitated coping with disorders of body and mind, as well as evil spirits" (Watson 1984, 3). Voodoo, like other manifestations of the African Living Belief System, required active participation in operating the material and non-material world to bring about the medical consequences of Ma'at.

CHAPTER 13

AFRICAN AGENCY IN THE CARE AND TREATMENT OF ILLNESS/DISEASE

> My mammy larned me a lot of doctorin what she larnt from old folkses from Africy, and some de Indians larnt her. . .All dese doctorin' things come clear from Africy, and dey allus worked for Mammy and for me, too.
>
> *Harriet Collins*

Enslaved Africans played an important role in the development of medicine in the antebellum South. Africans were active participants in the care and treatment of illness/disease; and in assisting Whites in maintaining their own general health care. African participation was an absolute necessity. Africans were more than aware of the various medical health risks inherent in the institution of enslavement. Despite the perception that enslaved Africans generally "loved" the slaveowner, according to one survivor of the Holocaust of Enslavement, Annie Hawkins:

> I never had no white folks that was good to me. We all worked jest like dogs, and had about half enough to eat, and got whupped for everything. Our days was a constant misery to us. I know lots of niggers that was slaves and had a good time, but we never did. Seems hard that I can't say anything good for any of my white folks, but I sho' can't (Mellon 1988, 242).

For many enslaved Africans of southeastern Louisiana having a "good time" in the slaveocracy could mean that the overseer didn't punish much; or the slaveowner whipped instead of the overseer; the feeding trough was filled daily (Wall 1990, 166); you didn't labor in agriculture; or perhaps, if you were female, you weren't pregnant during the busiest sugar or cotton labor months. Understanding the precarious nature of African existence during the slaveocracy, Africans participated as: 1) recipients of medical health care; 2) functioned as dispensers of medical health care; and 3) acted as diviners of medical health care (Harrison 1975–76, 547–560).

Many enslaved Africans from southeastern Louisiana describe the medical care and remedies they received. Catherine Cornelius, born about 1836 on Smithfield Plantation near Baton Rouge, Louisiana, remembered her plantation days:

> De plantation sat on de river. Dere was more dan a hundred slaves on it. De cabins was white, and dere was one family to a cabin. What did dey do for us when we was sick? Why, we had a nice hospital in de place with a Negro nurse and midwife. And not only Doctor Lyles, but a doctor from town tended us (Clayton 1990, 46).

Many enslaved Africans like Rebecca Fletcher recalled medical treatment: "old missis used to give us blue mass pills when we needed medicine. It sho did make us sick. We had to get sick to get well, old missis said" (Clayton 1990, 67). Elizabeth Ross Hite remembered that on Trinity Plantation there was a "house for children and a hospital. Grandma Delaite had charge of de hospital. . .dere was two nurses in de hospital to take care of de children" (Clayton 1990, 99). Daffney Johnson, born on the Miller Don Plantation in Gretna, Louisiana also related her medical health care experience with the mistress of the plantation:

> I worked around de house a long time 'fore de boss put me in de sugar cane fields. I knows one time when I was small, us had what dey called the seven-year-itch. De ole missis made my ma dig a pot of pokeroot and boil it and put us chaps in it. If us had been put in de fire, we would not have burned any worse, but it show did cure dat itch (Clayton 1990, 130).

Frances Lewis also stated:

> We didn't get sick much, but when we did old missis gave us blue mass pills and ipecac and sarsaparilla. She

took bark and made a tea out of it, and for flux she gave us sage tea (Clayton 1990, 160).

In the article "Health Status and Healing Practices: Continuations from an African Past," Ira E. Harrison asks the question, "Is there evidence of diviners, dispensers, and mid-wives in the literature on Africans in the New World?" He cites the traditional West African medical phenomena of the Babalawo and the Onishegun as the paradigms. The Babalawo among the Yoruba (in the Ifa tradition) has been referred to as "medicine man." The Babalawo is a healer of the body and mind. He has a clear function in the medical universe of the African to invoke the spirits and administer cures for healing. The Onishegun translates also as healer and physician. However, according to some scholars the Onishegun may/may not necessarily be a physical person; still, the Onishegun, once called upon, is responsible for invoking the spirits to promote healing in the individual. Regarding the antebellum medical experience of Africans, Harrison surmises that the plantation overseer "was the chief health officer" and that "blacks did not learn health-seeking behavior" or "how to use money to purchase medical services" (Harrison 1975–76, 557; Harrison and Harrison 1971, 178–79). However, utilizing the concepts of diviner and dispenser in the antebellum South, enslaved Africans exerted power (as well as exhibited attributes) similar to the Babalawo and Onishegun of the Yoruba and the Baomale (healer of the family) of the Dagara in Burkino Faso (Some' 1994).

For example, Warner Willis of Iberville Parish, Louisiana explained that enslaved Africans "In the old times...were our own druggist and doctor and cured ourself with roots and herbs and homemade remedies" (Clayton 1990, 215). Overarching the enslaved Africans' understanding of medicine is the holistic African worldview. Further, midwives are not viewed as a separate category (as in Harrison's work), but in this research they are included among the dispensers for the services they provide. Many indigenous African midwife practioners represented a high level of skill, "African midwives possessed a good understanding of some fundamental obstetric and pediatric principles including inducing oxytocin for uterine contractions and facilitating dilation and labor" (Finch 1990, 138).

Slavery and Medicine: Enslavement and Medical Practices in Antebellum Louisiana

According to Jan Knappert "All the words in African languages which are translated by 'medicine', also have the meaning of 'magic antidote' (Knappert 1990, 154). The Eurocentric analysis of traditional African medicine suggests that it is anti-scientific because it acknowledges no separation between the conceptual phenomena of God-man-nature-good-evil-temporal-spiritual. Antebellum observers of Africana culture comprehended and appreciated little that was not in the interest of the slaveocracy. To the African, illness, disease and injury all had deeper meanings than their physical manifestation suggested. Among Africalogists African cultural retentions stemming from enslaved Africans in north America are well documented (Holloway 1990, 1–18; Herskovits 1942, 1–32; Jahn 1989, 1–25; Asante and Asante 1990, 3–12; Ani 1980, 15–22; and Walker 1980, 25–36).

Dispensing medical care was a natural occupation among enslaved Africans (Goodson 1987, 198–203). Many enslaved Africans of southeastern Louisiana recounted dispensing experiences handed down from their mothers, fathers, grandmothers and grand-fathers. The pharmacopoeia of enslaved Africans included herbs, roots, leaves, bark, compounds, and to a limited extent, vegetables which were prepared in the form of soups, teas, tonics, poultices, etc. In addition, herbal medicines were often combined to effectuate cures. For example, pumpkinseed with Indian hemp was used for yellow fever (See Appendix C Selected Pharmacopoeia Used by Enslaved Africans in the Southeastern Parishes of Antebellum Louisiana). Verice Brown of St. James Parish, Louisiana recounted:

> I always use the things my ma told me about. I still use dem now. Just take [an] bush and make a tea out of it and bathe with it. Dat's all we ever did use for fever. The leaves are good to place on a sore or a swollen place. Jackvine is the best blood purify you can get. I have a piece dried. We always make tea out of it and eat [it] with our bread when us would be in de swamps (Clayton 1990, 37).

Melinda (no slave surname provided) of Baton Rouge, Louisiana noted:

> My ma and pa left early in the mornin' to work in the fields, and I remained with my grandma from sunrise to

SLAVERY AND MEDICINE: ENSLAVEMENT AND MEDICAL PRACTICES IN ANTEBELLUM LOUISIANA

> sunset. So it is that I was very fond of her and learned many useful things, for she knew the value of herbs and how to prepare remedies for almost every evil (Clayton 1990, 165).

Lizzie Chandler of Louisiana indicated that enslaved Africans did not always agree on the medical care provided by Whites:

> Old Miss was a great believer in quinine for 'most everythin'. When she wanted me to make some, I would say, 'Quinines all right for white folks but it ain't no good for niggers. Jimson weed [was] for us.'
>
> We made our own medicine when we needed any, but we wasn't sick much. Country people don't get sick like they do in the city (Clayton 1990, 43).

Mother Duffy of Louisiana recalled that to cure pneumonia "hog's hoofs" tea was required; and for an earache, "don't put no oil [in it], No, you split a pod of garlic and wrap it in cotton so it don't burn your ear. It sho will cure it, yes" (Clayton 1990, 64). Lindy Joseph, born in enslavement in Baton Rouge, Louisiana, also provided dispensing remedies:

> Coal oil and salt warmed is good for rheumatism/You can take rusty nails; put vinegar on dem; let stand; dat's good for worms. Drink about a half-glass at de time/Take castor oil; soak on cotton; put in the hollow of your throat; will stop hoarseness/Take Jacob bush and boil it; drink the tea. It's good for fever. I never is had a doctor for fever. Mole tea is good for fever too; just boil it/Sassafras tea is good to brak (break) out measles/Hot ashes and salt wet in vinegar is good for pains in de sides (Clayton 1990, 144–145).

John McDonald explained to the Louisiana Works Progress Administration interviewer that he could remember several dispensing remedies that are a part of the African materia medica:

SLAVERY AND MEDICINE: ENSLAVEMENT AND MEDICAL PRACTICES IN ANTEBELLUM LOUISIANA

> . . .we had plenty dem old-time cures, you know. De doctor give us quinine and bitters, but we used plenty [of] asafetida and rabbit foots to help out. We'd tie a bit of asafetida up in a rag, and put it 'round the baby's neck to keep colds away, and to help it when dey cuts teeth. . .Cure for measles? Well, now dere ain't none. Just keep your hands off dem poison bushes and be careful to stay indoors (Clayton 1990, 164–165).

Silas Spotfore, of Louisiana, was born in Fort Adams, Mississippi, and recalled dispensing remedies for rheumatism, chapped hands, colds, hoarseness, headaches, vomiting, flesh moles, warts, sty on eye, and "stomach trouble." His remedies included "horseradish for hoarseness" and "plenty [of] doses of burnt 'lasses (molassas) and lard for stomach trouble" (Clayton 1990, 196). Warner Willis provided additional dispensing strategies:

> Collard leaves we put on head for misery and again we made a poultice with them for boils. Once when I had a carbucle on the back of my neck and they said I was goin' to die, I cured myself with it. When we wanted to stop bleedin', we got a handful of soot out of the chimney, and it would quit. Cobwebs did the same thing. If you got a sprain, take clay, mix it with vinegar, bind it on the wrnch and it goes out. When children had worms they ma made a tea of Jersualey weed [Jerusalem artichoke], and it was a wormifuge [wormseed] that cured 'em. When [the] palate was down, all you had to do was to lift up a tuff of hair from top of [the] head and tie it with a cord. In three days it was all right (Clayton 1990, 215).

Probably the most misunderstood aspect of the African materia medica is the incidence of divining. The value of divining was dismissed as an aspect of medical health and healing, though its existence dates back to ancient Kemet (Dorman 1990, 1–6; Finch 1990, 121–168) and other ancient cities of Africa. In addition to herbal pharmacopoeia, aspects of divining also included a catalogue of observations of spirits and ghosts in addition to the magico-medical remedies. In every aspect of divining there was a lesson to be learned by the patient, including a deeper

SLAVERY AND MEDICINE: ENSLAVEMENT AND MEDICAL PRACTICES IN
ANTEBELLUM LOUISIANA

understanding of the nature of the origin of illness and disease. Slaveowners looked upon African divining as "primitive" African superstitions and defined all that they saw as "Voodoo".

There are two theories regarding the origin and development of Voodoo in antebellum Louisiana. The strong belief that Voodoo came to Louisiana through Haiti has gained acceptance among Voodoo scholars. The large transmigration of enslaved Africans and their owners from the plantations of Haiti to New Orleans in the 1800s, brought influential numbers of African practitioners of Voodoo into Louisiana. However, some researchers give credence to the idea that an original form of Voodoo was brought directly into Louisiana (by way of New Orleans) from West Africa. While there is support for both theories, the Haitian connection has been more substantially documented; and there is the possibility that both experiences did exist and at some point they intersected. However, in general, the existence of Voodoo in the United States, as previously mentioned, is most associated with New Orleans, Louisiana. Voodoo scholars provide a glimpse of the practice before the Civil War, yet most of the discourse on Voodoo is provided after the Civil War, with great attention focused on influential personages such as Marie Laveau and Papa John. So much attention has been placed on the Laveau phenomena that there are few scholarly attempts to examine the idea of Voodoo as part of the African diasporan understanding of the African Living Belief System (a notable exception is Bobby Joe Neeley's "Contemporary Afro-American Voodooism (Black Religion): The Retention and Adaptation of the Ancient African-Egyptian Mystery System"). To be sure, this Voodoo was such a threat to the slaveowners and overseers' power, that they eventually attempted to crush any perceived threat of it.

Slaveowners who began to uncover instances of Voodoo among enslaved Africans unwittingly discovered "priests," (male and female), "conjurors," "herbalists," "seers/signers" etc. To the European there was also the disturbing idea that this divining power, brought by various African ethnic groups, and subsumed under the label of "Voodoo," was also being linked to the Africans' understanding and interpretation of Christianity. Slaveowners attempted to inculcate in the African a fear of Voodoo, likening its existence to the concept of evil in Christianity. Notwithstanding this attempt, Africans were manifesting their own divining nature in the swamps, wooded areas and forests in secret; or with

Slavery and Medicine: Enslavement and Medical Practices in Antebellum Louisiana

their heads under buckets (used to muffle the sounds of singing, prayer, etc.). Enslaved Africans continued to explore their divining interests in the coded language and songs they cultivated during enslavement. They were dancing their divining nature in rural Louisiana during the plantation holidays and especially in Congo Square in New Orleans.

Congo Square (Circus Square, Place Publique, Place Congo) in New Orleans, Louisiana is a national symbol for the legacy of the "raw" African and the Africanisms brought to the Americas. From 1817 Louisiana laws allowed enslaved Africans to meet in Congo Square on Sunday evenings. Louisiana chronicler Lyle Saxon described the event in this way:

> The negroes held high carnival in Congo Square, as hour after hour they shuffled and stamped in their dances of old Africa, swaying and sweating in the afternoon sunshine while tom-toms thudded their eternal rhythm (Saxon 1929, 124)

White participant-observers saw that Africans exhibited the ethnically-specific dances and music of West Africa (*Daily Picayune* 1843, October 18). White reaction to the gathering at Congo Square varied. Some thought that the gathering of Africans was barbaric, some thought it was innocent fun for the slaves. Still others felt that it was a necessary enslavement tool in that it helped Africans "release tension." Slaveowners saw the event as a way to discourage unauthorized meetings of Africans which might lead to rebellion. Whites also witnessed Africans in their persistent manifestation of Africa's spirituality through Voodoo.

What is the connection between Congo Square, Voodoo and medicine among enslaved Africans of southeastern Louisiana? Through the forum of a Congo Square, enslaved Africans used Voodoo to practice the ritual aspects of their medical universe. Slaveowners knew that Voodoo was ever-present, and at times they watched the Africans in wonder. A small number of Whites participated in Voodoo rites and finally Whites came to fear the pervasiveness and power that they represented. Ultimately they suppressed the cultural-spiritual practices of the Africans at Congo Square. However, this did not eliminate the preponderance and practice of Voodoo among enslaved Africans in the state of Louisiana.

SLAVERY AND MEDICINE: ENSLAVEMENT AND MEDICAL PRACTICES IN ANTEBELLUM LOUISIANA

Given the persistence of Voodoo, as well as the slaves' engagement of Christianity, former enslaved Africans of southeastern Louisiana described a complex divining system. Divining is often linked to the organized religious experience of many enslaved Africans. According to Lizzie Chandler: "People don't seem to have the religion that they once had. Each generation it seems to be passing, and they don't get close to God now and have visions. In my ma's time it was better" (Clayton 1990, 42). They often include remedies and rituals. For example Verice Brown of St. James Parish, Louisiana recalled:

> . . . another that will take all the rheumatism, and dat is find you a old dilapidated dog almost dead. Tie his feet and put a over his mouth and lay your feet across him. 'Course dat dog will soon die. When he do, all your pains is gone. De dog draws dem out.
>
> I have got a good-luck bone I carry with me all [the] time. It is out a black cat. You know how you get it? Well, just go to the forks of the road and build your fire. Put de pot on and put the black cat in dere and boil it good. When all de meat come off of de bones, the lucky bone will fall. Den take dat with you for your luck. It will charm off evil too (Clayton 1990, 37).

Edward De Buiew of Lafourche Parish, Louisiana, who "joined de church" before getting married, discussed a deep belief in spirits.

> Oh, yes, I believes in de spirits and see dem very often. . .We used to go and dig for treasure, and de spirits would get to us. I know one night we were diggin' and come to the top of de box. The spirit was so bad—till we run—dat one of de mens fell dead. We had to go back after him de next day. You know, miss, de reason money is so hard to find when dey bury it? Dey always take somebody with dem, and dey kill him and put him in dere with de money (Clayton 1990, 48–49).

Slavery and Medicine: Enslavement and Medical Practices in Antebellum Louisiana

Sally Snowden, born in Geneva Georgia and later brought to Louisiana, discussed remedies that fall in the realm of divining:

> Dere's many a remedy dat I knows too. A man must come in de house before a woman in de mornin' or you will surely have bad luck. If a person comes in de house, dey must come in and go out de back or front door, never through de same door. Dese old yellow top weeds is mighty fine for de fever (Clayton 1990, 194).

In continental African and African diasporan mythology there is the belief that being born with a veil or caul (the amniotic sac) over one's face will provide the person with supernatural powers throughout their life time. These "veiled" people are purported to be endowed diviners who receive future knowledge, perceive ghosts/spirits and experience visions. Francis Doby discussed the concept of spirits in the context of a veil:

> You see, I was born wid a veil, so I see ghostses. Dey come in and dey go out, in de house and in de yard. Dey just knock on de wall like dat, three times—boom, boom, boom; but me, I never bother 'em. Dey got deir worry and I got mine. T'aint no use to bother 'em (Clayton 1990, 54).

Like Francis Doby, Wilkinson Jones, born in Jefferson Parish, Louisiana had a divining experience with a veil:

> De spirit comes around me all [the] time now. My ma always told me I was born with a veil. I guess dat's the reason I is always seeing something. I see a woman right here all [the] time with no head. When you go to dig treasure, if you ain't never seen any, you sure will then. They used to walk with me all [the] time. Some I see sure do look natural. I seen one jump on my dog one day in the swamp and kilt him dead. I knows dat was a spirit for it sure did scream (Clayton 1990, 142).

Peter Hill of Meeker Plantation in Lecompte, Louisiana provided a detailed account of his experiences with "ghosts."

SLAVERY AND MEDICINE: ENSLAVEMENT AND MEDICAL PRACTICES IN
ANTEBELLUM LOUISIANA

> Sho I knows about ghosts. One day me and my wife was on de bridge, and she pulled me right quick. I ax her what was de matter, and she told me she just pulled me outen de way of de spirits. She said dey come by, and some had bodies and no heads.

Another time a woman died terrible in a house, and nobody could stay in it 'cause at night de ghosts would knock down de planks from de ceilin'. One time it thundered and lightened so much we couldn't go to work, and Mr. Walker come after me. I wouldn't go, and he turned and shooked his fist at the clouds. Dem spirits knocked him clean offen his horse, and in one week he died. He was so crooked-up dat de men had to come and straighten him out after he was dead (Clayton 1990, 97).

Hill went on to describe how ghosts/spirits "passes you, it is just like a hot steam goin' by." He then talked about spirits guarding buried treasure; and that they "will come to your bed and ride you in your sleep" (Clayton 1990, 97). Furthermore, Francis Doby continued to discuss what constituted "luck", a popular concept among enslaved Africans:

> Dis is call 'basilique' [basil]. T'is good luck to keep it on you or around your house. Dey got two kind of basilique: Dem dat's got de long thin leaf, dat's de papa plant; and dem dat's got thick round leaf, dat's de mama plant. You got to put de both of 'em de ground to make dem grow. When you got dat in your yard, you sho got good luck to you all de year around (Clayton 1990, 56).

N. H. Hobley described himself as a "Divine Healer":

> . . . a Divine Healer is one who heals all bodily, temporal, and spiritual ills by prayer faith, the laying on of hands, and the use of certain herbs and vegetation; also [by] Christian Science, ritualism of the Catholic Church, and occult reasoning (Clayton 1990, 115).

Equella Wheeler provided a story of a successful Louisiana diviner or "two-headed" person:

Slavery and Medicine: Enslavement and Medical Practices in Antebellum Louisiana

Dis man what I'm going to tell you about is one of the best kind of two-headed persons I ever knowed. He was born somewhere in or around Zachary, Louisiana a few years before peace was declared and we was set free. Of course, he was born of slave parents, and when dey was freed, he was freed wid dem. I might say dat we was all born on de same plantation. Dis plantation was owned by a man by de name of Mr. Ed Young who was very good to us at all times.

Now Pap, even when we was coming up, was very different from de rest of us children, and always said dat he could see things of de other world and talk to dem just as dat he could talk to us. He got so dat he could tell us things about ourselves dat happened at us homes at night when he was nowhere around. When we was about de age of twelve years, he explained to us dat dis was brought to him by de spirit (Clayton 1990, 210).

Hannah Kelly was born into slavery in Louisville, Kentucky and after the war she moved to Texas and then to Louisiana. Kelly stated that "I never believed in spirits or things like that" however she provided a few "omens" in her Louisiana oral testimony. Her omens included prophetic "signs" which allowed her to perceive and control the positive energy (luck) in the home and gave her some indication of future events:

> If you bump your elbow, somebody strange is coming. Don't never bring a[n] ax in the house; dat's bad luck too. If dere is a circle around de moon, it will rain (Clayton 1990, 148).

Silas Spotfore also provided information on omens or signs:

> When a rooster crows with his head toward de door, a stranger is coming. If he looks a-far off and crows, sad news [is coming] (Clayton 1990, 196).

Finally, according to John McDonald spirits also entered the bodies of animals:

> Folks say when a body dies wid things on deir mind, deir spirit goes in a dog, or hog, or any animal near-by. The spirit in this animal then acts on the thing in folks'

mind when they dies. If you don't have no worries on your mind when you dies, the spirit rests. I's seen rabbits with spirits what ain't act noway natural (Clayton 1990, 165)

In the African cultural-spiritual experience, especially in reference to Voodoo, Gris-Gris (also Gri-Gri and Gree-Gree) is defined as "the placing and removing of curses" (Mulira 1990, 56). Gris-Gris is in most cases an object described as an African "charm." According to Laura Porteus in "The Gri-Gri Case," the word was used and accepted in a 1773 criminal trial (involving Africans in a conspiracy to murder the master and overseer for cruel treatment) in New Orleans "to designate the crocodile concoction as though it were poison" (Porteus 1934, 50). In addition, one of the African defendants in the Gri-Gri Trial was thought to have "associated it in his mind with a "charm" for working one's will on another" (Porteus 1934, 50). While Gris-Gris is a word generally considered by most to be of African origin, Ron Bodin stated in his glossary in *Voodoo Past and Present* that Gris-Gris (according to an Vermillion Parish, Louisiana informant) was "from the French word for gray—a potion or conjo to ward off bad luck or to cross another. Often a bag filled with hair, nail-clippings, etc." (Bodin 1990, 95). Former enslaved African Melinda of Baton Rouge, Louisiana spoke of her experience in making Gris-Gris so that the young mistress of the plantation would not experience visits from an unwanted suitor:

> Well, dat man come back again—dat 'Merican from dat place call Chicago—but I done took no chances. I done made so many gris-gris on him for my little missis not to care for him, dat, sure enough, in de next spring we had a big weddin' right on dat plantation. . .'If my eyes ain't foolin' me, it's dat same man, de 'Merican from dat place, Chicago'. . .I left. A-grumblin' to myself I says, 'Where dat gris-gris I made last year to chase him away' And when I brought de coffee and de biscuits, I sprinkle dat powder right under his rocker for him to never come back no more (Clayton 1990, 168–169).

Ceceil George described the significance of emergency dispensing and divining with reference to yellow fever and her slaveowner:

Slavery and Medicine: Enslavement and Medical Practices in Antebellum Louisiana

> De yaller fever come along and he sweat. He used to keep his money in a iron chest, and ease out just enough money to run de house on to Mrs. Jerry, dat was his wife and a good woman, den she get sick.
>
> De yaller fever was ragin'; every day coffins [were] goin' to de graveyard. So he sent for a special doctor for Mrs. Jerry. His name was Dr. Levere, and he had a crippled foot. Well, de doctor, he took sick. Mrs. Jerry, she call me to her bed. She say, 'Oh, Ceceil, I'm sick, I'm scart, de doctor sick and de medicine don't do no good. My husband must not know, but can't you make me some tea? Do something. But I was scart of Mr. Green, so I just prayed over her, and something said, 'Trust God. Make dat tea.' I went out, got de grass, got some Indian root, put it on to boil, and I get some whiskey. I say, 'For God's sake, I don't want to be killed.' I give her de tea and she don't sweat, so I cover her up. I go get de guts out of a pumkin and boil it with whiskey and give it to her and she sweat de fever out. Her clothes were yaller, but wid God's help I got her on her feet (Clayton 1990, 85–86).

George, like so many dispensers of the antebellum period, made no distinction between the sacred and the secular. In this case, God was implored, and utilized along with the necessary herbal remedies. Like dispensing, the divining experience also demonstrates the power enslaved Africans possessed in a system where they are thought to have held no power at all.

SUMMARY AND CONCLUSION

> Yes, sah! I sho does come from dat old stock who had de misfortune to be slaves, but who decided to be men, at one and de same time, and I's right proud of it.
>
> *George Cato*

Enslavement in Louisiana, especially southeastern Louisiana, is considered somewhat different from enslavement as practiced in other parts of the lower South. It is suggested that this difference is a result of the colonizing cultures of the French and Spanish and of the large numbers of free people of color in New Orleans, Louisiana. The gens de la coleur libre of New Orleans were the descendants of some of these early French and Spanish colonizers and enslaved African women. New Orleans enslavement is thought to be unique because this large number of free people of color intermingled with enslaved Africans who worked as domestics, artisans, skilled craftspersons and agricultural laborers. Some of the free people of color married enslaved Africans. However, as their culture began to develop, the gens de la coleur libre did not necessarily consider themselves "Negro," "Black," or "African." Contemporary scholars on the issue of race during the antebellum period often confuse racial ancestry with an accepted and cherished identity. Therefore, many "Black firsts" in southeastern Louisiana, including the area of medicine, are attributed to some free people of color who, in their time, would not have considered themselves Black or African; especially given the harshness of bondage, the social stigma of enslavement and the negative perceptions of the continent of Africa.

The continuing problem of "Black Firsts," or isolated incidences of Africans operating outside of the antebellum norm, continues to be presented as significant marks of achievement or as aberrations from the enslaved African masses. For example, there are numerous references to James Derham, the first African American physician in the United States. There is also discussion of Andrew Durnford, previously mentioned, and Coincoin (Marie Therese Metoyer), who are characterized as Black ("Negro") slave/plantation owners in Louisiana. The problem with these historical revelations is that they erroneously reinterpret the history of the enslaved African population. They often give the impression of an important pattern emerging (such as "Black slaveowners") which attempts to obfuscate the actual antebellum conditions and absolve historiographers from discussing areas of enslavement that are considered too polemic for serious academic review.

Despite the challenges of a distinctive slaveocracy and the persistence of hegemonic scholarship, the purpose of this research was not to argue the effectiveness of the cures and remedies offered by enslaved Africans and the White slaveowner; but to assert that the role of the African, as a central agent-participant in antebellum medical care, was much more substantial than we have previously been led to believe. The traditional focus of enslavement and medicine studies has been to prove or support the thesis that Africans were treated "well" in the slaveocracy; that slaveowners cared something about the African's humanity, and that this caring phenomena can be quantified. An important proof used to support this thesis is the fact that slaveowners sought medical care for enslaved Africans. Slaveowners did indeed provide medical care to enslaved Africans as a part of their "slave management" operations on the farms and plantations. In addition, the issue of brutality and medical health care is generally not addressed by enslavement and medicine scholars. According to the oral histories and narratives, brutality against Africans must have caused significant medical health care problems which often went untreated.

Despite efforts to ignore or diminish the presence of Africans in the development of medical care in the antebellum South, medical management, practices and the hospital experience demonstrate that Africans were a central focus of the antebellum medical world. Africans who were enslaved in the antebellum South suffered constant medical health risks by virtue of their

SLAVERY AND MEDICINE: ENSLAVEMENT AND MEDICAL PRACTICES IN ANTEBELLUM LOUISIANA

status. Notwithstanding the oppressive nature of the slaveocracy Africans made important contributions to the development of medicine in the United States. Still scholars failed to acknowledge the medical risks, and minimized the Africans' contributions to medicine, largely because their studies about enslaved Africans focus on the experiences of Whites, particularly White males in the slaveocracy. Therefore, they enhance and forward some of the same traditional negative and false "objective" ideas about the culture of enslaved Africans.

Many scholars avoid the discourse on "slave medicine" and the "Negro/Slave Diseases" because of the obvious racial supremacist implications; and because of their pseudo-scientific nature. Disease devoid of racial connotations was a major medical risk enslaved Africans faced. The significant aspect of antebellum morbidity was the racial connotation applied where Africans were concerned. The ideologies of "Negro/Slave Diseases" attempted to apply a racial supremacist answer to illnesses and conditions which were said to demonstrate symptoms that were physical and more importantly, psychological. "Negro/Slave Diseases" included: Negro Consumption, Cachexia Africana, Dysaesthesia Aethiopica and Drapetomania. Other diseases/illnesses that Africans suffered from, with a limited amount of racial supremacist connotation, included dysentery, cholera, yellow fever, diarrhea, etc. Slave medicine is an example of the scientific and philosophical foundations of racism in the lower South. It represents a pseudo-scientific inquiry which was ultimately used to foster a bio-medical rationale for the maintenance of White supremacy and the slaveocracy in general.

Slaveowners sought at all times to protect their slave property. Government and social systems assisted them in this effort. The Black (Slave) Codes, like Le Code Noir in Louisiana, protected the interests of the slaveowner, rarely addressing the medical needs of enslaved Africans. A major contributor to the medical health issues of enslaved Africans was slave labor. Most Africans performed

SLAVERY AND MEDICINE: ENSLAVEMENT AND MEDICAL PRACTICES IN ANTEBELLUM LOUISIANA

difficult labor which often put them at risk, especially where the use of machines/equipment was concerned. They worked long hours on the large farms and plantations; and the literature demonstrates that inadequate housing and nutrition, and frequent exposure to the natural environmental elements were great concerns. Labors related to the health status of Africans included the work in sugar and cotton; other labors which affected the health of African women were breeding and concubinage.

From an Afrocentric perspective, breeding and concubinage represent slave labor functions, and possess similar labor requirements and characteristics as agricultural or domestic enslavement labor. Breeding and concubinage required mandatory/forced or coerced performance. There was a reward/punishment system in place to address the performance aspect of breeding and concubinage. And finally, the results of breeding/concubinage labor was most often verifiable (except in cases where enslaved women could not reproduce, prevented pregnancies or performed abortions). Therefore, breeding/concubinage yielded a "cash crop" of enslaved persons who, of course, followed the condition of their mother.

The complex nature of enslavement and medicine in the old South included the questions about African humanity. The human/subhuman issue suggested that people of African descent were not human beings, though some slaveocracy scholars conceded that Africans might represent a human species different from Whites. Disorders about the so-called "subhumanity" of Africans assisted the slaveocracy in defining and defending the institution of enslavement. Slaveowners utilized a medical management system which included the use of folk medicine on African people, the development and use of plantation and city hospitals and infirmaries, and the use of licensed and experienced medical doctors to help maintain the slave labor force. Medical, industrial and agricultural journals and pamphlets provided physicians and slaveowners with information and instructions regarding their own medical care and the perceived "special" medical care needs of people of African descent.

Many southern antebellum hospitals, like Touro Infirmary of New Orleans, supported the needs of the slaveocracy by opening their facilities to enslaved Africans, and providing affordable rates to slaveowners. Enslaved Africans were the victims of medical experimentation, treatments, surgical procedures and post-mortem examinations. Records do not reveal, nor was there a social precedent for, enslaved Africans having been asked permission to have experimental or emergency procedures performed on them. The field of obstetrics/gynecology is indebted to the countless numbers of African women who were made available by their slaveowners to have some of these procedures performed and perfected.

African medicine was not acknowledged in the antebellum South. Despite the significant exposure of southeastern Louisiana physicians to the medical legacies from France, (and the Hippocratic model from Greece) the idea of African medicine was a rudimentary notion among White European/ Americans. What Whites knew of African medicine, religion, and philosophy was subsumed under the label "Voodoo." Voodoo was a major threat to the slaveocracy because it empowered enslaved Africans. In addition, if left to develop, slaveowners feared that Africans would reject and supplant the religious indoctrinations of the slaveowners. In essence Africans did reject traditional European/American Christian indoctrinations by changing their relationship to it. The African practitioners of Voodoo wielded respect, power and influence over believers and non-believers. Given the human/subhuman factor, it was impossible for Whites to explore, acknowledge and understand the legacy of African medicine among enslaved Africans. African perceptions of medicine in the antebellum South varied. Enslaved Africans acknowledged that the slaveowner and the mistress provided medical care. They also state that physicians were called in to provide care. In southeastern

SLAVERY AND MEDICINE: ENSLAVEMENT AND MEDICAL PRACTICES IN
ANTEBELLUM LOUISIANA

Louisiana in the parishes surrounding New Orleans, the oral histories of enslaved Africans do not state that they were brought in significant numbers to the city hospitals. However, the Touro Infirmary Admission records reveal for 1855 to 1860 that Africans represented almost half of the hospital's clientele. Enslaved Africans also understood why they received medical care and cited the economic importance of being the chattel property of the slaveowner as the underlying factor.

Legacies from the traditional African worldview influenced Africana medicine in the antebellum South. The African worldview is evident in the persistence of African based "religious" structures, better termed, the African Living Belief System. Traditional scholars failed to see the relationship between African "religion" via the African Living Belief System, the African worldview and medicine. African views toward medicine continued to be characterized as acts of "barbarism" and manifestations of "the savage primitive." Survivals such as Voodoo, notwithstanding the preponderance of syncretization, is demonstrative of some of the characteristics inherent in the African Living Belief System. Africans participated in the care and treatment of illness/disease as dispensers and diviners of medical care. As dispensers, Africans administered medicines the slaveowner, mistress and physician provided. They also prepared and dispensed botanical remedies of their own making. As diviners Africans provided medical care by incorporating a magico-religious-medical structure intended to bring the body to holistic healing.

Much more important than traditional contributionist history, enslaved African people impacted the development of medicine in the United States, particularly in the lower South. Contrary to the findings of contemporary enslavement and medicine scholars, Africans were exposed to numerous medical health risks by virtue of their slave status. Medical health risks were higher for Africans, not just because they shared a harsh environment and climate with Whites, but because of the arbitrary nature of enslavement. The

Slavery and Medicine: Enslavement and Medical Practices in Antebellum Louisiana

arbitrary nature of enslavement was a major risk factor that cannot necessarily be quantified, yet it can be seriously considered because we can document its existence in the oral histories and narratives of Africans who survived the Holocaust of Enslavement.

There is a need for scholars to employ diverse research methods and perspective in the social scientific study of enslavement and medicine in the United States, the West Indies and other parts of the African diaspora. Each territory of the slaveocracy possesses information on medicine and enslavement which has not yet been uncovered and interpreted. Private and public records regarding enslavement and medicine may be challenging to procure, not necessarily because of the risks of surviving antebellum documents; but because some records reveal painful insights regarding medical care, experimentation and post-mortem examinations of enslaved Africans. Many private descendant-keepers of surviving antebellum documents do not wish to share the data with the general public. Existing hospitals with roots in the antebellum period, on the other hand, may not readily appreciate the importance, or know the whereabouts of surviving materials related to medicine and enslavement.

The call for a dispassionate discourse regarding the African world experience is another attempt to deny the centrality of the African in his own historiography. It suggests that objectivity in historical analysis actually prevails in the interpretive record. However, the ante- and post-bellum literature demonstrates that what is offered as objective analysis is actually a subjective historical discourse based on the history and culture of Europeans and chronicled by many contemporary scholars. A scholarly historical and cultural analysis of enslavement and medicine demonstrates, as former enslaved African Mary Reynolds stated, that the overwhelming reality of enslavement were "things past tellin'" (Mellon 1988, 18). However, an interpretation based on an African centered methodology and perspective reveals the complexities of the African's survival of the Holocaust of

SLAVERY AND MEDICINE: ENSLAVEMENT AND MEDICAL PRACTICES IN ANTEBELLUM LOUISIANA

Enslavement; and the congruency and development of the African Living Belief System. While the system of enslavement provided a multitude of medical health risks, Africans recreated a complex medical universe in the diaspora in an attempt to maintain the optimal continuity of human life.

BIBLIOGRAPHIC ESSAY

Primary Sources

Our information on enslavement and medicine is revealed through numerous primary and secondary source documents. The primary source documents include: slave narratives/interviews/oral histories, ship records/logs, antebellum medical/science journals, plantation books (or farm) records (journals, letters, diaries, logs), the Black Codes, anti-slavery (abolitionist) documents, hospital/infirmary records, medical records/bills, municipal records, traveler's logs/letters, newspaper articles and advertisements. The secondary sources include: scholarly/historical articles, books, monographs, unpublished papers, master's thesis and doctoral dissertations. Primary source documents, with the exception of many of the oral histories and narratives of enslaved Africans, tend to support the views and experience of the slaveowners. The primary source documents on enslavement and medicine follow the themes of instruction and edification to the slaveowning class—teaching them how to care for Africans. Whites were instructed fully—from the slaveholding cells of the West African forts and castles, on the slaving ships bound for the Caribbean islands and through the enslavement experience in north and south America. Slaveowners developed and shared information about their own medical needs and counseled one another about the medical maintenance of Africans.

In "A Philadelphia Surgeon on a Slaving Voyage to Africa, 1749–1751," the slave surgeon meticulously documented the hazards of slave ships in general and noted that many doctors were employed on slave ships to care for the crew and the cargo of African people. He also noted that medical care of Africans began in the slave castles and on the docked slave ships as they waited to fill the ship's hold. Slave ship doctors handled major medical issues onboard the ships from contagious diseases to "mania." The mania that would have affected enslaved Africans on slave ships was described in 1811 as a condition which "originates from an encreased excitement of the brain" and is a "deranged state of the intellectual system" (Ralston 1811, 143). More often slave ship physicians handled routine medical issues en route. Doctors also performed surgical procedures onboard slave ships upon African men, women and children (Wax 1968, 465–493).

In 1817 Richard Harland presented another view of enslavement and medicine on slave ships in "Observations on Long Voyages." Harland

SLAVERY AND MEDICINE: ENSLAVEMENT AND MEDICAL PRACTICES IN ANTEBELLUM LOUISIANA

confirmed that lengthy voyages took place without significant on-board medical attention from doctors. He suggested that ship owner/investors did not want the expense of employing shipboard doctors—eliminating this expense allowed them to further increase their profit potential on each enslaved African. But crew members could not escape some of the same debilitating diseases that claimed the lives of Africans. In 1817 the crew of the ship, the William Savery, suffered from "dysenteries, diarrheas, hernias, fracture, luxation, hemorrhoids, wounds, furunculus, bilious fevers, sarcocele, hepatitis, dropsey, enteritis, rheumatism, paralysis. . ." (Harland 1817, 11).

Advertisements and announcements for the sale of enslaved Africans contain valuable information about the social status of slaves in the United States. They also provide information about age, racial categorization (negro, mulatto, etc.), marital status, children, language/linguistic skills, occupation (skills and abilities), disposition (psychological) and medical health status. Nearly all enslaved Africans were guaranteed by law to be medically fit for slave labor. The Hewlett and Bright sale of slaves scheduled for May 16, 1835 in New Orleans, Louisiana included the notation: "All the above named Slaves are acclimated and excellent subjects," they were "warranted against all vices and maladies prescribed by law" (Hewlett and Bright 1835). This was important since sellers could be sued for knowingly selling "defective" Africans. Bills of sale indicate that many Africans were sold "fully warranted" and any prior medical conditions that existed were disclosed. Enslaved Africans deemed to be "defective," were sold below cost, usually "repaired" and resold for a significant profit. In this same advertisement, we also find an example of an enslaved woman who served as nurse among her other tasks: "SARAH, a mulatress, aged 45 years, a good cook and accustomed to house work in general, is an excellent and faithful nurse for sick persons, and in every respect a first rate character" (Hewlett and Bright 1835).

Some scholars of enslavement and medicine have suggested that the school of thought which promoted a separate line of human development and physiology for Africans and Europeans was a southern medical phenomena. Gary Puckrein in "Climate, Health and Black Labor in the English Americas" showed that English colonial attitudes toward health, labor and enslaved Africans was similar to their southern counterparts. English colonists also developed the idea that Africans were better suited to intensive labor than White Europeans. This theme of the African's supposed "fitness" to the institution of enslavement rested in the notion that health was related to specific racial characteristics, environmental preferences and the race's ability to acclimate (Puckrein 1979, 179–193).

Africans were shown to have contracted the same diseases and debilities as Whites, and yet certain "maladies" were said to be uniquely African in origin. In 1799 W. M. Harvey and John Lindesay in their "Account of the Cachexia Africana" forwarded the idea of specific illnesses that only Africans contracted among themselves. One which survived to the Civil War was Cachexia Africana, better known as "dirt eating." Harvey and Lindesay offered a diagnoses of Cachexia Africana and looked at some of the initial symptoms, which included actual dirt eating and emotional distress such as sadness and depression (Harvey and Lindesay 1799, 282–284). Dr. P. Tidyman in "A Sketch of the Most Remarkable Diseases of the Negroes of the Southern States," discusses the physical differences between Africans and Europeans. According to Tidyman: "We must by a careful investigation endeavor to trace the physical peculiarities which are ascribed to the Aethiopian, and serve to distinguish him from the white man" (Tidyman 1826, 306). Tidyman asserts that skin color is a major factor of difference, which also allowed Africans to withstand hot, humid temperatures. Africans were perceived to be better suited to intensive labor because they sweated profusely and this sweat assisted in their adaption. Like many physicians of the early 1800s, Tidyman offered numerous remedies for medical conditions affecting Africans. Tidyman also notes that experiments were conducted upon enslaved Africans regarding skin color and the sun's rays. The physicians of Tidyman's time concluded that Africans were stronger than Whites when it came to surgeries—that Africans could better withstand the pain. Tidyman also asserted that Africans often consulted other African "quacks" regarding their remedies to their various illnesses. At the same time Tidyman noted that there were Africans who were knowledgeable about some medical cures (Tidyman 1826, 333).

Other doctors like Samuel A. Cartwright also pursued the course of a "peculiar" race of people (the African) and attempted to delineate that race's diseases and illnesses. Very much like Tidyman, Cartwright not only identified the specific diseases of the African, he also provided information on treatment. Cartwright identified "Negro Consumption" as being in no way related to the consumption condition experienced by the

SLAVERY AND MEDICINE: ENSLAVEMENT AND MEDICAL PRACTICES IN ANTEBELLUM LOUISIANA

White race. Cartwright went further to distinguish "Negro Consumption" as being caused by the superstitious beliefs held by Africans that they had been somehow "poisoned." Cartwright also discussed the disease entitled "Drapetomania"—"The disease causing Negroes to run away." Africans afflicted with Drapetomania were thought to be generally disobedient and predisposed to destroying crops and equipment (Cartwright 1851, 331–337). Cartwright is considered unabashedly racist by contemporary scholars who often apologize for his attitudes or attempt to distance themselves by quickly pointing out that not all White ante-bellum physicians, especially northern doctors, agreed with "mixing politics (enslavement of Africans) with medicine."

Antebellum letters also give insight into the attitudes of slaveowners, and more often, into the role of Africans regarding medical care and enslavement. Rachel O'Connor was an antebellum plantation owner in Louisiana, and she ran one of the largest plantations—enslaving 77 Africans. Allie Webb's editing of *The Mistress of Evergreen Plantation, Rachel O'Connor's Legacy of Letters 1823–1845*, indicates that sickness was a major preoccupation of plantation life. The letters provide a catalog of remedies and cures plantation owners used to keep Africans healthy enough to perform the labor. It should also be noted that in the "Who's Who" in Rachel O'Connor's life by Allie Webb, no Africans are listed; while the letters reveal that there were several Africans close to O'Connor who assisted the widow tremendously in the health care and general maintenance of the plantation (Webb 1983, 291–293).

White American and European travellers to the South often presented a different picture of enslavement and the medical health of Africans. In "A Letter From a Yankee Bride in Ante-Bellum Louisiana," Emma Lay Lane was impressed with the care and treatment of enslaved Africans on her father-in-law's plantation in 1857. Regarding food she noted that "The Negroes all have all the milk and butter they want" (Anderson 1960, 246). Lane was convinced of the good health of enslaved Africans and also that they were happy, docile people who were acclimated to the heat:

> They are just as merry a set of beings as ever you saw. I asked Peggy one day if she wasn't warm picking cotton in the hot sun. "Bless your putty eyes, Missy," said she, "taint too hot," and sure enough one of these

cooler days, here she comes with yarn stockings, freezing to death. I please them, asking who wants to go home with me (to Connecticut) and tell them awful stories about the cold, at which they roll their white eyes in horror and scream out, "Laws, Missy, don't take me, please don't" (Anderson 1960, 248).

The letters of another visitor, Frances Anne Kemble, provide a less than idyllic view of the health status of enslaved Africans. Frances found an infirmary on Butler's Island for enslaved Africans which contained immense sickness and disease including lockjaw, "inflammation of the lungs," "rheumatism", "falling (of the) womb" and a skin rotting condition (similar to yaws) which infected a fourteen year old girl. An enslaved African woman, Harriet had been "horsewhipped" because she told Kemble that the women did not have the time to properly clean their own children (Rose 1976, 420–423).

The Slave or Black Codes are important documents in understanding the connection between medical health issues and the institution of enslavement. The Black Codes defined slavery for the African—it specified in detail the limitations on his life. Conversely, the Black Codes highlighted the rights and privileges of slaveowners and other members of the White population. The Black Codes protected Whites and gave them the power to punish enslaved Africans for a variety of offenses; and often stipulated for example, the number of lashes for a specific offense. Africans were punished for offenses such as leaving/entering plantations without permission, assembling with other Africans, preaching to other slaves, running away, possessing weapons, etc. While the codes were meticulously outlined, less attention was given to the medical treatment of enslaved Africans. Yet some Black Codes contained rules and regulations regarding the "care and feeding" of African people. For example, the South Carolina Slave Codes for 1850 stated:

> It is the settled law of this State, that an owner cannot abandon a slave needing either medical treatment, care, food or raiment. If he does, he will be liable to any one who may furnish the same. . .The slave lives for his master's service. His time, his labor, his comforts, are all at his master's disposal. The duty of humane

SLAVERY AND MEDICINE: ENSLAVEMENT AND MEDICAL PRACTICES IN
ANTEBELLUM LOUISIANA

treatment and of medical assistance (when clearly necessary) ought not be withholden ("Slave Laws. . ." 1850, 182).

In addition to detailing how Africans would be fed, housed and punished by slaveowners, the Black Codes generally denied Africans the opportunity to testify in a court of law against a slaveowner he/she considered neglectful, harsh and/or abusive (Rose 1976, 176–178; Gayarre 1903, 531–540).

Abolitionists frequently pointed out the abuses of the medical field with regard to enslaved African people. In *American Slavery As It Is: Testimony of a Thousand Witnesses*, Theodore Weld and the American Anti-Slavery Society compiled numerous examples of the medical professions use (and abuse) of enslaved Africans. There are instances were enslaved Africans were diagnosed with disease, and placed under the care of a physician or surgeon; if the slave lived the doctor was paid by the slaveowner, if the slave died, the doctor was not necessarily paid. Enslaved Africans were not protected from inhumane treatment at the hands of doctors or surgeons. Africans were used in experiments and operations even if the procedures were not relevant to curing their ailment. In addition there were reported cases that when Africans informed the slaveowner about sickness, they were whipped and made to labor because the slaveowner or overseer refused to believe them. Many slaveowners believed that Africans generally, as a race of people, were given to lying and immoral behavior. There are also numerous cases of enslaved Africans being left alone in their slave quarters with illnesses left untreated. However, when physicians were sought they usually pursued a course of purging, blood-letting and/or administering salts to Africans since this was also the state of medical care for Whites at the time, a legacy from the Hippocratic model's four humors.

The medical health of slaves was extremely important to the large and small slaveowners. Since enslaved Africans represented a significant financial investment for many, slaveowners had a great concern for protecting their property. Louisiana established and maintained many hospitals during the antebellum period both urban and rural (plantation). According to Walter M. Burnett in *Touro Infirmary*, among the New Orleans hospitals were the Royal Military Hospital (1722), Charity Hospital of Louisiana (1736), Hotel Dieu (1859), New Orleans Mental

SLAVERY AND MEDICINE: ENSLAVEMENT AND MEDICAL PRACTICES IN
ANTEBELLUM LOUISIANA

Health Institute (1861) and Touro Infirmary (1854) (Burnett 1979, 89). Charity hospital not only contained medical and surgical wards, but also a chapel, a Lunatic Asylum and a Dead House ("Historical Sketch. . ." 1844, 72–77). Regarding the significance of hospitals and enslaved Africans, William D. Postell noted in *The Health of Slaves on Southern Plantations*:

The operation of hospitals was undoubtedly a profitable business. A slave's life was too valuable for the planter to risk, and if hospitalization would add to a Negro's chance of recovery, the planter did not hesitate to commit him to a hospital maintained by reputable physicians (1951, 140). Surviving antebellum hospital records involving enslaved Africans are often rare. "The Admission Book of the Touro Infirmary" for 1855 to 1860 is an important example of an undiscovered primary source record left by an antebellum hospital which speaks to the medical lives of enslaved African's in Louisiana.

An important antebellum journal to enslavement and medicine was *The New Orleans Medical and Surgical Journal* (NOMSJ). According to medical historian John Duffy the journal is "one of paramount importance." The journal first began publication in 1844 as the *New Orleans Medical Journal*. A year later it changed its name to the *New Orleans Medical and Surgical Journal*. After 1953 the journal became the *Journal of the Louisiana State Medical Society*. An important feature of the journal was its treatment of African medical/ health issues. Samuel Cartwright spearheaded the discourse on the differences between African and European physiology; including discussions on Drapetomania (running away), Cachexia Africana (dirt-eating) and other diseases said to be specific to African people. Duffy demonstrates the strength of Cartwright's arguments regarding African inferiority and European superiority from his articles which appeared in the *New Orleans Medical and Surgical Journal* (Duffy 1957, 3–24).

Antebellum medical journals such as the *New Orleans Medical and Surgical Journal*, the *Charleston Medical Journal*, etc., while written for White physicians and slaveowners, provide examples of the proactive involvement of enslaved Africans in medical health cases. For example, a short excerpt in the 1854–55 edition of the *New Orleans Medical and Surgical Journal* explains how an African midwife performed a cesarian section on another young African woman. The baby was healthy and the mother recovered quickly (Dowler 1854–1855, 19). The author, Bennett Dowler goes on to say that even though many midwives lacked even the most basic elementary anatomical instruction, they were often more successful than doctors (Dowler 1854–55, 19–21).

The primary source data regarding the enslaved African's impression of, and his participation in, medical care is revealed in the narratives of his life, oral histories and letters. There is significant concern over the use of oral testimonies of enslaved Africans (Phillips 1929, 219) particularly the narrative genre because so many were prepared by or with the assistance of Whites and often reflect their perspective, culture, values, etc. on a system that they themselves did not experience as slaves. However, Norman Yetman in "Ex-Slave Interviews and the Historiography of Slavery" argues for the significance of oral history regarding the institution of enslavement (Yetman 1984, 189). According to B. A. Botkin, regarding his work with the "Slave Narrative Collection of the Federal Writers' Project," the "slave narratives and interviews" are used in "two main fashions: for serious historical and sociological documentation. . .or for nostalgic character and local-color sketches of old times" (Botkin 1945, xxxvi). Ronnie W. Clayton in *Mother Wit, The Ex-Slave Narratives of the Louisiana Writers' Project* indicates how the narratives of Louisiana were controlled and framed by White researchers (especially Lyle Saxon), who developed the guidelines as to what questions would be asked of Africans and what data would be included in final projects (Clayton 1990, 1–12; Clayton 1978, 327–335). *Mother Wit* also demonstrates the biases of the interviewers towards subjects who speak of the enslavement experience with fondness and praise. Many of the formerly enslaved Africans expressed profound sentiments, a wealth of information and an overwhelming desire to be heard: "you got to listen, chile, with all the 'tention you got in your head, and you better remember it too. I ain't tellin' you dis for you to forget it and get it clean out of your head. You got to remember all dis, you hear me?" (Clayton 1990, 167)

Former enslaved Africans commented upon the state of medical care and their own participation during the institution of enslavement. Many Africans in Botkin's *Lay My Burden Down* give us such insight. For example, Ellen Betts who was born approximately 1853 near Opelousas, St. Landry Parish, Louisiana and enslaved in Louisiana, stated: "I nurse the sick folks too. Sometime I dose with blue mass pills, and sometime Dr. Fawcett leave rhubarb and ipecac and calomel and castor oil and such" (Botkin 1945, 126). There is also the legacy of "conjure" doctors

SLAVERY AND MEDICINE: ENSLAVEMENT AND MEDICAL PRACTICES IN ANTEBELLUM LOUISIANA

during the institution of enslavement. Conjuring, "a system of belief, a way of perceiving the world which placed people in the context of another world no less 'real' than the ordinary one" (Raboteau 1978, 275), was used for such illnesses as mumps, smallpox and snakebites. The incidence of conjuring is evidence that White doctors and hospitals were not wholly accepted by enslaved Africans. The conjure doctor provided a medical treatment alternative to the health and peace-of-mind of the enslaved African.

Secondary Sources

Enslavement and medicine has not been taken seriously as a popular or important topic in United States history. Standard university texts in African American history and culture more often fail to include any information on the important issue of medicine during the institution of enslavement. Eurocentric historians have consistently failed to look at the correlation between enslavement and medicine and brutality and labor; however they do focus primarily on the following factors: general health care, legal mandates, property management, "slave diseases," experimental treatments, procedures and surgeries, the role of lay and licensed physicians, and sectional conflict regarding "slave medicine." These issues were important to the institution of enslavement in southern Louisiana because of the duality of its brand of enslaving Africans and maintaining a notable free African population; and because of its economic, geographic and cultural significance to the old South.

Since the experience of enslaved Africans has been viewed as peripheral to the overall analysis of the scheme of slaveocracy studies, there are to date, no Afrocentric treatments of enslavement and medicine in Louisiana or any other part of the United States. The research on enslaved Africans and medicine is presented in the primary and secondary source research regarding general health, disease and the development of medicine in the antebellum South. Not only does the research fail to place enslaved Africans at the center of the analysis, they often offer a defense of the system of enslavement and present slanted views of the role of slaveowners. However, while antebellum and contemporary scholars were not Afrocentric in their treatment, much of their work is important for Afrocentric analysis of enslavement and medicine. There are numerous secondary source documents which address the issue of general medical health of enslaved Africans in the antebellum United States,

SLAVERY AND MEDICINE: ENSLAVEMENT AND MEDICAL PRACTICES IN
ANTEBELLUM LOUISIANA

particularly the South (Adams 1989, 259–278; Duffy 1959, 53–72; Marshall 1942, 52; and Mitchell 1944, 424–446). Discussions of enslavement and medicine are usually found in the research on the development of the medical field in the United States and specifically in the antebellum South.

R. H. Shryock in "Medical Sources and the Social Historian" suggests that historiographers were concerned with whether or not enslaved Africans were treated well by the slaveowners. In doing so historians found that free Africans demonstrated a higher mortality rate than enslaved Africans. This supported the theory that enslavement was a better condition for Africans than freedom (Shryock 1936, 458–473). William D. Postell in "The Health of Slaves on Southern Plantations" suggested that enslaved Africans essentially had the same health status of Whites. According to Postell:

> ... it seems that the health of slaves was comparable to the public health of that era. The medical care and treatment rendered the slaves was in accordance with the accepted practices of that day, and the failures were the failures of the times. The over-all picture of slave health is simply a picture of health conditions in the United States, and their health status was no better and no worse than that of the populace as a whole for that period (Postell 1951, 164).

Howard Mahorner continues the traditional apologist position regarding the institution of enslavement and medicine in "The History of Medicine in Louisiana." In this transcript of a paper presented to the Louisiana Historical Society in 1973, Mahorner supplies general information regarding medical care in the city of New Orleans during the antebellum period, including the role of the doctor and the environmental factors that influenced the health care of Whites and enslaved Africans (Mahorner 1973, 49–67). Elizabeth Keeney in "Unless Powerful Sick: Domestic Medicine in the Old South," describes the difference between "Folk and Domestic" medicine. Folk medicine refers to those health care practices not agreed upon by the professional medical community, such practices considered by lay people administering medical care. Domestic medicine refers to "professional" medicine as advocated by trained and licensed physicians. Keeney discusses the theme of "Domestic" medicine as being unique to the South and suggests that southerners adapted medicine to their own needs, which particularly focused on enslaved Africans (Keeney 1989, 276–294).

There is rarely a discussion regarding the impact of labor and the medical health status of enslaved Africans. V. Alton Moody, in his doctoral dissertation entitled "Slavery on Louisiana Sugar Plantations" emphasized that dangerous labor performed by, and brutality perpetrated against, enslaved Africans was prohibited by law, but made no other connection between brutality, enslavement and the need for medical care. Moody notes that plantation labor included clearing the land for cultivation; and that in general, the sugar plantations required long, arduous hours by enslaved Africans. He also notes that most slaveowners provided medical care for enslaved Africans; and that they cared for old and disabled Africans by hiring doctors and establishing, on most of the large plantations, hospitals and infirmaries (Moody 1924, 271–275). Kenneth Stampp acknowledged the connection between labor and medical care in *The Peculiar Institution Slavery in Ante-Bellum South*. Stampp also notes the "crude diagnoses" and "vague names" given to illnesses including those applied to Africans; and in addition, he mentions that many enslaved Africans were in need of dental care (Stampp 1956, 295–321).

John Duffy in "Medical Practice in the Antebellum South," provides an overview of antebellum medicine noting that the physicians and lay people of the time had little understanding of disease, particularly epidemics. Like many scholars, Duffy in this work does not acknowledge the significance of brutality and enslavement regarding the medical care of African people (Duffy 1959, 53–72). Further, in "A Note on Antebellum Southern Nationalism and Medical Practice," Duffy presents a major theme of enslavement and medicine in the antebellum south—that White doctors thought that Africans required special medical care. White doctors based this theory on other assumptions about and observations of African physiology. They felt that Africans were resistant to certain diseases (such as yellow fever and malaria), but more susceptible to respiratory illnesses. Because of the idea that Africans were significantly different from White Europeans, the South developed a distinctive medical practice based on racial theories (Duffy 1968, 266–276). In "Slavery and Slave Health in Louisiana" Duffy provides a general outline of the health status of enslaved Africans, detailing the threats to their health, which included disease, "hard manual labor, a restricted diet, and the psychological impact of slavery" (Duffy 1967, 6). "The Negro and the Southern Physician: A Study of Medical and Racial Attitudes" by John Haller recounts the various "slave diseases" of the South. He also notes that the planter, his wife and overseer were the actual "physicians" of the old South. According to Haller, planters rarely used doctors to treat the diseases of Africans; they "physicked" the enslaved Africans using the various books of medicine that they purchased and those they catalogued themselves (Haller 1972, 238–253).

Another important theme of enslavement and medicine has to do with the "profit motive" of slaveowners. In "Medical Care of Slaves: Louisiana Sugar Region and South Carolina Rice District," David O. Whitten discusses the connection between the hazardous health conditions that enslaved Africans were forced to work in. Because of the health threat of labor (especially that of sugar production), slaveowners provided medical care as a necessary aspect of product (slave) maintenance. Enslaved Africans represented valuable property, an investment which had to be maintained in order to realize a future profit (Whitten 1977, 153–180). While most researchers do not attempt to address the profit motive and the issue of punishment and brutality, Theodore Rosengarten in *Tombee: Portrait of a Cotton Planter* acknowledges the connection between punishment and brutality and the enslaved Africans need for medical care (Rosengarten 1986, 184–185). However, like Duffy, Whitten does not address the issue of brutality as a medical health factor for enslaved Africans.

The "profit motive" is also a signature feature in discussions regarding the trade in enslaved Africans and such issues as insurance. Benjamin Quarles notes the meticulous manner in which slave traders conducted their business:

> They inspected their potential wares with great care, examining a slave's teeth for signs of age and looking for whip scars that would indicate unruliness. When the slave's distinctive qualities were not observable, such as a male's labor skills or a female's ability to produce offspring, the auctioneer called attention to them (Quarles 1964, 64).

SLAVERY AND MEDICINE: ENSLAVEMENT AND MEDICAL PRACTICES IN ANTEBELLUM LOUISIANA

In the article "Bernard Kendig and the New Orleans Slave Trade," Richard Tansey shows how slave dealers sold "defective" (diseased or wounded) slaves and conducted illicit sales of Africans (kidnapped free Africans). The slave dealers were responsible for housing and feeding the slaves, yet the literature does not indicate that they took a real medical interest in enslaved Africans unless their ailments were obvious. However, Judith Kelleher Schafer noted in "'Guaranteed Against the Vices and Maladies Prescribed by Law': Consumer Protection, the Law of Slave Slaves, and the Supreme Court in Antebellum Louisiana" that there was a profitable business in buying sick Africans, clearing up any medical/health conditions the African possessed and then reselling him/her at a higher profit (Schafer 1987, 306–321). Slave dealers like Kendig were embroiled in litigation for selling "defective" and "illicit" Africans; demonstrating that their primary interest was in making a profit (Tansey 1982, 159–178). In 1942 Thomas Gowan asked the question "Was Plantation Slavery Profitable?" In this article he concluded that despite the efforts to suggest that it was not, that plantation slavery was indeed most often profitable to slaveowners, especially the larger class of slaveowners in the United States (Gowan 1942, 513–535). Finally, Eugene Genovese surveyed the sources regarding the insurance and medical costs of maintaining enslaved Africans in the old South (Genovese 1960, 141–155).

Like John Duffy, Todd Savitt has provided significant scholarship which addresses enslavement and medicine in the South. In "The Use of Blacks for Medical Experimentation and Demonstration in the Old South," Savitt focuses on Africans as helpless victims of medical mistreatment by Whites, especially regarding experiments and demonstration for medical schools. In other major work Savitt presents scholarship on the health care of enslaved Africans on Virginia plantations. Savitt continues to note that "slave health" made southern society distinctive and provided the medical rationale for the enslavement of Africans. Savitt also suggests that Africans participated in their own medical health care matters (Savitt 1989, 327–355).

In "The Use of Blacks for Medical Experimentation and Demonstration in the Old South," Savitt gives accounts of the use of enslaved Africans by antebellum medical colleges. During the antebellum period, a medical college's success depended largely on it's ability to obtain enslaved Africans, freedmen and poor Whites as subjects. The establishment of a medical school in Louisville, Kentucky was possible due to the "large black (as well as transient white) population." These subjects were often used in lecture classes. At the Atlanta Medical College Infirmary, an African suffering from hepatic abscess was lectured upon for several weeks to medical students. At the Medical College of the State of South Carolina, Africans in need of surgery were admitted to the "Colored Ward" of the hospital and cared for exclusively by student doctors. Savitt points out that it was easy to secure enslaved Africans for experimental procedures, or their deceased bodies for dissection because White society generally frowned upon the practice and African people could not refuse or protest (Savitt 1989, 327–355).

Enslavement and medicine scholars often discuss the issue of medical experimentation upon enslaved Africans. In "Body Snatchers and Anatomy, Professional Medical Education in Nineteenth Century Virginia," James O. Breeden discusses the impact, significance and challenges inherent in securing bodies for medical education. Medical schools needed cadavers to teach students about the internal workings of the human body, and medical school students often selected schools based on the number of available bodies. Enslaved Africans were used for this purpose, especially those in areas of the country with significant African populations (Breeden 1975, 321–345). According to Duffy, New Orleans, Louisiana, was an accessible port to the medical professionals seeking bodies for dissection (Duffy 1979, 169).

F. N. Boney in "Slaves as Guinea Pigs: Georgia and Alabama Episodes," compares the medical experiments of Nazi Germany on Jews to those practices of antebellum Southern doctors upon enslaved Africans. These "Black Guinea Pigs" included men, women and children. Boney discusses one of the better known surgical cases involving enslaved African women and the physician J. Marion Sims. Sims, with the permission of the slaveowner, conducted years of painful research upon enslaved African women in order to learn how to repair the rupture between the bladder and the vagina, a condition known as vagico-fistula (vesico-vaginal fistula or vaginal fistula) (Boney 1984, 45–51). A discussion of Sims work which seeks to address the voicelessness of the enslaved African women patients comes from Diana Axelson in her article "Women as Victims of Medical Experiments: J. Marion Sims Surgery and Slave Women, 1845–1850." Axelson notes that it was not uncommon for enslaved African women to be the subject of gynecological surgical experiments by doctors like Sims; and that Whites

SLAVERY AND MEDICINE: ENSLAVEMENT AND MEDICAL PRACTICES IN
ANTEBELLUM LOUISIANA

did not recognized their own insensitivity toward the enslaved women, who had no freedom of choice regarding the surgical procedures (Axelson 1985, 10–12). Finally, Duffy, in *The Healers* notes that in Louisiana, all cesarian section procedures of the antebellum South were performed on enslaved African women (Duffy 1979, 141–143). Duffy concludes that medical risk and social status influenced antebellum physicians decision to perform new surgical procedures upon enslaved African women (Duffy 1979, 142).

In the area of African American bio-historical research and historical archeology several scholars have provided evidence regarding the relationship between medical health and occupational status. For example Jennifer Kelley and J. Lawrence Angel, using the research sites of Maryland, Virginia and the Carolinas, presents the "Life Stresses" concept whereby external forces (enslavement) and internal forces (physiological) combine to determine the age of the African at death. They note the differences between urban and rural enslaved Africans and how these venues determine life stresses (Kelley and Angel 1987, 199–211). Furthermore, Douglas Owsley (et al.) in "Demography and Pathology of an Urban Slave Population," concludes that urban Africans in New Orleans led a better lifestyle, probably due to the dependence upon Africans to perform in domestic occupations (Owsley et al. 1987, 185–197). Finally, in the area of historical archeology, analysis of historic sites confirms the various environments in which enslaved Africans labored as in the case of *Elmwood: The Historic Archeology of a Southeastern Louisiana Plantation* (Goodwin et al. 1984, 44–51). John Otto and Augustus Burns in "Black Folks and Poor Buckras, Archeological Evidence of Slave and Overseer Living Conditions on an Antebellum Plantation" excavated from plantation sites physical evidence regarding the medicines used by enslaved Africans and overseers (Otto and Burns 1983, 192–193, 195).

Racist assumptions which pervade some Eurocentric scholarship operate from the premise that the various people brought from the African continent (and their descendants), were no longer African after reaching the shores of the Caribbean and North and South America. Ulrich B. Phillips championed the school of thought that Africans were savages who ceased being African (but retained their savagery) once having been taken from Africa; that they became a new breed of person they called Negroes. Phillips states:

Slavery and Medicine: Enslavement and Medical Practices in Antebellum Louisiana

> These negroes when brought in from Africa were heathen savages accustomed only to precarious tribal existence in the jungles. To be fitted for life in civilized, Christian, industrial society, they had to be drilled, educated in a measure, and controlled (Phillips 1968, 26).

Stanley M. Elkins in *Slavery a Problem in American Institutional and Intellectual Life* addressed the "African culture argument." Elkins also attempted to give currency to the concept of the culturally alienated African. According to Elkins there is a:

> ... vast gulf between African culture and Negro life in North America...the gulf between Africa and America is even wider than we imagined. We can suppose that the pseudo-anthropologists of the early 1900's must have begun, in their reasoning, not with Africa but with the depressed state of Negro existence in this country. They were thus prepared a priori, in their efforts to make connections, to find something comparable in the original tribal state. They were most sensitized, in short, not to sophistication or complexity, but rather to crudity, depravity, and primitivism (Elkins 1959, 92).

And then Elkins concludes: "Something very profound, therefore, would have had to intervene in order to obliterate all this and to produce, on the American plantation, a society of helpless dependents" (Elkins 1959, 98). In his survey of plantation society Phillips echoes Elkins' thesis regarding the supposed insignificance of the cultural retentions among transplanted Africans. Phillips presented his ideas on "the American negro" in this way:

> While produced only in America, the plantation slave was a product of old-world forces. His nature was an African's profoundly modified but hardly transformed by the requirements of European civilization. The wrench from Africa and the subjection to the new discipline while uprooting his ancient language and customs had little more effect upon his temperament than upon his complexion. Ceasing to be Foulah,

SLAVERY AND MEDICINE: ENSLAVEMENT AND MEDICAL PRACTICES IN
ANTEBELLUM LOUISIANA

> Coromantee, Ebo or Angola, he became instead the American negro. The Caucasian was also changed by the contact in a far from negligible degree; but the negro's conversation was much the more thorough, partly because the process in his case was coercive, partly because his genius was imitative (Phillips 1966, 291).

This "negro" illusion, as Asante describes it, is important in understanding why, for example, the African materia medica has not been seriously considered (Asante 1990, 132–135) in the scholarship on enslavement and medicine.

Eurocentric discussions regarding the African's participation in his/her medical health are categorized as either magico-religious (Voodoo) or folk herbalism. The African is rarely seen as a proactive participant in or a progenitor of his own medical care issues. "Negro Folklorists" have written extensively about African religious beliefs with reference to the antebellum South. Research similar to Louis Pendleton's "Notes on Negro Folk-Lore and Witchcraft in the South," discuss Africana concepts regarding myth, nature, nommo and conjuring as the cultural manifestations of "savage tribes" (Pendleton 1890, 201–207). Some contemporary scholars have also made attempts to raise the issue of African medicine in north America. Albert Raboteau in *Slave Religion: The "Invisible Institution" in the Antebellum South* posits an African worldview involving spirituality, conjuring and herbalism. He notes that west African "magic" was important to enslaved Africans with conjuring being the African's traditional form of "magic" (Raboteau 1978, 275–288). Juliane Crete' in *Daily Life in Louisiana 1815–1830* provides some information, under the magico-religious category, regarding African materia medica (Crete' 1978, 159–179). There are scholars who have discussed African "conjurers" during the antebellum period and suggest that they exercised some power over the institution of enslavement (Gorn 1989, 295–326). Wilbur Watson, editor of *Black Folk Medicine* discusses the relationship between African beliefs, medical treatments and the African based religious/spiritual structures of Voodoo, Shango, Santeria, and Curandero (Watson 1984, 1–11; 24–27) in the Americas.

Afrocentric scholarship which seeks to initiate a discourse on the continental African's legacy in the medical field include Frederick

SLAVERY AND MEDICINE: ENSLAVEMENT AND MEDICAL PRACTICES IN ANTEBELLUM LOUISIANA

Newsome's "Black Contributions to the early History of Western Medicine," and Charles S. Finch's *The African Background to Medical Science*. Newsome asserts that the Africans of the Nile Valley provided the medical precedent for the western foundations of medical science. Newsome challenges contemporary scholarship's need to address African contributions to the medical field (Newsome 1986, 127–139). Finch also postulates a Nile Valley (Kemetic) origin of medical science, predating the Hippocratic model, and details the various medical traditions contained on the continent of Africa. According to Finch:

> . . . the traditional doctors of Africa from the earliest times had a high level of medical and surgical skill, certainly much more than they have been given credit for. It is to be hoped that more substantive and careful investigations will be carried out among the traditional healers of Africa before Western-style medicine supplants them entirely (Finch 1990, 140).

Molefi Kete Asante notes that "in traditional African societies medicine, ethics, and rhetoric are connected." This is an extension of the Nile Valley Ma'atic concepts of justice, truth, harmony, etc. (Karenga and Carruthers 1986, 19–20). Among the diversity of continental Africans are similar notions of Ma'at; and many African ethnicities share this ancient, traditional concept outside of the African continent into the African diaspora (Asante 1990, 83). Another author, Janheinz Jahn addressed the issue of African medicine in his work *Muntu, African Culture and the Western World*. Jahn asserts that western European medical ideas clashed with indigenous African concepts largely because Europeans could not accept the Africans holistic (mind-body-spirit) approach to curing ailments and disease (Jahn 1989, 127–132). Despite this, Gwendolyn Midlo-Hall in *Africans in Colonial Louisiana* notes that "Slaves were commonly used as medical doctors and surgeons. . . ." in antebellum Louisiana (Midlo-Hall 1993, 126). Midlo-Hall also examines African religious beliefs including charms, superstitions and sorcery (Midlo-Hall 1993, 162–165). Beverly J. Robinson in "Africanisms and the Study of Folklore," commented on the African worldview regarding medical healing and the art of healing itself. Johnson also noted that the African view of "medicine" involved both body and mind treatment (Robinson 1990, 211–224). Martha Graham Goodson asserted that enslaved Africans left a legacy of curative plants to the medical practices of the old South and that enslaved African women

SLAVERY AND MEDICINE: ENSLAVEMENT AND MEDICAL PRACTICES IN ANTEBELLUM LOUISIANA

in particular made important contributions to medical science in general (Goodson 1987, 198–203). According to Ira E. Harrison's "Health Status and Healing Practices: Continuations from an African Past," there were three groups of traditional medical practitioners of Africa (diviners, dispensers and midwives) who were retained as important medical caregivers by enslaved Africans in the diaspora (Harrison 1975–76, 547–560). Marimba Ani in her discourse on nommo posits that nommo, as a significant African retention in the diaspora, was important to (and during), the institution of enslavement. According to Ani nommo "is the street call of the vendor in New Orleans. Nommo is the "mumbo-jumbo" of the conjure-man. His incantation calls forth spirits to perform 'magic.' The Rootman uses the power of Nommo to energize the herbs, roots, and potions he prescribes so that they will heal" (Ani 1980, 40). Asante posits that nommo is "the generative and productive power of the spoken word" (Asante 1980, 17) acknowledging the traditional Africans use of the spoken word in the holistic healing of the human being. Like Asante, Ani's scholarship also affirms the mind-body-spirit nature of traditional Africana medicine. Their work demonstrates how the cultural phenomena of healing is a major feature of the African cultural continuum; and how the African materia medica manifested itself in the Black diaspora.

APPENDICES

APPENDIX A

A LIST OF RELATED RISK FACTORS TO MEDICAL HEALTH AMONG ENSLAVED AFRICANS OF SOUTHEASTERN LOUISIANA

CAPTURE
Chains
Disease
Brutality

MAAFA
Chains
Sanitation
Disease
Brutality
Rape

SEASONING
Acclimation
Disease
Brutality
Labor

LABOR
Disease
Brutality
Diet/Nutrition
Clothing
Housing
Hygiene
Injury
Hours/Intensity
Environmental

BREEDING
Pregnancy
Difficult Births
Abortion
Gestation and Intensive Labor

PREGNANCY
Frequent Births
Abortion
Gestation and Intensive Labor

BIRTH
Abortion
Post-Partum Complications
Multiple Births

RAPE
Pregnancy
Gestation and Labor
Gestation and Brutality
Abortion
Psychological Impact

DIET/NUTRITION
Vitamin Deficiencies
Malnutrition
Food/Water Contamination

CLOTHING
Inadequate clothes/shoes

MEDICAL TREATMENT/ EXPERIMENTAL PROCEDURES
Painful procedures
Recovery risks

DISEASE/ILLNESS
Contagions

INJURY
Labor injuries
Labor intensity
Labor hours
Punishment
Breeding
Rape

SLAVERY AND MEDICINE: ENSLAVEMENT AND MEDICAL PRACTICES IN ANTEBELLUM LOUISIANA

ENVIRONMENTAL
Disease
Acclimation
Housing
Labor

PUNISHMENT
Containment
Devices
Whipping
Mutilation
Branding
Infections
Psychological Impact

APPENDIX B

ADMISSION BOOK OF THE TOURO INFIRMARY 1855–1860, ENSLAVED AFRICANS[1]

Entry Format:
No.[Patient Number]—Name/Place of Birth/Occupation/Last Place From/Residence in New Orleans/Date of Admission/Hour of Admission/Date of Discharge/Date of Death/Age/Whose Account/Deposit/Rate Per Day/Malady/How Long Sick/Single or Married/No. of Ward/Total No. of Days/Amount/Remarks[2]

Key:
NA = Date of Death Not Applicable
NL = Not Listed in the Admission Book of the Touro Infirmary
NR = No Remarks

1855

12—Alfred/Virginia/Slave/NL/Born in New Orleans/Jan 9/10AM/March 23/NA/28/Mr. M.C. Quick/NL/$1.00/ Dysentery/2 Weeks/Single/NL/73 Days/$73.00/NR

27—Jane Lankerser/Maryland/Slave/New Orleans/2 Months/February 2/10AM/March 5/NA/18/George

---

[1]The Admission Book records patients from 1855 through 1860. After 1859 slaves were not listed, only individuals listed as servants, without racial designation. These are not included among the listing of enslaved Africans. Thus, this transcription of the Admission Book of the Touro Infirmary reflects enslaved Africans through 1859.

[2][Only five deposits (out of 680 cases) were listed for enslaved Africans in the "Deposit" category; an asterisk "*" notes the date of death recorded by the Infirmary; the "Rate Per Day" for enslaved Africans was consistently $1.00, except in the cases of patients 549, 552, 649, 650 and 657 which were $2.00; and patient 666 which was $3.00. The Admission Book does not indicate the admittance of free Africans or the gens de la coleur libre.]

SLAVERY AND MEDICINE: ENSLAVEMENT AND MEDICAL PRACTICES IN ANTEBELLUM LOUISIANA

Davis/NL/$1.00/Syphilis/ NL/Single/ NL/31/ 31.00/Paid
28—David/South Carolina/Slave/New Orleans/2 Years/February 2/9 AM/March 1/NA/26/Wm. H. Paxton/NL/$1.00/Typhoid Pneumonia/8 Days/Single/NL/26/$26.00/Paid/NR
29—Bill/Florida/Slave/New Orleans/NL/ February 5/4 PM/March 11/NA/28/Haskell /NL/$1.00/Secondary Syphilis/5 Months/Single /NL/6 Days/$6.00/Paid
30—Choice/Georgia/Slave/New Orleans/NL/February 5/4 PM/ March NL/NA/30/Pendegrast/NL/$1.00/Typhoid Pneumonia/3 Weeks/Single/NL/23 Days/$23.00/Paid
31—Hannah/Louisiana/Slave/New Orleans/NL/February 7/9 AM/ March 7/NA/35/Stadeker/NL/$1.00/Int. Fever/8 Days/Married/ NL/30 Days/$30.00/NR
32—Jerry/Florida/Slave/New Orleans/NL/February 10/NL/ February 19/NA/19/Mrs. Harrell/NL/$1.00/Typhoid Fever/3 Days/Married/NL/9 Days/$9.00/Paid
35—Henrietta/Virginia/Slave/New Orleans/NL/February 15/ 5PM/March 1/NA/15/M. M. Simpson/NL/$1.00/Gonorrhea/NL/ Single/NL/14 Days/$14.00/Paid
36—Louis/Virginia/Slave/New Orleans/4 Years/February 16/9AM/March 2/NA/35/Henry Brown/NL/$1.00/Bronchitis/2 Weeks/Married/NL/14 Days/$14.00/Paid
37—Maria/Louisiana/Slave/New Orleans/NL/February 5/NL/March 5/NA/21/Daniel Blocks/NL/$1.00/Prolapsus Uterus/2 Days/ Married/NL/30 Days/$30.00/NR
40—Rosetta/Virginia/Slave/Florida/ NL/February 23/5PM/ March 8/NA/23/G. W. Pinchard/NL/$1.00/Dysmenorrhea/14 Days/ Married/NL/14 Days/ $14.00/Paid
42—Solomon/Not known/Slave/New Orleans/NL/February 26/ 4PM/March 2/NA/31/Hall and Street/NL/$1.00/Catarrh/4 Days/Married/NL/4 Days/$4.00/Paid

47—Erin/NL/Slave/NL/NL/March 9/5PM/April 1/NA/23/R. Condon/NL /$1.00/Typhoid Pneumonia/4 Days/Single/ NL/22 Days/$22.00/NR
51—Mary Ann/NL/Slave/NL/NL/March 27/12AM/May 16/NA/38/J. L. Bein/NL/$1.00/Fracture of Leg/NL/ Married/NL/47 Days/$47.00/ Paid
53—Washington/Virginia/Slave/New Orleans/4 Years/March 30/10AM/April 9/NA/21/ Dominique Madden/NL/ $1.00/ Gastritis/3 Days/Single/NL/11 Days/$1.00/Paid
58—James/Maryland/Slave/New Orleans/NL/April 10/11AM/ April 23/NA/16/W. L. Campbell/NL/ $1.00/Diarrhea/ NL/Single/NL/13 Days/$13.00/Paid
59—Hannah/Maryland/Slave/New Orleans/NL/April 13/10AM /May 19/NA/19/Lionel Levy/NL/$1.00/Prolapsus Uterus/36 Days/ Single/NL/36 Days/$36.00/Paid Surgical Extra $15.00
60—Clara/Virginia/Slave/New Orleans/NL/April 20/11AM/ May 17/NA/40/Mrs. B. Cook/NL/ $1.00/Undetermined /NL/Married/NL/27 Days/$27.00/Paid
64—Daniel Brooks/Virginia/Slave/New Orleans/1 Year/April 24/11AM/May 15/36/H. J. Ranney/NL/$1.00/Puncture Wound/1 Day/NL/NL/21 Days/$21.00/Paid
66—Mary/Louisiana/Slave/New Orleans/3 Days/May 3/10AM/May 12/NA/36/T. J. Casey/NL/$1.00/ Eczema/ NL/Married/NL/10 Days/ $10.00/Paid
68—Richard/NL/Slave/New Orleans/NL/May 1/NL/May 6/NA/22/J. Mitchell/NL /$1.00/Scrotal Hernia/NL/Single /NL/6 Days/$6.00/Paid
69—Choice/Georgia/Slave/New Orleans/1 Year/May 8/NL/June 23/NA/21/Richard Pendergast/NL/$1.00/ Ulcer of Rectum/4 Weeks/Single/NL/46 Days/ $46.00/Paid
73—Andrew/NL/Slave/New Orleans/NL/May 14/2PM/June 12/ NA/35/G. P. Parker/NL/$1.00/Eruption Disease/2 Weeks/NL/NL/ 37 Days/$37.00/Paid

74—Ralph/NL/Slave/New Orleans/1 Year/May 14/2 PM/June 12/NA/40/W. W. Allen/NL/$1.00/Ascites/2 Months/ NL/NL/37 Days/$37.00/Paid
76—Martha/Virginia/Slave/Virginia/2 Months/May 20/10 PM/July 29/NA/22/O.G. Donnella/NL/$1.00/ Hysteria/2 Weeks/Single/NL/70 Days/$70.00/Paid
78—William/Louisiana/Slave/New Orleans/NL/May 22/4PM/May 28/NA/16/John Mitchell/NL/$1.00/ Convulsions/NL/NL/NL/6 Days/$6.00/Paid
81—William/Maryland/Slave/Lake(?)/2 Days/May 24/1PM/June 14/NA/30/Mrs. Weims/NL/$1.00/Typhoid Pneumonia/4 Days/ Single/NL/20 Days/$20.00/Paid
83—Matilda/Maryland/Slave/New Orleans/NL/May 31/7PM/June 13/NA/35/D. Madden/NL/$1.00/ Cholera/2 Weeks/Single/NL/12 Days/$12.00/Paid
86—Melvinia/Maryland/Slave/New Orleans/8 Months/June 6/4PM/July 21/NA/21/W.G. Stevens/NL/$1.00/ Syphilitic Eruptions/2 Weeks/Single/NL/45 Days/$45.00/Paid
88—Anderson/Virginia/Slave/New Orleans/2 Years/June 12/ 10AM/July 18/NA/25/Thomas Finney/NL/$1.00/ Diarrhea/2 Months/Single/NL/6 Days/$6.00/Paid
89—Maria/Louisiana/Slave/New Orleans/NL/June 12/12PM/ September 3/NL/NL/Daniel Blocks/NL/$1.00/ Pregnancy and Prolapsus Uterus/2 Weeks/Married/ NL/83 Days/108.00/$25 for delivery.
90—Leah/Virginia/Slave/New Orleans/NL/June 18/NL/July 6/NA/NL/R. W. Davis/NL/$1.00/Ulceration of Rectum/2 Weeks/Married/NL/18 Days/$18.00/Paid
95—Peter/South Carolina/Slave/New Orleans/9 Months/June 21/NL/July 2/NA/21/John Mitchell/NL/$1.00/Injury of Foot/5 Days/Single/NL/10 Days/$10.00/NR
100—Harriet/Virginia/Slave/New Orleans/4 Years/June 22/ NL/July 18/NA/30/H. T. Lousdale/NL/$1.00/Typhoid Fever/2 Weeks/Single/NL/25 Days/$25.00/Paid

SLAVERY AND MEDICINE: ENSLAVEMENT AND MEDICAL PRACTICES IN ANTEBELLUM LOUISIANA

102—Adam/Kentucky/Slave/New Orleans/5 Months/June 28/ NL/NL/NL/NA/26/B. Kendig/NL/$1.00/Eryrated Tumor with Hernia/6 Years/NL/79 Days/$133.00/Paid Operation $50.
103—Martha/Florida/Slave/New Orleans/3 Weeks/June 30/NL/July 2/NA/19/Post-L Mel/NL/$1.00/ Pregnancy/3 Days/Married/NL/2 Days/$2.00/Paid
112—William Banks/Kentucky/Slave/New Orleans/26 Years/July 12/5PM/July 20/NA/28/Daniel Blocks/NL/$1.00/ Retention of Urine/2 Weeks/Married/NL/8 Days/$8.00/NR
114—Margaret/NL/Slave/New Orleans/NL/July 16/6PM/July 25/NA/24/H. Hassman/NL/$1.00/Prolapsus Uterus/NL/ Single/NL/10 Days/$10.00/Paid
116—Jerry/Virginia/Slave/New Orleans/6 Weeks/July 17/ 4PM/July 21/NA/35/D. Madden/NL/$1.00/ Phlegmanns Abscess/3 Weeks/Single/NL/14 Days/$14.00/Paid
120—Herod/Virginia/Slave/New Orleans/NL/July 22/11AM/ August 1/NA/22/Henry Brown/NL/$1.00/ Dysentery/2 Weeks/Single/NL/10 Days/$10.00/Paid
122—Edmond/Kentucky/Slave/Attakapas/1 Week/July 25/ 3PM/August 20/NA/25/W.G. Stevens/NL/$1.00/ Phycosis/1 Week/Single/NL/26 Days/$36.00/Paid Operation $10.00
123—Harriet/Kentucky/Slave/Attakapas/1 Week/July 25/ 3PM/July 27/NA/20/W.G. Stevens/NL/$1.00/Diarrhea /1 Week/Single/NL/3 Days/$3.00/Paid
128—Mitchell/Virginia/Slave/New Orleans/3 Years/July 26/1PM/July 31/NA/22/D. Madden/NL/$1.00/Yellow Fever/8 Days/Single/NL/5 Days/$5.00/Paid
130—George/Virginia/Slave/New Orleans/3 Months/July 27/2PM/August 13/NA/22/O.J. Donnella/NL/ $1.00/Yellow Fever/20 Hours/Single/NL/17 Days/$17.00/Paid

139—Jimbo/Tennessee/Slave/New Orleans/10 Months/August 2/2 PM/NL/August 15*/24/T. Hassman/NL/$1.00/Gastro Enteritis/2 Weeks/Single/NL/13 Days/$13.00/Paid

153—Ellen/Virginia/Slave/New Orleans/12 Months/August 12/10AM/August 30/NA/14/O. J. Donnella/NL/$1.00/Yellow Fever/12 Hours/Single/NL/19 Days/$19.00/Paid

165—Martha/Missouri/Slave/New Orleans/3 Years/August 17/9 AM/September 18/NA/25/H. J. Ranney/NL/$1.00/Abortion/3 Days/Married/NL/33 Days/$33.00/Paid

166—Harriet/Kentucky/Slave/New Orleans/6 Months/August 17/11AM/August 27/NA/25/Mr. Hogan/NL/$1.00/Yellow Fever/4 Hours/Married/NL/11 Days/$11.00/Paid

177—William/New Orleans/Slave/New Orleans/21 Years/August 24/1PM/September 10/NA/21/Mrs. E. M. Israel/NL/$1.00/ Secondary Syphilis/3 Weeks/Single/NL/18 Days/$18.00/NR

180—Robert/Georgia/Slave/New Orleans/2 Years/August 26/11AM/October 12/NA/26/Mr. Key/NL/$1.00/Injury/10 Days/NL/NL/47 Days/$97.00/Paid Operation $50.00

182—Henry/Virginia/Slave/New Orleans/6 Years/August 27/PM/August 31/NA/33/Mr. Intosh/NL/$1.00/Yellow Fever/6 Hours/Married/NL/5 Days/$5.00/Paid

190—Woodruff/Maryland/Slave/New Orleans/7 Years/August 4/11AM/September 18/NA/19/H. J. Ranney/NL/$1.00/ Fistulous Abscess/2 Days/Single/NL/15 Days/$15.00/Paid

191—John/Alabama/Slave/New Orleans/4 Years/September 8/9AM/September 13/NA/12/R. Condon/NL/$1.00/Yellow Fever/24 Hours/Single/NL/6 Days/$6.00/NR

212—Charles/New Orleans/Slave/New Orleans/22 Years/October 4/1 PM/October 11/NA/22/D. Sidle/

NL/$1.00/Yellow Fever/26 Hours/NL/NL/8 Days/$8.00/Paid

213—Ellen and Child/New Orleans/Slave/New Orleans/21 Years/October 5/11AM/November 21/NA/21/R.M. Davis/NL/ $1.00/Prolapses Vagina/10 Months/Married/NL/48 Days/ $58.00/Paid $10.00 Extra

214—Daniel Young/Kentucky/Slave/Natchez/NL/October 5/12 Noon/NL/NA/36/W. J. Key/NL/$1.00/Injury/3 Hours /Married/NL/NL/ NL/NR

215—William/New Orleans/Slave/New Orleans/21 Years/ October 8/10AM/October 12/NA/21/Mrs. Israel/ NL/$1.00/Constipation/3 Days/Single/NL/5 Days/$5.00/Paid

219—Rose/Louisiana/Slave/NL/NL/October 10/12 Noon/ December 14/NA/10/Harvey/NL/$1.00/Paraplegia /NL/Single/NL/66 Days/ $66.00/Paid

221—John/Maryland/Slave/New Orleans/8 Years/October 15/6 PM/October 28/NA/28/D. Madden/NL/$1.00/ NL/NL/ Married/NL/14 Days/$14.00/Paid

222—Jacob/Louisiana/Slave/New Orleans/25 Years/October 19/6PM/October 20/NA/25/Mr. Key/NL/$1.00/ Gonorrhea/4 Days/Single/NL/2 Days/$2.00/NR

223—Emma/Louisiana/Slave/New Orleans/17 Years/October 20/4 PM/November/NA/17/B. Kendig/NL/$1.00/ Abortion/3 Weeks/ Single/NL/17 Days/$17.00/NR

226—Perry/Tennessee/Slave/New Orleans/18 Months/October 26/1PM/January 3, 1856/NA/30/J. M. Bell/NL/$1.00/ NL/18 Months/Single/NL/NL/$70.00/Paid

230—Peter/Louisiana/Slave/New Orleans/2 Years/November 8/11AM/November 9/NA/23/B. Kendig/NL/ $1.00/Necrosis/5 Months/Single/NL/NL/$2.00/NR

231—Ben/Louisiana/Slave/New Orleans/14 Years/November 8/10 AM/November 21/NA/39/G.M. Pinchard/NL/ $1.00/ NL/NL/3 Months/ NL/Nl/14 Days/$14.00/Paid

235—Lavinia/Louisiana/Slave/New Orleans/18 Years/November 28/12AM/December 13/NA/18/George Jonas/NL/

$1.00/Abortion/1 Day/Married/NL/16 Days/ $16.00/Paid

238—Washington/Maryland/Slave/Louisiana/3 Years/November 29/1PM/December 28/NA/19/Dr. Clark/NL/$1.00/ Dirt-Eating/3 Months/Single/NL/30 Days/$30.00/Paid

239—Sophia/Maryland/Slave/Louisiana/2 Days/November 29/1PM/NL/December 4*/21/Dr. Clark/NL/$1.00/ Anasarca/4 Months/Married/NL/6 Days/$6.00/Paid

240—Joe/New Orleans/Slave/New Orleans/25 Years/December 3/4 PM/December 8/NA/25/D.S. Graham/NL/$1.00/ Catarrh/5 Days/ Married/NL/6 Days/$6.00/Paid

241—Daniel Brooks/Virginia/Slave/New Orleans/1 Year/ December 10/3 PM/December 18/NA/36/H. J. Ranney/NL/$1.00/ Hemorrhoids/4 Days/Married/NL/9 Days/$9.00/Paid

244—Jerry/Virginia/Slave/New Orleans/NL/December 12/ 7PM/December 19/NA/25/D. Madden/NL/$1.00/ Gastrodynia/ 3 Days/Single/NL/8 Days/$8.00/Paid

245—Harry/S. Carolina/Slave/New Orleans/1 Year/December 13/4 PM/December 31/NA/20/John Mitchell/NL/$1.00 /Bubo/1 Day/Single/NL/19 Days/$19.00/NR

247—Ben/Virginia/Slave/New Orleans/15 Years/December 18/5 PM/NL/December 31*/34/G.M. Pinckard/NL/ $1.00 Asthma/6 Months/Single/NL/14 Days/ $14.00/Paid

248—John/Virginia/Slave/New Orleans/32 Years/December 18/ 5PM/December 29/NA/67/G.M. Pinckard/NL/$1.00/ Dysentery/2 Months/Single/NL/12 Days/$12.00/Paid

254—Bill/Maryland/Slave/New Orleans/9 Years/January 5, 1856/8AM/January 7/NA/26/D. Madden/NL/$1.00/ Diarrhea/1 Days/Single/NL/2 Days/$2.00/Paid

255—Henry/Baltimore/Slave/New Orleans/1 Year/January 5/2 PM/February 20/NA/30/W. J. Key/NL/$1.00/Ulcer/2 Weeks/ Single/NL/46 Days/$46.00/NR

1856

256—Toby/Charleston/Slave/New Orleans/1 Year/January 6/10AM/January 23/NA/35/John Mitchell/NL/$1.00/Pleurisy/1 Day/Single/NL/18 Days/$28.00/$10.00 Extra (Certificate) Pleurisy from Injury
262—Jessie/Virginia/Slave/New Orleans/5 Years/January 24/4PM/February 1/NA/28/Capt. Ure/NL/$1.00/Inguinal Hernia/1 Week/Single/NL/7 Days/$7.00/NR
265—Isaac/North Carolina/Slave/New Orleans/14 Years/January 30/11AM/February 10/NA/28/S. Jamison/NL/$1.00/Pleuro-Pneumonia/18 Hours/Single/NL/12 Days/$12.00/Paid
266—George/North Carolina/Slave/New Orleans/8 Years/January 9/7PM/June 2/NA/26/S. Jamison/NL/$1.00/Fracture of Cranium/7 Hours/Single/NL/145 Days/$195.00/$50 Operation Paid
267—Burrell/Virginia/Slave/New Orleans/2 Years/February 1/5PM/March 8/NA/22/W. J. Key/NL/$1.00/Syphilis/1 Week/ Single/NL/36 Days/$36.00/NR
268—George/Alabama/Slave/New Orleans/3 Years/February 3/10AM/February 1/NA/44/T.J. Casey/NL/$1.00/Indurated Fistula/3 Weeks/Single/NL/4 Days/$4.00/Paid
269—Jerry/Maryland/Slave/New Orleans/25 Years/February 6/10AM/February 10/NA/35/J. McIntosh/NL/$1.00/Pleurisy/1 Week/Married/NL/5 Days/$5.00/Paid
270—William/Virginia/Slave/New Orleans/30 Years/February 13/8AM/February 17/NA/60/D. Sidle/NL/$1.00/Injury/3 Days/ Single/NL/5 Days/$5.00/Paid
273—Fleming/Nashville/Slave/Nashville/1 Day/February 17/9AM/Feb. 20/NA/26/Mr. Edgar/NL/$1.00/Psous(?) Abscess/9 Months/Married/NL/4 Days/$4.00/NR
274—Hester/Tennessee/Slave/New Orleans/20 Years/February 18/12 Noon/March 28/NA/40/H. A. Fassman/NL/$1.00/Hysteritis/4 Weeks/Married/NL/40 Days/$40.00/Paid

275—Malinda/NL/Slave/New Orleans/NL/February 19/11 AM/ NL/February 26*/35/Mrs. Felger/NL/$1.00/ Typhoid Fever/NL/ NL/NL/7 Days/$7.00/Paid
276—John/Maryland/Slave/New Orleans/3 Years/February 22/ 10AM/March 1/NA/22/James Calder/NL/$1.00/ Pleurisy/2 Days/ Single/NL/9 Days/$9.00/Paid
281—James/Louisville/Slave/New Orleans/16 Years/March 4/7PM/March 12/NA/32/D. Sidle/NL/$1.00/Injury/1 Day/ Single/NL/9 Days/$9.00/Paid
282—Tom/Virginia/Slave/New Orleans/3 Years/March 5/ 10AM/March 14/NA/45/W. J. Key/NL/$1.00/Injury/6 Days/ Single/NL/10 Days/$10.00/NR
283—Toby/S. Carolina/Slave/New Orleans/26 Years/March 5/4 PM/April 3/NA/45/H. J. Ranney/NL/$1.00/Injury/6 Days/ Single/NL/30 Days/$30.00/Paid
284—Eliza/Tennessee/Slave/Tennessee/1 Day/March 8/5PM/June 14/NA/26/G. W. Cook/NL/$1.00/ Pneumonia/3 Weeks/Single/NL/99 Days/$99.00 Paid
285—Joe Diggs/Maryland/Slave/Maryland/1 Month/March 12/10AM/March 21/NA/24/James Calder/NL/$1.00/ NL/1 Week/ Single/NL/10 Days/$10.00/Paid
286—Bob/Louisiana/Slave/New Orleans/6 Years/March 18/9AM/March 25/NA/22/D. Sidle/NL/$1.00/NL/3 Weeks/ Single/NL/8 Days/$8.00/Paid
288—James/Louisiana/Slave/NL/NL/March 21/5PM/April 26/NA/27/W. P. Poitevent/NL/$1.00/Injury/3 Hours/ Single/NL/57 Days/$57.00/$20.00 Extra for Surgery Paid
303—Bob/Louisiana/Slave/New Orleans/6 Years/March 31/9AM/March 5/NA/22/D. Sidle/NL/$1.00/NL/NL/ Single/NL/6 Days/$6.00/Paid
307—Stephen/Washington/Slave/New Orleans/6 Years/April 3/5PM/April 16/NA/25/Brown/NL/$1.00/Injury/1 Day/Single/ NL/14 Days/$14.00/Paid
308—Frank/Louisville/Slave/New Orleans/4 Years/April 8/10AM/April 11/NA/33/McKelvery Agent/NL/$1.00/ Syphilis/2 Months/Single/NL/NL/NL/NR

309—Henry/Louisiana/Slave/New Orleans/10 Years/April 8/10 AM/April 20/NA/15/A. Marks/NL/$1.00/Injury/NL/Single/NL/13 Days/$13.00/Paid

311—Priscilla/Virginia/Slave/New Orleans/7 Years/April 9/9AM/May 19/NA/30/J. Davis/NL/$1.00/Pneumonia/1 Day/Single/NL/41 Days/$41.00/Paid

312—Daniel/Alabama/Slave/New Orleans/2 Months/April 15/NL/April 28/NA/15/Thomas A. Glass/$100.00/$1.00/NL/5 Years/Single/NL/14 Days/$49.00/$35 Extra for surgery Paid

313—Philis/Alabama/Slave/New Orleans/2 Months/April 15/NL/May 26/NA/35/Thomas A. Glassman/NL/$1.00/ Scrofulous Tumor/9 Months/Married/NL/42 Days/$94.50/Extra for Surgery Paid

314—Georgiana/Mississippi/Slave/New Orleans/6 Months/April 18/4 PM/May 23/NA/26/Mrs. Bustamente/NL/$1.00/Histeria/2 Years/Single/NL/36 Days/$36.00/Paid

317—Robert/S. Carolina/Slave/New Orleans/13 Years/April 23/10AM/July 10/NA/40/George Purvis/NL/$1.00/Fistula on Arm/10 Days/Married/NL/69 Days/119.00/Paid

318—Jerry/Virginia/Slave/New Orleans/4 Months/April 24/2 PM/April 28/NA/25/D. Madden/NL/$1.00/Diarrhea/NL/Single/NL/5 Days/$5.00/Paid

320—Mary Ann/N. Carolina/Slave/New Orleans/1 Year/April 28/3 PM/NL/May 29*/27/Bernard/NL/$1.00/Phthisis/2 Years /Single/NL/82 Day/$212.00/Burial Paid

321—Joe Diggs/Maryland/Slave/New Orleans/2 Months/April 30/7AM/May 12/NA/24/James Calder/NL/$1.00/Diarrhea/ NL/ Single/NL/13 Days/$13.00/Paid

322—Frank Johnson/Virginia/Slave/New Orleans/29 Years/May 2/4PM/May 14/NA/30/J. McIntosh/NL/$1.00/Pneumonia/3 Weeks/ Single/NL/13 Days/$13.00/Paid

324—John Dorsen/Maryland/Slave/New Orleans/5 Months/May 4/2 PM/May 10/NA/21/John Calder/NL/$1.00/Injury/14 Hours/Single /NL/7 Days/$7.00/Paid

SLAVERY AND MEDICINE: ENSLAVEMENT AND MEDICAL PRACTICES IN ANTEBELLUM LOUISIANA

325—Harriett/Louisiana/Slave/New Orleans/NL/May 6/11AM/July 19/NA/19/G. H. Lyons/NL/$1.00/Burn /4 Days/Married/NL/75 Days/$75.00/NR
329—Andrew Henderson/New Orleans/Slave/New Orleans/20 Years/May 20/10AM/June 25/NA/20/G. Anjele Blass/NL/$1.00 /Syphilis/16 Days/Single/NL/35 Days/$35.00/Paid
333—Bob/Louisiana/Slave/New Orleans/15 Years/May 26/ 11AM/June 3/NA/15/D. O. Sullivan/NL/$1.00/Gen. Debility/3 Weeks/Single/NL/9 Days/$9.00/Paid
335—William/Mississippi/Slave/New Orleans/2 Weeks/May 27/9AM/June 4/NA/18/B. Kendig/NL/$1.00/ Pleurisy/3 Days/ Single/NL/9 Days/$9.00/Paid
336—Jack/New Orleans/Slave/New Orleans/NL/May 27/6PM/July 5/NA/20/H. J. Ranney/NL/$1.00/ Injury/1 Day/Single/NL/40 Days/$40.00/Paid
337—Henderson/Tennessee/Slave/New Orleans/5 Weeks/May 28/6PM/June 16/NA/18/B. Kendig/NL/$1.00/ Anemia/7 Days/ Single/NL/20 Days/$20.00/Paid
338—Tom/Alabama/Slave/New Orleans/5 Weeks/May 28/6PM/June 9/NA/17/B. Kendig/NL/$1.00/ Diarrhea/3 Days/Single/NL/12 Days/$12.00/Paid
339—Mathilda/Maryland/Slave/New Orleans/10 Years/May 29/6AM/June 8/NA/25/D. Madden/NL/$1.00/ Hysteria/1 Day/ Single/NL/11 Days/$11.00/Paid
342—Maria Levy/S. Carolina/Slave/New Orleans/4 Years/May 30/11AM/June 15/NA/9/L. Levy/NL/$1.00/ Blenorrhagia/1 Day /Single/NL/17 Days/$17.00/Paid
343—Ann Maria/Tennessee/Slave/New Orleans/3 Years/May 30/6PM/June 8/NA/27/J. Cohen/NL/$1.00/ Amenorrhea/2 Months/ Married/NL/10 Days/ $10.00/Paid
344—Fred/S. Carolina/Slave/Tennessee/6 Weeks/May 31/ 10AM/June 9/NA/16/T. J. Pipkin/NL/$1.00/Diarrhea /3 Days/ Single/NL/10 Days/$10.00/Paid

347—Henry/Arkansas/Slave/New Orleans/5 Weeks/June 1/ 9AM/June 9/NA/30/B. Kendig/NL/$1.00/Diarrhea/4 Weeks/ Single/NL/9 Days/$9.00/Paid
349—George/Tennessee/Slave/New Orleans/12 Years/June 7/ 11AM/NL/June 7*/32/Bell and Boyd/NL/$1.00/Injury /12 Hours/ Single/NL/NL/$5.00/Paid
350—Henry/Arkansas/Slave/New Orleans/6 Weeks/June 10/ 8PM/June 22/NA/30/B. Kendig/NL/$1.00/Diarrhea/ NL/Single/ NL/13 Days/$13.00/Paid
351—Louis/Virginia/Slave/New Orleans/38 Years/June 8/12 Noon/NL/NA/48/Knapp/NL/$1.00/Hemiplegia/3 Years/Single/ NL/NL/NL/NR
352—Alley/Georgia/Slave/New Orleans/1 Day/June 14/6PM/ NL/June 20*/15/B. Kendig/NL/$1.00/Phthisis/3 Months/Single/ NL/7 Days/$7.00/NR
354—Nelson/NL/Slave/New Orleans/NL/June 18/5PM/NL/ June 18*/48/Belleville Iron Works/NL/$1.00/ Injury/NL/NL/NL/ NL/$5.00/NR
355—Lydia Ann/Kentucky/Slave/Kentucky/5 Months/June 19/ 10AM/August 14/NA/22/B. Kendig/NL/$1.00/ Hysteria/6 Months/ Married/NL/47 Days/$470.00/NR
356—Eliza/Mississippi/Slave/Natchez/4 Months/June 19/ 10AM/June 28/NA/29/B. Kendig/NL/$1.00/ Amenorrhea/1 Year/ Married/NL/10 Days/$10.00/Paid
358—Carter/Virginia/Slave/New Orleans/7 Years/June 25/ 9AM/July 12/NA/NL/McIntosh/NL/$1.00/Pleuro-Pneumonia/14 Days/Married/NL/18 Days/$18.00/Paid
359—Aaron/Alabama/Slave/New Orleans/2 Years/June 26/NL/June 30/NA/14/R. Condon/NL/$1.00/Diarrhea /2 Days/Single/NL/5 Days/$5.00/NR
360—Lawery/Missouri/Slave/Missouri/14 Days/June 28/10AM/ July 19/NA/26/Horrell Gayle and Co./NL/$1.00/ Cholera/12 Days/Single/NL/22 Days/$22.00/Paid
362—Rachael/Florida/Slave/New Orleans/4 Years/July 2/ 4PM/July ?/NA/24/B. Kendig/NL/$1.00/Pregnancy/8 Months/ Married/NL/53 Days/$78.00/Paid $25.00 Extra

SLAVERY AND MEDICINE: ENSLAVEMENT AND MEDICAL PRACTICES IN ANTEBELLUM LOUISIANA

365—Daniel Brooks/N. Carolina/Slave/New Orleans/13 Years/July 7/10AM/July 11/NA/50/H. J. Ranney/NL/ $1.00/ Diarrhea/1 Day/Married/NL/5.00/$5.00/NR

367—Charles/Louisiana/Slave/New Orleans/1 Year/July 10/ 10AM/NL/NA/18/J. P. Abrams/NL/$1.00/Phthisis/3 Months/ Single/NL/29 Days/$41.00/Paid $12.00 Extra

368—Washington/Virginia/Slave/New Orleans/5 Years/July 11/8AM/July 14/NA/21/D. Madden/NL/$1.00/Int. Fever/6 Days/Single/NL/4 Days/$4.00/Paid

369—Alfred/Georgia/Slave/New Orleans/10 Weeks/July 11/ 1PM/July 23/NA/24/B. Kendig/NL/$1.00/Diarrhea/5 Days/ Single/NL/13 Days/$13.00/Paid

370—Eliza/Virginia/Slave/New Orleans/2 Months/July 11/ 6PM/NL/NA/NL/B. Kendig/NL/$1.00/Amenorrhea/4 Weeks/ Single/NL/44 Days/$44.00/Paid

371—Ann Eliza/Mississippi/Slave/New Orleans/NL/July 12/ 11AM/NL/NA/NL/B. Kendig/NL/$1.00/Ascites/2 Months/ Single/NL/26 Days/$26.00/Paid

372—Aleck/Tennessee/Slave/New Orleans/14 Years/July 15/ 11AM/July 21/NA/27/M. Carson and Patterson/NL/ $1.00/Fever/3 Days/Married/NL/7 Days/$7.00/Paid

373—Dennis/Maryland/Slave/New Orleans/10 Years/July 16/ 8AM/NL/NA/30/D. Donnovan/NL/$1.00/Dysentery/ 5 Weeks/ Married/NL/10 Days/$10.00/Paid

375—Reuben/Kentucky/Slave/New Orleans/6 Years/July 20/ 5PM/NL/NA/26/Capt. Ure/NL/$1.00/Injury/2 Hours/Single/NL/31 Days/$56.00/$25 Extra

376—Bob/Louisiana/Slave/New Orleans/15 Years/July 21/ 9AM/July 24/NA/15/D. O. D. Sullivan/NL/$1.00/ Debility/ NL/Single/NL/4 Days/$4.00/Paid

377—Bob/New Orleans/Slave/New Orleans/21 Years/July 21/ 10AM/NL/NA/21/Stevenson & Co./NL/$1.00/ Gonorrhea/7 Weeks/ Single/NL/36 Days/$36.00/Paid

378—Lafayette/Kentucky/Slave/New Orleans/4 Months/July 21/1 PM/NL/NA/28/B. Kendig/NL/$1.00/ Dysentery/8 Days/Single/NL/15 Days/$15.00/Paid

SLAVERY AND MEDICINE: ENSLAVEMENT AND MEDICAL PRACTICES IN
ANTEBELLUM LOUISIANA

379—Jim Porter/Virginia/Slave/New Orleans/14 Years/July
24/6PM/July 25/NA/44/Dubois and Mish/NL/$1.00/
Cholera Morbus/1 Day/Married/NL/5 Days/$5.00/Paid
380—Bob/Louisiana/Slave/New Orleans/15 Years/July 28/
10AM/NL/NA/28/S. J. Pipkin/NL/$1.00/Injury/1
Day/ Single/NL/22 Days/$32.00/Paid $10.00 Extra
381—Amistead/Louisiana/Slave/New Orleans/5 Years/July
28/4PM/NL/NA/26/J. M. Ure/NL/$1.00/Tonsillitis/3
Weeks/ Single/NL/17 Days/$17.00/NR
382—Abraham/Virginia/Slave/New Orleans/5 Months/July 29/
11AM/NL/NA/25/G. M. Pinchard/NL/$1.00/General
Debility/2 Months/Single/NL/60 Days/$60.00/Paid
383—John Shotman/Virginia/Slave/Bayou Sara/15 Years/July
31/10AM/NL/NA/23/J. H. Ure/NL/$1.00/Injury/36
Hours/ Single/NL/37 Days/$62.00/$21.00 Extra
384—Fanny/Virginia/Slave/Bayou Sara/16 Years/July 31/12
Noon/NL/NA/22/Ricketts/NL/$1.00/Gastritis/6
Days/Married/ NL/17 Days/$17.00/Paid
385—Alexander/Virginia/Slave/Bayou Sara/13 Years/July 31/3
PM/NL/NA/29/McCann & Patterson/NL/$1.00/
Dysentery/2 Weeks/ Married/NL/5 Days/$5.00/Paid
386—George Johnson/Maryland/Slave/Bayou Sara/11 Years/
August 1/8AM/NL/NA/35/Dennis Donnovan/NL/
$1.00/NL/3 Weeks/ Married/NL/18 Days/$18.00/Paid
387—Lewis Davis/Virginia/Slave/Bayou Sara/11 Years/August
1/9AM/NL/NA/37/Dennis Donnovan/NL/
$1.00/NL/NL/Married/NL/4 Days/$4.00/Paid
389—(St. ?) John/New Orleans/Slave/New Orleans/40 Years/
August 4/2PM/NL/NA/40/S. J. Pipkin/NL/$1.00/
Injury/4 Hours/ Married/NL/4 Days/$4.00/Paid
390—Wolford/Maryland/Slave/New Orleans/8 Years/August 5/
9AM/NL/NA/42/H. J. Ranney/NL/$1.00/
Dysentery/1 Day/Married/ NL/11 Days/$11.00/NR
392—Oliver/Texas/Slave/Texas/4 Days/August
6/10AM/NL/NA/ 22/B. Kendig/NL/$1.00/

Dislocation of Thumb/3 Weeks/Single/ NL/25 Days/$25.00/Paid
394—Anderson/Tennessee/Slave/New Orleans/5 Years/August 7/10AM/NL/NA/30/T. J. Pipkin/NL/$1.00/ Diarrhea/3 Months/ Single/NL/12 Days/$12.00/Paid
396—Thomas/Virginia/Slave/New Orleans/3 Years/August 9/3PM/NL/NA/24/T. J. Pipkin/NL/$1.00/ Gonorrhea/1 Month/ Single/NL/2 Days/$2.00/Paid
399—John/Virginia/Slave/New Orleans/7 Years/August 11/ 3PM/August 17/NA/26/T. J. Pipkin/NL/$1.00/NL/8 Days/ Single/NL/7 Days/$7.00/Paid
400—Lafayette/Kentucky/Slave/New Orleans/4 Months/August 11/4PM/NL/August 25*/28/B. Kendig//$1.00/ Typhoid Fever/8 Days/Single/NL/15 Days/$27.00/ Paid/Burial $12.00
404—Maria/Tennessee/Slave/New Orleans/NL/August 21/ 10AM/September 8/NA/9/L. Levy/NL/$1.00/ Blenorrhagia/2 Days/Single/NL/19 Days/$19.00/Paid
405—Henry/Maryland/Slave/New Orleans/4 Years/August 21/4PM/August 27/NA/30/T. J. Pipkin/NL/$1.00/ Pleurisy/1 Day/Single/NL/7 Days/$7.00/Paid
407—William/Virginia/Slave/New Orleans/NL/August 23/1 PM/October 9/NA/29/D. Sidle/NL/$1.00/Injury/2 Hours/ Married/NL/48 Days/$145.00/Paid/$100.00 Extra
408—Anne/Virginia/Slave/New Orleans/22 Years/August 25/11 AM/August 31/NA/40/R. Tisdale/NL/$1.00/ Hysteria/3 Months/ Married/NL/7 Days/$7.00/Paid
409—William/S. Carolina/Slave/New Orleans/3 Months/August 25/4PM/August 30/NA/27/B. Kendig/NL/$1.00/ Fever/10 Days/ Single/NL/6 Days/$6.00/Paid
411—George/Virginia/Slave/New Orleans/15 Years/August 26/10 AM/November 10/NA/28/M. Finch/NL/$1.00 /Fracture Patilla/1 Hour/Married/NL/77 Days/ $127.00/Paid $50.00 Extra

412—Jerry/Georgia/Slave/New Orleans/8 Months/August 27/3 PM/August 30/NA/23/D. Madden/NL/$1.00/ Diarrhea/14 Days/ Single/NL/4 Days/$4.00/Paid
413—[Skipped Number in the Record]
414—Anne/N. Carolina/Slave/New Orleans/15 Years/August 27/1 PM/September 29/NA/57/John Blenderman/ NL/$1.00/ Dropsy/3 Months/Married/NL/33 Days/$32.50/Paid
416—Mary/Virginia/Slave/New Orleans/2 Months/August 30/10 AM/September 16/NA/34/B. Kendig/NL/$1.00/ B. R. Fever/15 Days/Married/NL/18 Days/$18.00/Paid
417—Pennington/Texas/Slave/New Orleans/7 Months/August 31/11 AM/September 8/NA/19/Henderson, Terry/NL/ $1.00/ Intermit Fever/7 Days/Married/NL/9 Days/ $9.00/Paid
418—Jack William/N.Carolina/Slave/New Orleans/9 Months/ August 31/11 AM/NL/September 4*/36/James Calder/ NL/ $1.00/Typhoid Fever/8 Days/Single/NL/5 Days/ $5.00/Paid
419—Eva/New Orleans/Slave/New Orleans/15 Years/ September 1/2 PM/November 12/NA/15/D. Edwards/NL/$1.00/Syphilis/4 Weeks/Single/NL/73 Days/$73.00/Paid
420—Charles/Kentucky/Slave/New Orleans/6 Months/ September 1/11 AM/September 8/NA/30/B. Kendig/NL/$1.00/Pneumonia/8 Days/Single/NL/8 Days/$8.00/Paid
421—Levy/Maryland/Slave/New Orleans/2 Years/September 2/10 AM/September 20/NA/50/T. J. Casey/NL/$1.00/ Injury/12 Months/ Married/NL/19 Days/$19.00/Paid
422—Jack/Kentucky/Slave/New Orleans/4 Years/September 3/2 PM/September 6/NA/16/T. J. Casey/NL/$1.00/Injury/ 1 Day/ Single/NL/4.00/$4.00/Paid
423—Louis Davis/Virginia/Slave/New Orleans/11 Years/ September 4/4 PM/September 12/NA/37/D.

SLAVERY AND MEDICINE: ENSLAVEMENT AND MEDICAL PRACTICES IN ANTEBELLUM LOUISIANA

Donnovan/NL/ $1.00/Dysentery/NL/NL/NL/10 Days/$10.00 Paid

425—Billy/Virginia/Slave/New Orleans/35 Years/September 6/8 AM/September 9/NA/62/H. J. Ranney/NL/$1.00/ Pleurisy/1 Day/ Married/NL/4 Days/$4.00/Paid

426—Emanuel/Maryland/Slave/New Orleans/10 Years/September 6/11 AM/September 15/NA/24/H. J. Ranney/NL/$1.00/Diarrhea/12 Hours/Single/NL/4 Days/$4.00/Paid

427—Joseph/New Orleans/Slave/New Orleans/18 Years/ September 6/12 AM/September 9/NA/18/B. Kendig/ NL/$1.00/Intermittent Fever/1 Day/Single/NL/4 Days/$4.00/Paid

428—Martha/Mississippi/Slave/New Orleans/5 Years/September 7/4 PM/September 23/NA/26/H. J. Ranney/NL/$1.00/ Abortion/1 Day/Married/NL/17 Days/$17.00/Paid

429—William/Virginia/Slave/New Orleans/5 Years/September 8/1 PM/September 11/NA/25/Pipkin/NL/ $1.00/ Diarrhea/1 Day/ Single/NL/4 Days/$4.00/Paid

430—Henry/Virginia/Slave/New Orleans/22 Years/September 10/10 AM/September 12/NA/43/R. Condon/NL/ $1.00/Constipation /1 Day/Married/NL/2 Days/ $2.00/NR

431—Hyman/Virginia/Slave/New Orleans/8 Years/September 13/2 PM/September 28/NA/30/Belleville Iron Works/ NL/$1.00/ Rheumatism/1 Week/Married/NL/16 Days/$16.00/Paid

432—Bob/Louisiana/Slave/New Orleans/28 Years/September 17/ 11AM/September 21/NA/35/T. J. Pipkin/NL/ $1.00/Remit. Fever/4 Days/Single/NL/5 Days/ $5.00/Paid

436—Henry/Virginia/Slave/New Orleans/3 Years/September 19/ 10 AM/September 26/NA/25/Luther Holmes/NL/ $1.00/Diarrhea/2 Days/Single/NL/8 Days/$8.00/Paid

437—John/Maryland/Slave/New Orleans/9 Years/September 22/2 PM/September 27/NA/25/D. Madden/NL/$1.00/ Injury/5 Days/ Married/NL/6 Days/$6.00/Paid

438—Billy/Virginia/Slave/New Orleans/35 Years/September 22/ 2 PM/September 29/NA/62/H. J. Ranney/NL/$1.00/ Pleurisy/1 Day /Married/NL/8 Days/$8.00/Paid

439—Eliza/New Orleans/Slave/New Orleans/21 Years/ September 24/1 PM/October 17/NA/21/H. J. Ranney/NL/$1.00/Rheumatism/4 Days/Single/NL/24 Days/$24.00/Paid

440—Peter/Virginia/Slave/New Orleans/1 Day/September 24/10 AM/September 26/NA/42/Cuddy, Brown & Co./NL/$1.00/Cataract/3 Weeks/Married/NL/3 Days/$3.00/Paid

442—Jack Leroy/N. Carolina/Slave/New Orleans/14 Years/ September 25/11 AM/September 29/NA/58/H. J. Ranney/NL/ $1.00/Cholic/1 Day/Single/NL/5 Days/$5.00/Paid

444—Jim/New Orleans/Slave/New Orleans/6 Years/September 26/10AM/September 29/NA/20/H. J. Ranney/NL/ $1.00/Remit. Fever/2 Days/Single/NL/4 Days/ $4.00/Paid

445—Bob/Louisiana/Slave/New Orleans/15 Years/September 26/ 4PM/October 17/NA/21/Stevenson & Co./NL/ $1.00/Cystitis/2 Weeks/Single/NL/22 Days/$22.00/Paid

446—Toby/Virginia/Slave/New Orleans/8 Years/September 29/ 3PM/October 2/NA/24/H. J. Ranney/NL/$1.00/ Constipation/4 Days/Single/NL/4 Days/$4.00/Paid

447—Rachael/Louisiana/Slave/New Orleans/NL/September 9/ 11AM/September 30/NA/44/P. H. Morgan/NL/$1.00/ Injury/1 Day/ Single/NL/21 Days/$21.00/Paid

448—Zaccharia/Virginia/Slave/New Orleans/NL/October 14/11AM/October 7/NA/51/H. J. Ranney/NL/$1.00/ Rheumatism/3 Days/Single/NL/7 Days/$7.00/Paid

450—Lewis Davis/Virginia/Slave/New Orleans/11 Years/October 4/3PM/October 31/NA/37/D.

Donnovan/NL/$1.00/Dysentery/10 Days/Single/NL/28 Days/$28.00/Paid

452—Primus/Virginia/Slave/New Orleans/18 Years/October 7/ 10AM/October 14/NA/60/D. C. Labat/NL/$1.00/ Dysentery/4 Days/Married/NL/8 Days/$8.00/Paid

453—Levi/Maryland/Slave/New Orleans/4 Days/October 7/ 11AM/November 22/NA/52/Cuddy, Brown/NL/$1.00/ Enteritis/2 Months/Single/NL/47 Days/$47.00/Paid

454—Jacob/Virginia/Slave/New Orleans/5 Months/October 10/ 4PM/October 22/NA/44/O. M. Lisk/NL/$1.00/ Injury/1 Day/ Married/NL/13 Days/$13.00/Paid

455—William/Alexandria, S.C./Slave/New Orleans/NL/October 12/11AM/October 26/NA/29/McCann & Patterson/ NL/$1.00/ Ground Itch/5 Days/Single/NL/15 Days/ $15.00/Paid

456—Joe/Kentucky/Slave/New Orleans/18 Years/October 12/ 5PM/October 30/NA/27/Magee/NL/$1.00/Scalp Wound/1 Day/ Single/NL/19 Days/$34.00/$15.00 Extra

457—Peyton/Virginia/Slave/New Orleans/12 Years/October 15/ 9AM/October 27/NA/28/Eaton & Henderson/NL/ $1.00/ Constipation/4 Weeks/Single/NL/13 Days/ $13.00/Paid

459—Dennis/Maryland/Slave/New Orleans/10 Years/October 20/8 AM/October 31/NA/30/D. Donnovan/NL/$1.00/ Dysentery/1 Week/ Single/NL/12 Days/$12.00/Paid

460—Lewis/Virginia/Slave/Louisiana/20 Years/October 21/9AM/ November 2/NA/42/H. Brown/NL/$1.00 /Orchitis/1 Day/Single/ NL/13 Days/$13.00/Paid

461—Ned Johnson/Virginia/Slave/Louisiana/9 Months/October 21/11AM/October 28/NA/25/A. Hagan/NL/$1.00/ Remit. Fever/3 Days/Single/NL/8 Days/$8.00/Paid

462—Lewis/Virginia/Slave/Louisiana/7 Years/October 22/10AM/October 31/NA/40/W. J. Poitevent/NL/ $1.00/ Hemorrhoids/3 Years/Single/NL/10 Days/ $30.00/Paid $20.00 Extra

463—George Smith/Maryland/Slave/Louisiana/15 Years/ October 22/6PM/November 19/NA/22/W. A. Elmore/NL/$1.00/Bronchitis/8 Months/Single/NL/29 Days/$29.00/Paid
464—Perkins/N. Carolina/Slave/Louisiana/13 Years/October 22/7PM/January 19/NA/36/H. J. Ranney/NL/ $1.00/Fracture of Ulna/1 Day/Single/NL/NL/NL/Paid
465—Eliza/New Orleans/Slave/Louisiana/21 Years/October 24/9AM/November 26/NA/21/H. J. Ranney/NL/$1.00/ Rheumatism/1 Month/NL/NL/ 34.00 Days/$34.00/Paid
469—Jackson/North Carolina/Slave/Pearl River/9 Days/October 29/2PM/November 24/NA/30/W. J. Poitevent/NL/ $1.00/ Hemorrhoids/6 Months/NL/NL/27 Days/$52.00 /Paid/$25 Extra
470—Julia/Virginia/Slave/New Orleans/8 Years/November 1/ 11AM/November 19/NA/28/J. S. Levy/NL/ $1.00/ Varicosella/3 Months/NL/NL/19 Days/$19.00/NR
471—Tom/Virginia/Slave/New Orleans/6 Years/November 3/10 AM/November 12/NA/34/H. J. Ranney/NL/ $1.00/Int. Fever/4 Days/NL/NL/10 Days/$10.00/Paid
474—Ned Turner/Virginia/Slave/New Orleans/4 Years/ November 5/10AM/November 9/NA/38/Thomas Finney/NL/$1.00/Rheumatism/4 Days/Single/NL/5 Days/$5.00/Paid
476—Ann/Virginia/Slave/New Orleans/NL/November 10/ 10AM/November 24/NA/40/N. O. J. Tisdale/NL/ $1.00/Diarrhea/4 Days/Married/NL/15 Days/ $15.00/Paid
478—Harriet/Mississippi/Slave/Mississippi/1 Day/November 15/4 PM/November 24/NA/17/Capt. Poitevent/ NL/$1.00/NL/2 Weeks/Single/NL/10 Days/ $10.00/Paid
479—Adam/NL?/Slave/Louisiana/2 Years/November 17/12AM/ NL/November 18*/52/S. O'Rourk/

NL/$1.00/ Pneumonia/4 Days/ Single/NL/2 Days/ $12.00/Paid Burial $10.00

480—Susan/Baltimore/Slave/New Orleans/NL/November 17/ 10AM/ December 6/NA/42/Mr. Forsyth/NL/$1.00/ Bronchitis/ 4 Months/ Married/NL/20 Days/ $20.00/Paid

481—Joe/Kentucky/Slave/New Orleans/18 Years/November 24/ 5PM/December 6/NA/27/Mr. Macgee/NL/$1.00/ Injury/40 Days/ Single/NL/13 Days/$13.00/NR

482—Howard/Virginia/Slave/New Orleans/5 Years/November 26/ 12 Noon/November 30/NA/21/H. J. Ranney/ NL/$1.00/Int. Fever/8 Days/Married/NL/5 Days/$5.00/Paid

483—Horace/Virginia/Slave/New Orleans/8 Years/November 27/ 10AM/December 11/NA/19/H. J. Ranney/NL/ $1.00/ Epilepsy/7 Months/ Single/NL/15 Days/ $15.00/Paid

484—William/Alexandria/Slave/New Orleans/NL/November 27/ 3PM/December 9/NA/29/McCann & Patterson/ NL/$1.00/ Debility/2 Days/Single/NL/12 Days/ $12.00/Paid

485—Jefferson/Mississippi/Slave/New Orleans/9 Years/ November 22/11 AM/December 12/NA/25/J. E. Caldwell/NL/$1.00/ Rheumatism/4 Weeks/Single/ NL/21 Days/$12.00/Paid

486—Tom/Mississippi/Slave/New Orleans/NL/November 28/ 4PM/December 12/NA/35/A. Levy/NL/$1.00/ Cholera/3 Days/ Single/NL/14 Days/$14.00/Paid

488—Fanny/NL/Slave/New Orleans/NL/November 30/9AM/December 31/NA/20/G. Patterson/NL/$1.00/ Abortion/2 Days/Married/NL/32 Days/$32.00/Paid

490—Bill/Virginia/Slave/New Orleans/10 Years/December 5/ 8AM/December 8/NA/27/D. Madden/NL/$1.00/ Debility/1 Month/ Single/NL/11 Days/$11.00/Paid

491—Mary/Virginia/Slave/New Orleans/NL/December 5/3PM/ December 18/NA/41/Capt. Grant/NL/$1.00/ Abortion/NL/ Married/ NL/[14 Days]/$14.00/Paid
492—Zack/Virginia/Slave/New Orleans/NL/December 8/11AM/ December 11/NA/NL/H. J. Ranney/NL/ $1.00/Hernia/NL/Single/ NL/4 Days/$4.00/Paid
495—Rachael/Florida/Slave/New Orleans/4 Years/December 17/ 10AM/NL/April 3*/24/F. J. Frisby/NL/$1.00/ Dropsy/NL/ Married/NL/105 Days/NL/Paid
496—Jefferson/Mississippi/Slave/New Orleans/9 Years/ December 17/4PM/January 25/NA/25/Caldwell & Lisk/NL/$1.00/ Syphilitic Pneumonia/4 Weeks/Single/ NL/40 Days/$40.00/Paid
497—Chloe/Virginia/Slave/New Orleans/30 Years/December 18/ 4PM/May 16/NA/50/Capt. Bowdich/NL/$1.00/ NL/15 Years/Married /NL/150 Days/$200.00/$50.00 Extra
500—Bob/Louisiana/Slave/New Orleans/15 Years/December 25/ 5PM/December 31/NA/15/D. O. D. Sullivan/NL/ $1.00/ Tonsillitis/1 Day/Single/NL/7 Days/$7.00/Paid
501—Marcus/Tennessee/Slave/New Orleans/4 Years/December 27/ 10AM/February 16/NA/17/H. A. Fassman/NL/ $1.00/Ulcers on Legs /1 Year/Single/NL/52 Days/ $52.00/Paid
503—Mary/Virginia/Slave/New Orleans/3 Years/December 30/ 8AM/Jan 26, 1857/NA/37/Andrews (?)/NL/$1.00/ Amenorrhea/6 Weeks/Married/NL/28 Days/ $28.00/Paid
504—Nicholas/Opelousas/Slave/New Orleans/3 Weeks/ December 31/2PM/February 5/NA/18/C. M. Bradford/ NL/$1.00/Ulcers on Leg/1 Day/Single/NL/57 Days/ $57.00/Paid

1857

SLAVERY AND MEDICINE: ENSLAVEMENT AND MEDICAL PRACTICES IN ANTEBELLUM LOUISIANA

506—Zac/NL/Slave/New Orleans/NL/Jan 10/3PM/Jan 31/NA/NL/H. J. Ranney/NL/$1.00/ Cholic/ NL/Single/NL/22 Days/$22.00/Paid
508—Jonas/N. Carolina/Slave/New Orleans/3 Years/Jan 11/ 2PM/Jan 12/NA/38/Andrews & Co./NL/$1.00/ Epilepsy/1 Day/ Married/NL/3 Days/$3.00/Paid
511—William Thomas/Virginia/Slave/New Orleans/NL/Jan 17/12 Noon/Jan 26/NA/25/H. J. Ranney/NL/$1.00/ Pneumonia/1 Week/ NL/NL/10 Days/$10.00/Paid
512—Daniel/Virginia/Slave/New Orleans/15 Years/January 20/ 11AM/March 5/NA/29/H. Brown/NL/$1.00/Injury/1 Month/Single/ NL/45 Days/$45.00/Paid
513—Thomas/Virginia/Slave/New Orleans/3 Years/January 23/ 6PM/April 22/NA/22/P. Fortier/NL/$1.00/NL/15 Days/Married/ NL/90 Days/$125.00/$35.00 Extra Paid
515—Washington/Virginia/Slave/New Orleans/4 Years/January 28/11AM/Jan 31/NA/27/M. Nicolea (?)/NL/$1.00/ Tonsillitis/3 Days/Married/NL/4 Days/$4.00/Paid
516—John Bell (?)/N. Carolina/Slave/New Orleans/1 Day/ January 29/12 Noon/February 27/NA/16/Cuddy Brown & Co./NL/ $1.00/Node on Tibia/2 Years/Single/NL/30 Days/$30.00/Paid
519—Pat/Virginia/Slave/New Orleans/NL/February 4/10 AM/ February 16/NA/22/J. Armstrong/NL/$1.00/Syphilis/2 Weeks/ Married/NL/13 Days/$13.00/Paid
521—Harriet/Louisiana/Slave/New Orleans/NL/February 5/ 4PM/May 25/NA/18/G. M. Bayley/NL/$1.00/ Hysteria/NL/Single/ NL/110 Days/$112.00/Paid
524—Judy/Georgia/Slave/New Orleans/NL/February 11/8PM/ NL/February 16*/36/J. S. Andrews/NL/$1.00/NL/5 Days/Married /NL/6 Days/$6.00/Paid
526—January/Mississippi/Slave/Mississippi/1 Day/February 14/3 PM/February 26/NA/23/J. L. Moore/NL/$1.00/ Diarrhea/3 Days/Single/NL/13 Days/$13.00/Paid

SLAVERY AND MEDICINE: ENSLAVEMENT AND MEDICAL PRACTICES IN ANTEBELLUM LOUISIANA

527—George/Mississippi/Slave/Mississippi/1 Day/February 14/3 PM/February 26/NA/57/J. L. Moore/NL/$1.00/ Bronchitis/2 Days/Single/NL/13 Days/$13.00/Paid
528—Louis/Mississippi/Slave/Mississippi/1 Day/February 14/3 PM/February 26/NA/21/J. L. Moore/NL/$1.00/ Bronchitis/4 Days/ Single/NL/13 Days/$13.00/Paid
529—Philip/Mississippi/Slave/Mississippi/1 Day/February 14/3 PM/February 26/NA/28/J. L. Moore/NL/$1.00/ Diarrhea/5 Days/Single/NL/13 Days/$13.00/Paid
531—Howard/Virginia/Slave/New Orleans/5 Years/February 14/ 2PM/February 25/NA/26/H. J. Ranney/NL/$1.00/ Pneumonia/2 Days/Married/NL/12 Days/$12.00/Paid
532—Charles/Kentucky/Slave/Kentucky/5 Months/February 15/1 PM/March 5/NA/29/B. Kendig/NL/$1.00/ Diarrhea/2 Weeks/ Married/NL/83 Days/$83.00/NR
533—Loomus/Louisiana/Slave/New Orleans/NL/February 15/12 Noon/NL/April 10*/NL/H. J. Ranney/NL/$1.00 /Scrofula/NL/ Single/NL/55 Days/NL/NR
534—John Badger/Georgia/Slave/Georgia/1 Day/February 15/5 PM/March ?/NA/24/J. Johnson/NL/$1.00/ Gonorrhea/8 Weeks/ Single/NL/17 Days/$17.00/Paid
535—Abraham/Virginia/Slave/New Orleans/2 Days/February 16/6 PM/March 2/NA/23/T. J. Pipkin/NL/$1.00/ Bronchitis/2 Weeks/ Single/NL/12 Days/$12.00/Paid
536—Jack/Louisiana/Slave/New Orleans/NL/February 17/10 AM/March 1/NA/14/B. Kendig/NL/$1.00/Diarrhea/1 Week/Single/ NL/13 Days/$13.00/NR
537—Marcus/Tennessee/Slave/New Orleans/NL/February 18/10 AM/May 2/NA/17/H. A. Fassman/NL/$1.00/ Ulcer on Leg/1 Year/ Single/NL/74 Days/$74.00/Paid
541—Charles/Louisiana/Slave/New Orleans/2 Years/February 27/6 PM/NL/NA/22/Mrs. Collins/NL/$1.00/Ulcers from ?/5 Years/Single/NL/NL/NL/NR
542—Nicholas/Opelousas/Slave/New Orleans/3 Months/ February 28/5 PM/March 8/NA/18/C. M. Bradford/NL

SLAVERY AND MEDICINE: ENSLAVEMENT AND MEDICAL PRACTICES IN ANTEBELLUM LOUISIANA

/$1.00/Pneumonia/1 Week/Single/NL/9 Days/ $9.00/Paid
543—Charles/Alabama/Slave/New Orleans/4 Weeks/March 2/9 AM/March 8/NA/30/A. O. Sibley/NL/$1.00/ Pneumonia/3 Days/ Single/NL/7 Days/$7.00/NR
544—Sam/S. Carolina/Slave/New Orleans/1 Year/March 2/9 AM/March 8/NA/21/A. O. Sibley/NL/$1.00/ Pneumonia/2 Weeks/ Single/NL/7 Days/$7.00/NR
545—Sharper/S. Carolina/Slave/New Orleans/3 Weeks/March 2/9 AM/March 8/NA/25/A. O. Sibley/NL/$1.00/ Diarrhea/2 Days/ Single/NL/7 Days/$7.00/NR
546—Alfred/Virginia/Slave/New Orleans/3 Weeks/March 2/9 AM/March 7/NA/25/A. O. Sibley/NL/$1.00/ Diarrhea/1 Week/ Single/NL/6 Days/$6.00/NR
547—George/Mississippi/Slave/New Orleans/1 Month/March 2/2 PM/March 12/NA/57/J. L. Moore/NL/$1.00/ Diarrhea/1 Day/ Single/NL/11 Days/$11.00/Paid
548—January/Mississippi/Slave/New Orleans/2 Weeks/March 2/2 PM/March 12/NA/25/J. L. Moore/NL/$1.00/ Diarrhea/1 Day/ Single/NL/11 Days/$11.00/Paid
549—Sarah/Kentucky/Slave/New Orleans/12 Years/March 2/6 PM/March 15/NA/12/Mr. Graham/NL/2.00/Measles/1 Day/Single/NL/13 Days/$26.00/Paid
550—Abraham/Virginia/Slave/New Orleans/1 Month/February 3/9 PM/March 7/NA/25/A. O. Sibley/NL/1.00/ Pneumonia/3 Weeks/ Single/NL/5 Days/$5.00/NR
551—Lewis/Mississippi/Slave/New Orleans/3 Weeks/March 3/9 AM/March 15/NA/21/J. L. Moore/NL/$1.00/ Diarrhea/1 Day/ Single/NL/13 Days/$13.00/Paid
552—Delia/Mississippi/Slave/New Orleans/2 Weeks/March 3/6 PM/March 11/NA/17/NL/ NL/[2.00]/Measles/3 Days/Single/NL/9 Days/$18.00/NR
553—John Badger/Georgia/Slave/New Orleans/3 Weeks/March 4/5 PM/March 31/NA/20/NL/NL/$1.00/Gonorrhea/3 Months/Single/NL/ 28 Days/$28.00/Paid

SLAVERY AND MEDICINE: ENSLAVEMENT AND MEDICAL PRACTICES IN
ANTEBELLUM LOUISIANA

554—Philip/Mississippi/Slave/New Orleans/3 Weeks/March 5/7 PM/March 12/NA/25/J. ? Moore/NL/$1.00/Diarrhea/3 Days/ Single/NL/8 Days/$8.00/Paid
555—Randall/Mississippi/Slave/New Orleans/1 Month/March 5/9 AM/March 7/NA/26/A. O. Sibley/NL/$1.00/ Pneumonia/3 Days/ Single/NL/3 Days/NL/NR
556—Eppes/Virginia/Slave/New Orleans/4 Weeks/March 6/7 PM/March 31/NA/24/T. E. Matthews/NL/$1.00/ Pneumonia/1 Day/ Single/NL/26 Days/$26.00/Paid
557—Eugene/N. Orleans/Slave/New Orleans/2 Weeks/March 7/7 PM/March 7/NA/19/T. Foster/NL/$1.00/ Pneumonia/1 Day/Single/ NL/11 Days/$11.00/NR
558—Peter/Carolina/Slave/New Orleans/1 Year/March 10/9AM/ March 21/NA/45/A. O. Sibley/NL/$1.00/ Pneumonia/2 Days/Single /NL/12 Days/$12.00/NR
559—Ann/Carolina/Slave/New Orleans/6 Years/March 20/9AM/ NL/NA/38/J. McLanathan/NL/$1.00/ Pleurisy/4 Weeks/Married/ NL/11 Days/$11.00/Paid
560—Alfred/Virginia/Slave/New Orleans/6 Weeks/March 11/10 AM/March 20/NA/25/A. O. Sibley/NL/$1.00/ Diarrhea/5 Days/ Single/NL/10 Days/$10.00/NR
561—Bob/Virginia/Slave/New Orleans/4 Weeks/March 15/NL/NL/ NA/26/A. O. Sibley/NL/$1.00/ Tonsillitis/3 Days/Single/NL/5 Days/$5.00/NR
562—Huldah/Louisiana/Slave/New Orleans/2 Weeks/March 17/12 Noon/April 10/NA/35/J. B. Robertson/NL/$1.00 /Typhoid Fever/3 Days/Married/NL/31 Days/ $31.00/Paid
563—Abraham/Virginia/Slave/New Orleans/1 Month/March 12/10 AM/March 29/NA/25/A. O. Sibley/NL/$1.00/ Diarrhea/3 Weeks/ Single/NL/18 Days/$18.00/NR
564—Sam/S. Carolina/Slave/New Orleans/1 Year/March 12/10 AM/April 18/NA/26/A. O. Sibley/NL/$1.00/ Diarrhea/2 Days/ Single/NL/37 Days/$37.00/NR

565—January/Mississippi/Slave/New Orleans/2 Weeks/March 15/4 PM/March 30/NA/23/T. J. Moore/NL/$1.00/ Dysentery/1 Days/Single/NL/16 Days/$16.00/Paid
566—Randall/Mississippi/Slave/New Orleans/6 Weeks/March 16/9 AM/March 22/NA/20/A. O. Sibley/NL/$1.00/ Diarrhea/2 Days/Single/NL/7 Days/$7.00/NR
567—Daniel/Louisiana/Slave/New Orleans/NL/March 16/6 PM/ March 23/NA/29/H. Brown/NL/$1.00/ Rheumatism/4 Days/Single/ NL/8 Days/$8.00/Paid
568—Horace/Louisiana/Slave/New Orleans/8 Years/March 18/12 Noon/April 29/NA/19/H. J. Ranney/NL/$1.00/ Epilepsy/NL/ Single/NL/43 Days/$43.00/Paid
570—George/Mississippi/Slave/New Orleans/6 Weeks/March 19/12 Noon/March 12/NA/57/J. L. Moore/NL/$1.00/ Diarrhea/2 Days/Single/NL/4 Days/$4.00/Paid
571—Mary Jane/Mississippi/Slave/New Orleans/6 Weeks/March 21/11 AM/April 20/NA/24/F. Foster/NL/$1.00/Pleuro Pneumonia/1 Day/Single/NL/41 Days/NL/NR
572—Moses/Mississippi/Slave/New Orleans/4 Weeks/March 21/1PM/April 5/NA/22/A. O. Sibley/NL/$1.00/Int. Fever/1 Day/Single/NL/16 Days/$16.00/NR
574—Mary/Virginia/Slave/New Orleans/3 Years/March 5/7AM/ March 22/NA/37/J. S. Andrews/NL/$1.00/NL /4 Days/Married/ NL/18 Days/$18.00/Paid
575—Amy/Louisiana/Slave/New Orleans/NL/March 24/5 PM/April 15/NA/12/F. Foster/NL/$1.00/NL/NL/ NL/NL/23 Days/$23.00/NR
576—Peter/Carolina/Slave/New Orleans/?/March 24/5PM/April 5/NA/45/A. O. Sibley/NL/$1.00/ Diarrhea/NL/NL/NL/13 Days/ $13.00/NR
578—Sharper/S. Carolina/Slave/New Orleans/1 Month/March 26/9 AM/April 5/NA/25/A. O. Sibley/NL/$1.00/ Diarrhea/3 Days/Single/NL/11 Days/$11.00/NR
579—Philip/Mississippi/Slave/New Orleans/1 Month/March 26/11AM/March 30/NA/28/J. L. Moore/NL/$1.00/ Diarrhea/2 Days/Single/NL/5 Days/$5.00/Paid

580—Isham/Mississippi/Slave/New Orleans/3 Weeks/March 26/4PM/NL/April 3*/NL/Dr. Bein/NL/$1.00/ Tetanus/1 Day/ Single/NL/NL/NL/NR

581—Philip/Tennessee/Slave/New Orleans/2 Weeks/March 28/4 PM/April 8/NA/26/F. Foster/NL/$1.00/ Diarrhea/4 Days/Single/ NL/12 Days/$12.00/NR

582—Matt/Alabama/Slave/New Orleans/6 Weeks/March 28/5PM/ April 13/NA/24/A. O. Sibley/NL/$1.00/ Diarrhea/3 Days/ Single/NL/17 Days/$17.00/NR

583—George/Mississippi/Slave/New Orleans/1 Month/March 28/6PM/March 30/NA/57/J. L. Moore/NL/$1.00/ Diarrhea/2 Days/Single/NL/3 Days/$3.00/Paid

[584—Mr. Weinstein, 21 Years old, from Germany is listed as a slave; no account holder is listed and no payment information is recorded.]

585—John/Virginia/Slave/Virginia/4 Years/March 31/9AM/April 4/NA/29/T. J. Pipkin/NL/$1.00/ Diarrhea/9 Days/Single/NL/5 Days/$5.00/Paid

586—William/Virginia/Slave/Virginia/7 Years/April 1/11AM/ April 4/NA/27/T. J. Pipkin/NL/$1.00/Diarrhea/5 Days/Single/ NL/4 Days/$4.00/Paid

587—Abraham/Virginia/Slave/Virginia/1 Month/April 1/3PM/ April 13/NA/35/A. O. Sibley/NL/$1.00/Diarrhea/3 Days/Single/ NL/13 Days/$13.00/NR

588—Allen/N. Carolina/Slave/New Orleans/25 Years/April 2/10AM/April 12/NA/34/F. Foster/NL/$1.00/ Rubeola/2 Days/ Married/NL/10 Days/$10.00/Paid

589—Sam/Mississippi/Slave/New Orleans/NL/April 3/2PM/April 16/NA/26/Capt. Poitevent/NL/$1.00/ Bubo/2 Weeks/Single/NL/14 Days/$14.00/Paid

590—Julice/Virginia/Slave/New Orleans/NL/April 4/4PM/May 9/NA/31/J. L. Levy/NL/$1.00/Pregnancy /NL/Married/NL/36 Days/ NL/NR

591—Bill/Virginia/Slave/New Orleans/2 Months/April 5/12 Noon/April 15/NA/25/A. O. Sibley/NL/$1.00/ Pneumonia/2 Days/ Single/NL/14 Days/$14.00/NR

593—Henry/Kentucky/Slave/New Orleans/3 Years/April 8/4PM/ April 28/NA/32/S. Johnson/NL/$1.00/ Syphilis/4 Weeks/Single/ NL/21 Days/$21.00/Paid
594—Amos/Virginia/Slave/New Orleans/1 Week/March 9/4PM/May 8/NA/28/F. Foster/NL/$1.00/Tonsillitis/3 Days/Single/NL/31 Days/$31.00/NR
595—Moses/Virginia/Slave/New Orleans/NL/April 10/9AM/May 4/NA/22/A. O. Sibley/NL/$1.00/ Diarrhea/5 Days/Single/NL/25 Days/$25.00/NR
596—Ned/Virginia/Slave/New Orleans/5 Days/April 10/9AM/ April 18/NA/21/A. O. Sibley/NL/$1.00/Injury/2 Days/Single/ NL/9 Days/$9.00/NR
598—Dan/N. Carolina/Slave/New Orleans/3 Months/April 10/ 9AM/April 8/NA/27/A. O. Sibley/NL/$1.00/Injury/2 Weeks/ Single/NL/9/$9.00/NR
599—Jane/Kentucky/Slave/Kentucky/3 Months/April 11/8AM/ April 20/NA/15/F. Foster/NL/$1.00/Diarrhea/1 Day/Single/ NL/10 Days/$10.00/NR
600—Sharper/S. Carolina/Slave/New Orleans/3 Months/April 13/9AM/April 18/NA/25/A. O. Sibley/NL/$1.00/ Diarrhea/5 Days/ Single/NL/6 Days/$6.00/NR
601—Daniel/Kentucky/Slave/New Orleans/3 Months/April 13/ 9AM/April 18/NA/26/A. O. Sibley/NL/$1.00/ Diarrhea/3 Days/ Single/NL/6 Days/$6.00/NR
602—Jacob/Kentucky/Slave/New Orleans/2 Weeks/April 13/ 9AM/April 18/NA/25/A. O. Sibley/NL/$1.00/ Diarrhea/4 Days/ Single/NL/6 Days/$6.00/NR
603—Jack/Virginia/Slave/New Orleans/7 Years/April 13/12 Noon/April 19/NA/36/T. J. Pipkin/NL/$1.00/ Dysentery/1 Week/Married/NL/7 Days/$7.00/Paid
605—Jim/Virginia/Slave/New Orleans/2 Weeks/April 15/5PM/ April 20/NA/21/F. Foster/NL/$1.00/Diarrhea/1 Week/Single/ NL/6 Days/$6.00/NR
606—Matt/N. Carolina/Slave/New Orleans/2 Weeks/April 15/ 5PM/May 2/NA/23/F. Foster/NL/$1.00/Diarrhea/2 Weeks/Single/ NL/18 Days/$18.00/NR

607—Matt/Alabama/Slave/New Orleans/3 Months/April 16/ 7AM/April 27/NA/24/A. O. Sibley/NL/$1.00/ Diarrhea/2 Days/ Single/NL/11 Days/$11.00/NR
608—Barney/Maryland/Slave/Maryland/5 Months/April 17/ 7AM/April 19/NA/37/Mr. Morton/NL/$1.00/ Diarrhea/10 Days/ Single/NL/3 Days/$3.00/NR
610—Dolly and Child/Virginia/Slaves/New Orleans/48 Days/ April 20/5PM/NL/NA/26/F. Foster/NL/$1.00/ Scrofula/4 Months/ Married/NL/NL/NL/NR
611—John/S. Carolina/Slaves/New Orleans/24 Days/April 21/ 7AM/May 14/NA/29/A. O. Sibley/NL/$1.00/ Diarrhea/14 Days/ Single/NL/25 Days/$25.00/NR
612—Sam/S. Carolina/Slaves/New Orleans/1 Year/April 21/7 AM/May 4/NA/21/A. O. Sibley/NL/$1.00/Diarrhea/4 Days/ Single/NL/14 Days/$14.00/NR
613—Jim/S. Carolina/Slave/New Orleans/2 Months/April 21/ 10AM/NL/NA/50/George R. King/NL/$1.00/NL/8 Weeks/Married/ NL/NL/NL/NR
614—Jim/Virginia/Slave/New Orleans/2 Months/April 22/10 AM/May 2/NA/17/A. O. Sibley/NL/$1.00/Perineal Abcess/1 Week/ Single/NL/11 Days/$11.00/Paid
615—Dan/Virginia/Slave/New Orleans/3 Months/April 22/5 PM/ May 4/NA/27/A. O. Sibley/NL/$1.00/Injury/4 Days/Single/NL/13 Days/$13.00/NR
616—Jane/Kentucky/Slave/New Orleans/3 Months/April 22/ 3PM/April 27/NA/15/F. Foster/NL/$1.00/Diarrhea/3 Days/ Single/NL/6 Days/$6.00/NR
617—Mary/Kentucky/Slave/New Orleans/6 Years/April 25/10 AM/ May 2/NA/20/F. Foster/NL/$1.00/Cararrh/1 Day/Single/NL/10 Days/$10.00/NR
619—Bill/Virginia/Slave/New Orleans/2 Months/April 25/7AM/ May 4/NA/25/A. O. Sibley/NL/$1.00/ Catarrh/2 Days/Single/ NL/10 Days/$10.00/NR
620—Abraham/S. Carolina/Slave/New Orleans/1 Month/April 25/7 AM/May 11/NA/25/A. O. Sibley/NL/$1.00/ Diarrhea/3 Days/ Single/NL/10 Days/$10.00/NR

621—Prince/S. Carolina/Slave/New Orleans/6 Weeks/April 25/
7AM/May 2/NA/50/A. O. Sibley/NL/$1.00/Diarrhea/1
Day/Single/ NL/8 Days/$8.00/Paid
622—Sam/S. Carolina/Slave/New Orleans/4 Weeks/April 25/
7AM/May 2/NA/38/A. O. Sibley/NL/$1.00/Diarrhea/4
Days/ Single/NL/8 Days/$8.00/NR
623—Arthur/Maryland/Slave/New Orleans/3 Years/April 25/11
AM/April 29/NA/35/H. J. Ranney/NL/$1.00/
Dysentery/8 Days/ Married/NL/5 Days/$5.00/Paid
624—Henderson/Maryland/Slave/New Orleans/10 Years/April
28/11 AM/May 5/NA/27/Mrs. Macgee/NL/$1.00/
Diarrhea/4 Weeks/ Single/NL/8 Days/$8.00/Paid
625—Charles/Alabama/Slave/Mobile/3 Weeks/April
30/9AM/May 6/NA/20/A. O. Sibley/NL/$1.00/
Diarrhea/2 Weeks/Single/NL/7 Days/$7.00/Paid
626—Allen/Alabama/Slave/Mobile/3 Weeks/April
30/9AM/NL/May 13*/NL/A. O. Sibley/NL/$1.00/
Dysentery/8 Days/Single/NL/14 Days/$26.00/NR
627—Austin/Virginia/Slave/New Orleans/2 Months/May
1/9AM/ May 13/NA/26/F. Foster/NL/$1.00/
Catarrh/NL/Single/NL/10 Days/$10.00/NR
629—George Smith/Maryland/Slave/New Orleans/15 Years/May
1/5 PM/May 6/NA/26/W. A. Elmore/NL/$1.00/
Catarrh/3 Days/ Single/NL/6 Days/$6.00/Paid
630—Robert/Virginia/Slave/New Orleans/12 Years/May
4/11AM/ May 7/NA/26/T. J. Pipkin/NL/$1.00/
Diarrhea/10 Hours/Single/ NL/4 Days/$4.00/NR
631—Letitia/Arkansas/Slave/New Orleans/3 Months/May
4/8AM/ May 8/NA/18/F. Foster/NL/$1.00/
Flatulence/3 Days/Single/NL/5 Days/$5.00/NR
632—Jacob/Kentucky/Slave/Kentucky/5 Weeks/May
4/9AM/May 14/NA/25/A. O. Sibley/NL/$1.00/
Diarrhea/5 Days/Single/NL/11 Days/$11.00/Paid
633—Henry/Virginia/Slave/New Orleans/4 Months/May 4/10
AM/ May 8/NA/17/F. Foster/NL/$1.00/Int. Fever/3
Days/Single/NL/5 Days/$5.00/NR

SLAVERY AND MEDICINE: ENSLAVEMENT AND MEDICAL PRACTICES IN ANTEBELLUM LOUISIANA

635—Milton/Kentucky/Slave/New Orleans/NL/May 6/12 Noon/May 9/NA/19/Yancy/NL/$1.00/Fistula in Arm/9 Months/Single/NL/4 Days/$4.00/NR

636—Horace/NL/Slave/New Orleans/NL/May 8/9AM/NL/NA/NL/H. J. Ranney/NL/$1.00/ Epilepsy/NL/Single/NL/NL/NL/NR

637—Alfred/New Orleans/Slave/New Orleans/NL/May 8/12 Noon/ May 13/NA/24/Leeds & Co./NL/$1.00/ Dysentery/3 Weeks/ Married/NL/6 Days/$6.00/NR

639—Maria/New Orleans/Slave/New Orleans/18 Years/May 9/ 5PM/May 16/NA/18/F. Foster/NL/$1.00/Hydro Pericarditis/ NL/Single/NL/10 Days/$10.00/NR

640—Sarah/Virginia/Slave/New Orleans/3 Weeks/May 9/5PM/ NL/May 16*/24/F. Foster/NL/$1.00/Int. Fever/NL/ Single/NL/8 Days/NL/NR

641—Morgan/Virginia/Slave/New Orleans/12 Years/May 10/11 AM/May 13/NA/28/Matt Breeden/NL/$1.00/Wen. Tumor/2 Years/ Single/NL/4 Days/$24.00/$20.00 Extra Paid

642—Turner/Georgia/Slave/Georgia/4 Weeks/May 12/9AM/May 15/ NA/38/F. Foster/NL/$1.00/Int. Fever/2 Weeks/Single/NL/7 Days/$7.00/NR

643—Mary Ann/Tennessee/Slave/New Orleans/3 Years/May 13/11 AM/NL/NA/12/Dr. (?) Bein/NL/$1.00/ Tonsillitis/2 Weeks/ Single/NL/NL/NL/NR

644—Frances/N. Carolina/Slave/New Orleans/2 Weeks/May 15/ NL/NL/NA/12/F. Foster/NL/$1.00/Rubeola/2 Days/Single/NL/ NL/NL/NR

645—Evaline/N. Carolina/Slave/New Orleans/NL/May 17/12 Noon/NL/NA/15/R. M. Harrison/NL/$1.00/ Hysteria/NL/Single/ NL/NL/NL/NR

648—Celia/Virginia/Slave/New Orleans/2 Weeks/May 18/PM/June ?/NA/30/F. Foster/NL/$1.00/Rubeola/3 Days/Single/NL/NL/NL/NR

649—Andy/Mississippi/Slave/Louisiana/2 Weeks/May 18/1 PM/June 1/NA/10/F. Foster/NL/NL/2.00/Rubeola/1 Day/Single/ NL/$26.00/NR
650—Kitty/Mississippi/Slave/New Orleans/NL/May 18/1PM/June 1/ NA/3/F. Foster/NL/NL/2.00/ Rubeola/ 1Day/Single/ NL/$24.00/NR
651—Aleck/Alabama/Slave/New Orleans/NL/May 20/11AM/May 22/NA/28/H. B. Philips/NL/$1.00/ Diarrhea/5 Days/Single/NL/3 Days/$3.00/Paid
652—Alfred/New Orleans/Slave/New Orleans/NL/May 21/7AM/June 1/NA/24/Leeds & Co./NL/$1.00/ Diarrhea/4 Days/Married/NL/11 Days/$11.00/NR
653—Esther/Virginia/Slave/New Orleans/2 Months/May 21/ 6PM/NL/June 2*/23/F. Foster/NL/$1.00/Typhoid Fever/4 Days/ Married/NL/13 Days/NL/NR
656—Nancy/Virginia/Slave/New Orleans/NL/May 26/5PM/ June 13/NA/30/NL/NL/$1.00/Rheumatism/2 Weeks/Married/NL/18 Days/$18.00/Paid
657—Julia/Louisiana/Slave/New Orleans/19 Weeks/May 28/ 7AM/June 4/NA/12/F. Foster/NL/2.00/Rubeola/8 Days/Single/ NL/12 Days/$12.00/NR
658—Mack/N. Carolina/Slave/New Orleans/1 Month/May 28/ 9AM/June 1/NA/24/F. Foster/NL/2.00/Diarrhea/2 Days/Single/ NL/5 Days/$5.00/NR
659—Amy/Virginia/Slave/New Orleans/4 Months/May 28/ 7AM/NL/NA/12/F. Foster/NL/$1.00/NL/1 Week/Single/NL/41 Days/$41.00/NR
660—Mary/Virginia/Slave/New Orleans/NL/May 28/7AM/June 7/NA/14/F. Foster/NL/$1.00/Intermit. Fever/1 Weeks/Single/ NL/11 Days/$11.00/NR
662—James Jackson/Virginia/Slave/New Orleans/1 Day/May 31/ 3PM/August 18/NA/32/NL/NL/$1.00/NL/2 Years/Married/NL/80 Days/$105.00/Paid
663—Jonas/N. Carolina/Slave/New Orleans/5 Years/June 3/ 7AM/July 11/NA/NL/NL/NL/$1.00/Arthritis/3 Days/Married/NL/39 Days/$39.00/Paid

664—James/Kentucky/Slave/New Orleans/3 Weeks/June
1/7AM/ June 11/NA/NL/F. Foster/NL/$1.00/Intermit.
Fever/2 Days/ Single/NL/11 Days/$11.00/NR
665—Barney/Maryland/Slave/New Orleans/32 Years/June 4/
11AM/June 8/NA/32/M. Morton/NL/$1.00/
Dysentery/3 Days/ Single/NL/5 Days/$5.00/Paid
666—Aaron/Alabama/Slave/New Orleans/3 Years/June
5/9AM/June 26/NA/15/R. Condon/NL/3.00/NL/2
Days/Single/NL/NL/$100.00/NR
667—John/Virginia/Slave/New Orleans/5 Years/June
6/7AM/June 13/NA/24/T. J. Pipkins/NL/$1.00/Umbil.
Hernia/1 Week/ Single/NL/8 Days/$8.00/NR
668—Woolford/Maryland/Slave/New Orleans/9 Years/June
6/6PM/June 10/NA/44/H. J. Ramsey/NL/$1.00/Remitt
Fever/5 Days/Married/NL/5 Days/$5.00/NR
670—Eliza/Virginia/Slave/New Orleans/2 Weeks/June 7/
10AM/June 11/NA/16/F. Foster/NL/$1.00/Abortion/3
Days/ Single/NL/5 Days/$5.00/NR
671—Williams/Virginia/Slave/New Orleans/14 Years/June
8/7AM/July 13/NA/30/Yancy/NL/$1.00/Amputation
Arm/1 Day/ Single/NL/36 Days/$36.00/NR
672—Lewis/Virginia/Slave/New Orleans/12 Years/June 9/11
AM/June 26/NA/35/Donnovan/NL/$1.00/Cholera/1
Day/Single/ NL/18 Days/$21.00/NR
673—Dennis/Maryland/Slave/New Orleans/10 Years/June
9/11AM/July 9/NA/37/Donnovan/NL
/$1.00/Cholera/1 Day/ Single/NL/31 Days/$34.00/NR
674—Philip/Mississippi/Slave/New Orleans/10 Weeks/June
10/11AM/June 23/NA/28/J. L. Moure/NL/$1.00/Injury
of Knee/1 Day/Single/NL/14 Days/$14.00/Paid
675—Henry/Baltimore/Slave/New Orleans/6 Years/June 10/
4PM/June 13/NA/30/T. J. Pipkins/NL/$1.00/Syphilis/1
Week/ Single/NL/21 Days/$21.00/NR
676—Edwards/New Orleans/Slave/New Orleans/6 Years/June
10/10AM/June 13/NA/20/T. J. Pipkins/NL/$1.00/
Diarrhea/4 Days/Single/NL/4 Days/$4.00/NR

677—Thomas/Virginia/Slave/New Orleans/12 Years/June 10/10AM/June ?/NA/25/T. J. Pipkins/NL/$1.00/ Diarrhea/4 Days/Single/NL/4 Days/$4.00/NR
678—Willis/New Orleans/Slave/New Orleans/27 Years/June 10/10AM/June 13/NA/27/T. J. Pipkins/NL/$1.00/ Injury of Shoulder/4 Days/Single/NL/4 Days/$4.00/NR
679—Phil/Virginia/Slave/New Orleans/8 Years/June 11/ 11AM/June 27/NA/37/H. B. Philips/NL/$1.00/ Syphilis/6 Weeks/Single/NL/17 Days/$17.00/Paid
680—Jack/Georgia/Slave/New Orleans/3 Months/June 11/ 2PM/June 18/NA/20/T. Johnstone/NL/$1.00/ Diarrhea/3 Days/ Single/NL/8 Days/$8.00/NR
682—Edger/Washington/Slave/New Orleans/22 Years/June 15/5AM/June 17/NA/29/Leeds & Co./NL/$1.00/ Diarrhea/1 Week/Married/NL/3 Days/$3.00/Paid
683—William/Virginia/Slave/New Orleans/6 Years/June 15/6PM/July 13/NA/23/T. J. Pipkin/NL/$1.00/ Rhumatism/4 Months/Single/NL/29 Days/$29.00/NR
684—Jack/New Orleans/Slave/New Orleans/25 Years/June 16/6PM/NL/June 18*/33/G. Andrews/NL/$1.00/ Pneumonia/5 Days/Single/NL/3 Days/$15.00/Paid
685—Martin Vanburen/N. Carolina/Slave/New Orleans/6 Months/June 17/10AM/July 5/NA/28/T. J. Pipkins/NL/ $1.00/Intermittent/3 Days/Single/NL/19 Days/$19.00/NR
686—Preston/Virginia/Slave/New Orleans/1 Year/June 17/10AM/June 20/NA/43/Tompkins/ NL/$1.00/ Neuralgez/3 Days/Single/NL/10 Days/$10.00/NR
687—Maria/Virginia/Slave/New Orleans/NL/June 19/4PM/July 9/NA/27/E. W. Carter/NL/$1.00/Constipation/3 Days/ Single/NL/21 Days/NL/$21.00 Paid
688—John/Virginia/Slave/New Orleans/7 Years/June 29/ 7AM/July 11/NA/36/T. J. Pipkin/NL/$1.00/Orchitis/5 Weeks/ Single/NL/13 Days/$13.00/NR

689—Herod/Virginia/Slave/New Orleans/7 Years/June 30/4 PM/July 3/NA/37/Henry Brown/NL/$1.00/Cholic/6 Days/Single/ NL/4 Days/$4.00/Paid
692—Robert/Virginia/Slave/Mobile/1 Day/July 4/9AM/July 24/NA/28/Capt. Grant/NL/$1.00/Anemia/3 Weeks/Single/NL/21 Days/$1.00/Paid
693—Jane/Virginia/Slave/New Orleans/2 Months/July 4/ 9AM/July 18/NA/23/S. C. Rehan/NL/$1.00/ Diarrhea/NL/1 Day/ Single/15 Days/$15.00/NR
694—Elijah/S. Carolina/Slave/Savannah/5 Days/July 7/ 10AM/October 28/NA/25/T. Johnstone/NL/$1.00/ Syphilis/3 Years/Single/NL/113 Days/$113.00/NR
695—Henry/Baltimore/Slave/New Orleans/6 Years/July 8/ 8AM/July 16/NA/30/T. J. Pipkin/NL/$1.00/Syphilis/10 Days/ Single/NL/9 Days/$9.00/NR
696—Charley/Kentucky/Slave/Paducah/6 Years/July 11/ 11AM/July 15/NA/26/T. J. Pipkin/NL/$1.00/ Dysentery/3 Days/ Single/NL/5 Days/$5.00/NR
697—David/New Orleans/Slave/New Orleans/50 Years/July 11/8AM/NL/August 21*/50/W. W. Kilpatrick/NL/ $1.00/Apoplexy/1 Day/Married/NL/43 Days/ $65.00/$12.00 Burial Paid
699—George/Florida/Slave/Texas/2 Weeks/July 20/4PM/ August 10/NA/18/T. L. Clarke/NL/$1.00/Syphilis/1 Week/Single/NL/21 Days/$1.00/Paid
700—Mary Anne/North Carolina/Slave/Pearl River/1 Day/July 21/1PM/September 5/NA/45/W. S. Peitevent/NL/ $1.00/ Ovarian Dropsy/2 Months/Married/NL/47 Days/$72.00/NR
702—Coleman/Virginia/Slave/New Orleans/20 Years/July 28/9AM/August 12/NA/68/H. J. Ranney/NL/$1.00/ Catarrh/2 Weeks/Single/NL/16 Days/$16.00/NR
703—Peter/Virginia/Slave/New Orleans/13 Years/July 28/9AM/August 12/NA/34/H. J. Ranney/NL/$1.00/ Erithema/4 Days/Married/NL/16 Days/$16.00/NR

SLAVERY AND MEDICINE: ENSLAVEMENT AND MEDICAL PRACTICES IN ANTEBELLUM LOUISIANA

704—Gilbert/Virginia/Slave/New Orleans/1 Year/July 31/12 Noon/August 25/NA/17/T. J. Pipkin/NL/$1.00/ Typhoid Fever/5 Days/Single/NL/26 Days/$26.00/NR
705—Emeline/Virginia/Slave/New Orleans/15 Years/July 31/12 Noon/August 3/NA/26/T. J. Pipkin/NL/$1.00/ Measles/1 Week/Single/NL/4 Days/$4.00/NR
706—Tom/Virginia/Slave/New Orleans/15 Years/August 5/7AM/August 10/NA/27/Thos. McKnight/NL/$1.00/ Neuralgia/1 Month/Single/NL/6 Days/$6.00/NR
711—Bob/Louisiana/Slave/New Orleans/16 Years/August 12/11AM/ August 14/NA/28/T. J. Pipkin/NL/$1.00/ Intermittent/2 Days/Single/NL/3 Days/$3.00/NR
713—William Atwood/Georgia/Slave/New Orleans/19 Years/ August 15/8AM/August 19/NA/40/H. J. Ranney/NL/ $1.00/Intermittent/4 Days/Single/NL/5 Days/$5.00/NR
714—William Thomas/Maryland/Slave/New Orleans/9 Years/ August 15/8AM/August 19/NA/28/H. J. Ranney/NL/ $1.00/Diarrhea /4 Days/Single/NL/5 Days/$5.00/NR
715—Charley/Kentucky/Slave/New Orleans/6 Years/August 17/10AM/August 21/NA/26/T. J. Pipkin/NL/$1.00/ Diarrhea/1 Week/Single/NL/5 Days/$5.00/NR
716—Jim/Kentucky/Slave/New Orleans/6 Years/August 17/3PM/ August 19/NA/35/T. J. Pipkin/NL/$1.00/ Indigestion/2 Weeks/ Single/NL/3 Days/$3.00/NR
719—Jim/Virginia/Slave/New Orleans/NL/August 20/8AM/ August 25/NA/38/H. J. Ranney/NL/$1.00/ Continuous Fever/6 Hours/ Single/NL/6 Days/ $6.00/NR
722—Abraham/Virginia/Slave/New Orleans/15 Years/August 25/11AM/August 28/NA/26/T.J. Pipkin/NL/$1.00/ Dysentery/2 Days/Single/NL/4 Days/$4.00/NR
723—John/Virginia/Slave/New Orleans/5 Years/August 25/ 4PM/August 30/NA/24/T. J. Pipkin/NL/$1.00/ Dysentery/2 Days/Single/NL/6 Days/$6.00/NR
724—Cyrus/Virginia/Slave/New Orleans/NL/August 26/5PM/August 30/NA/30/T. J. Pipkin/NL/$1.00/ Dysentery/2 Days/Single/NL/5 Days/$5.00/NR

SLAVERY AND MEDICINE: ENSLAVEMENT AND MEDICAL PRACTICES IN
ANTEBELLUM LOUISIANA

725—Jane/Louisiana/Slave/New Orleans/19 Years/August 27/8AM/September 16/NA/19/T. P. Abrams/NL/$1.00 /Hysteria/3 Days/Single/NL/21 Days/$1.00/Paid
726—Julia/Virginia/Slave/New Orleans/12 Years/August 27/11AM/September 11/NA/35/E. Boulware/NL/$1.00 /Anemia/5 Weeks/Single/NL/16 Days/$16.00/Paid
727—John/Virginia/Slave/New Orleans/6 Years/August 28/8AM/September 21/NA/27/T. J. Pipkin/NL/$1.00/ Diarrhea/3 Days/Single/NL/25 Days/$25.00/NR
728—Nathaniel/District of Columbia/Slave/Washington City/2 Days/August 29/12 AM/October 28/NA/18/T. Johnstone/NL/$1.00 /Syphilis/3 Months/Single/NL/60 Days/$60.00/NR
729—Willis/Louisiana/Slave/New Orleans/20 Years/September 7/11AM/September 9/NA/22/T. J. Pipkin/NL/$1.00/ Intermittent/ 4 Days/Married/NL/3 Days/$3.00/NR
730—Abraham/Virginia/Slave/New Orleans/15 Years/ September 8/9AM/September 13/NA/26/T. J. Pipkin/ NL/$1.00/Intermittent/ 3 Days/Married/NL/6 Days/$6.00/NR
732—Bob/Louisiana/Slave/New Orleans/16 Years/September 14/9AM/September 22/NA/28/T. J. Pipkin/NL/$1.00/ Continued Fever/4 Days/Single/NL/9 Days/$9.00/NR
737—Cyrus/Virginia/Slave/New Orleans/16 Years/September 15/12 Noon/September 18/NA/30/T. J. Pipkin/NL/ $1.00/Fever/3 Days/Married/NL/4 Days/$4.00/NR
742—Frank/Virginia/Slave/Virginia/4 Years/September 28/11AM/October 2/NA/40/T. J. Pipkin/NL/$1.00/ Dysentery/2 Weeks/Single/NL/6 Days/$6.00/NR
743—Abraham/Virginia/Slave/New Orleans/15 Years/September 28/11AM/October 2/NA/26/T. J. Pipkin/NL/$1.00/Dysentery/3 Days/Single/NL/6 Days/$6.00/NR
747—Coleman/Virginia/Slave/New Orleans/20 Years/October 3/4PM/October 28/NA/28/H. J. Ranney/NL/$1.00/ Bronchitis/ 12 Days/Married/NL/26 Days/$26.00/NR

751—Daniel/Virginia/Slave/New Orleans/15 Years/October 12/12 Noon/October 16/NA/30/H. Brown/NL/$1.00/ Delirium Tremens/6 Hours/Single/NL/5 Days/ $5.00/NR

752—Sam/Virginia/Slave/New Orleans/10 Years/October 14/9AM/October 17/NA/35/T. J. Pipkin/NL/$1.00/ Injury of Hip/2 Hours/Single/NL/4 Days/$4.00/NR

754—John/Virginia/Slave/New Orleans/7 Days/October 15/7PM/October 21/NA/25/T. J. Pipkin/NL/$1.00/ Dysentery/1 Day/Single/NL/7 Days/$7.00/NR

755—Henry/Virginia/Slave/Alabama/2 Months/October 16/4PM/November 2/NA/27/C. W. Rutherford & Co./NL/$1.00/ Dysentery/2 Months/Single/NL/18 Days/$18.00/NR

756—Jim Butler/South Carolina/Slave/New Orleans/27 Years/ October 7/2PM/NL/November 7*/50/City of New Orleans/NL/$1.00/NL/2 Months/Single/NL/22 Days/$22.00/NR

757—Bob/Louisiana/Slave/New Orleans/16 Years/October 18/2PM/October 22/NA/28/T. J. Pipkin/NL/$1.00/ Intermittent/1 Week/Single/NL/5 Days/$5.00/NR

758—Thomas/Alabama/Slave/New Orleans/10 Years/October 19/8PM/October 21/NA/24/T. J. Pipkin/NL/$1.00/ Diarrhea/9 Days/Single/NL/3 Days/$3.00/NR

761—Woolford/Maryland/Slave/New Orleans/10 Years/October 21/11AM/November 7/NA/44/H.J. Ranney/NL/$1.00/ Dysentery/4 Days/Married/NL/18 Days/$18.00/NR

762—Robert/Virginia/Slaves/New Orleans/17 Years/October 22/11AM/October 25/NA/26/T. J. Pipkin/NL/$1.00/ Diarrhea/3 Days/Married/NL/4 Days/$4.00/NR

763—NL/Missouri/Slave/Cap Gararado/5 Years/October 23/8AM/NL/NA/16/Horrel Gayle & Co./NL/$1.00/ Syphilis/2 Months/Single/NL/39 Days/$39.00/NR

764—Tobe/North Carolina/Slave/Mississippi/7 Years/October 24/8AM/October 31/NA/36/T. J. Pipkin/NL/$1.00/ Intermittent/2 Days/Single/NL/8 Days/$8.00/NR

765—Franke/Virginia/Slave/Virginia/4 Years/October
26/8AM/October 31/NA/30/T. J. Pipkin/NL/$1.00/
Intermittent Fever/3 Days/Single/NL/6 Days/$6.00/NR
766—Thomas/North Carolina/Slave/North Carolina/6 Years/
October 28/8AM/November 6/NA/45/T. J.
Pipkin/NL/$1.00/ Dysentery/2 Months/Single/NL/10
Days/$10.00/NR
768—Abraham/Virginia/Slave/Virginia/15 Years/October
29/8AM/October 31/NA/25/T. J. Pipkin/NL/$1.00/
Constipation/1 Day/Single/NL/3 Days/$3.00/NR
769—Peter/Carolina/Slave/Mississippi/1 Day/October
29/NL/November 7/NA/46/Mr. Rock/NL/$1.00/
Pericarditis/3 Months/Single/NL/10 Days/$10.00/NR
771—William/North Carolina/Slave/North Carolina/5
Days/October 31/NL/NL/November 2*/24/Mr.
Matthews/NL/$1.00/ Nostalgia/1 Day/Single/NL/3
Days/$3.00/NR
772—Frank/Virginia/Slave/Virginia/4 Years/November
2/NL/November 6/NA/30/T. J. Pipkin/NL/$1.00/
Dysentery/2 Days/Single/NL/6 Days/$6.00/NR
773—Zachariah/North Carolina/Slave/North Carolina/17
Years/November 3/NL/November 23/NA/58/H. J.
Ranney/NL/$1.00/ Indisposition/NL/Single/NL/21
Days/$21.00/NR
780—Harriet/Virginia/Slave/New Orleans/2 Years/November
12/NL/November 29/NA/23/J. M. Putman/NL/$1.00/
Pregnant/9 Months/Married/NL/18 Days/$43.00/NR
781—Sam/S. Carolina/Slave/South Carolina/1 1/2 Years/
November 14/NL/NL/November 18*/44/Rutherford &
Long/ NL/$1.00/Typhoid Pneumonia/3 Day/Single/NL
/5 Days/ $5.00/NR
782—Louisa/Kentucky/Slave/Kentucky/2 Days/November
14/NL/December 2/NA/19/Horrel Gayle & Co./NL/
$1.00/Abortion /6 Months 4 Days/Married/NL/19
Days/$19.00/NR

SLAVERY AND MEDICINE: ENSLAVEMENT AND MEDICAL PRACTICES IN ANTEBELLUM LOUISIANA

783—John (Black)/Virginia/Slave/Virginia/4 Years/November 16/NL/December 6/NA/26/T. J. Pipkin/NL/$1.00/ Injury/2 Days/Single/NL/21 Days/$1.00/NR
784—James/Kentucky/Slave/Kentucky/4 Years/November 17/NL/November 25/NA/27/T. J. Pipkin/NL/$1.00/ Orchitis/2 Days/Single/NL/9 Days/$9.00/NR
785—John (Yellow)/Virginia/Slave/New Orleans/7 Years/ November 17/NL/November 2/NA/24/T. J. Pipkin/NL/$1.00/ Dysentery/1 Day/Single/NL/7 Days/$7.00/NR
786—Coleman/Virginia/Slave/Richmond/NL/November 18/NL/December 4/NA/25/T. J. Matthews/NL/$1.00/ Pneumonia/1 Month/Single/NL/17 Days/$17.00/NR
787—Violet & Child/Georgia/Slave/Louisiana/1 Day/November 19/NL/December 13/NA/27/Hall, Rodd & Putman/NL /$1.00/Anemia/ 3 Weeks/Married/NL/30 Days/ $45.00/NR
788—Henry/Maryland/Slave/Baltimore/28 Years/November 19/NL/November 24/NA/32/McGinnies/NL/ $1.00/ Rheumatism/4 Months/Married/NL/5 Days/$5.00/NR
789—John/Virginia/Slave/Mobile/1 Day/November 21/NL/ November 30/NA/24/John Foster/NL/$1.00/NL/ NL/Married/NL/10 Days/$10.00/NR
790—Louisa Hester/Kentucky/Slave/Kentucky/7 Days/ November 24/NL/NL/November 29*/19/W. L. Campbell/NL/$1.00/ Peritonitis/NL/Married/NL/6 Days/$6.00/NR
791—Daniel Brown/NL/Slave/NL/NL/November 23/NL/ November 27/NL/NL/NL/NL/$1.00/ Injury/NL/NL/ NL / NL/$20.00/NR
792—Charley/Kentucky/Slave/New Orleans/6 Years/November 28/NL/December 9/NA/26/T. J. Pipkin/NL/$1.00/ NL/3 Weeks/Single/NL/12 Days/$12.00/NR
795—Frank/Virginia/Slave/Virginia/4 Years/December 8/NL/December 21/NA/30/T. J. Pipkin/NL/$1.00/NL /2 Days/Single/NL/14 Days/$14.00/NR

SLAVERY AND MEDICINE: ENSLAVEMENT AND MEDICAL PRACTICES IN
ANTEBELLUM LOUISIANA

796—Elizabeth/Virginia/Slave/Mobile/10 Years/December
   10/NL/December 29/NA/34/L. C. Levy/NL/$1.00/
   Injury/2 Days/NL/NL/20 Days/$20.00/NR
797—Marie/New Orleans/Slave/New Orleans/19 Years/
   December 14/NL/January 5, 1858/NA/19/William C.
   Macon/NL/$1.00/ Pregnant/9 Months/NL/NL/23
   Days/$48.00/NR
798—Isum/Virginia/NL/Mississippi/10 Years/December
   21/NL/December 23, 1857/NA/47/Denis Donovan/
   NL/$1.00/ Pneumonia/7 Days/NL/NL/3 Days/
   $3.00/NR
799—Eliza/New Orleans/NL/New Orleans/22 Years/December
   21/NL/January 13, 1858/NA/22/Jas. Stockton/NL/
   $1.00/ Pregnant/9 Months/NL/NL/24 Days/$49.00/NR
800—Arzeno/New Orleans/NL/New Orleans/40 Years/
   December 22/NL/NL/NA/NL/A. W. Walker/NL/
   $1.00/Chronic Diarrhea/2 Years/NL/NL/NL/NL/NR
801—Ben/Louisiana/Slave/New Orleans/50 Years/December
   22/NL/NL/NA/56/A. W. Walker/NL/$1.00/
   Frostbitten/NL/1 Month/NL/NL/NL/NR
802—Jerry/Georgia/Slave/Mobile/19 Months/December
   23/NL/December 25, 1857/NA/24/D. Madden/NL/
   $1.00/Catarrh/1 Week/NL/NL/3 Days/$3.00/NR
803—William/Virginia/Slave/Virginia/2 Years/December
   24/NL/January 10, 1858/NA/38/Dr. Holmes/NL/$1.00
   / Anemia/NL/NL/NL/18 Days/$20.30/NR
804—Jerry/Georgia/Slave/New Orleans/19 Months/December
   28/NL/January 1/NA/24/D. Madden/Diarrhea/
   NL/NL/5 Days/NL/NL/NL/NL/NR

SLAVERY AND MEDICINE: ENSLAVEMENT AND MEDICAL PRACTICES IN ANTEBELLUM LOUISIANA

1858

806—Abram/Virginia/Slave/Virginia/20 Years/January 1, 1858/NL/January 11, 1858/NA/25/T. J. Pipkin/ NL/$1.00/NL/3 Days/Single/NL/11 Days/NL/NR

807—Bob/Kentucky/Slave/Kentucky/30 Years/January 1/NL/January 23/NA/45/S. Boyd/NL/$1.00/Injury of Thumb/4 Days/Married/NL/25 Days/NL/NR

808—Shawney/Georgia/Slave/Georgia/1 Year/January 2/NL/February 20/NA/26/J. H. Longsfield/ NL/$1.00/Typhoid Fever/8 Months/Single/NL/50 Days/NL/NR

809—Jerry/Virginia/Slave/Virginia/5 Years/January 5/NL/ January 10/NA/30/D. Madden/NL/ $1.00/Injury/ NL/NL/NL/4 Days/NL/NR

811—Gilbert/North Carolina/Slave/North Carolina/17 Years/January 11/NL/February 4/NA/20/T. J. Pipkin/NL/$1.00/ Phthisis/2 Months/Single/NL/25 Days/NL/NR

812—Jerry/Georgia/Slave/Georgia/2 Months/January 16/NL/February 11/NA/24/D. Madden/NL/$1.00/ Typhoid Pneumonia/NL/Single/NL/27 Days/NL/NR

813—Eliza/Louisiana/Slave/New Orleans/22 Years/January 16/NL/January 18/NA/22/J. Stockton/NL/$1.00/ Indisposition/ NL/Single/NL/3 Days/NL/NR

816—Jim/Virginia/Slave/Virginia/30 Years/January 19/NL/NL/NA/55/Maj. Ranney/NL/$1.00/3 Days/Married/NL/14 Days/NL/NR

817—Cyrus/Virginia/Slave/Virginia/3 Years/January 21/NL/January 25/NA/30/T. J. Pipkin/NL/$1.00/4 Days/Single/NL/5 Days/NL/NR

818—Henry/South Carolina/Slave/South Carolina/11 Years/ January 27/NL/February 5/NA/32/T. D. Van Horn/NL/$1.00/NL/2 Months/Married/NL/10 Days/NL/NR

819—Tony/South Carolina/Slave/New Orleans/20 Years/January 30/NL/February 11/NA/42/H. J. Ranney/NL/$1.00/ NL/3 Days/ Married/NL/12 Days/NL/NR
820—Bob/Connecticut/Slave/New Orleans/5 Years/January 31/NL/NL/February 2*/30/H. H. Hansell/NL/$1.00/ Consumption/1 Year/Single/NL/3 Days/NL/NR
822—Jack/New Orleans/Slave/New Orleans/23 Years/February 6/NL/February 11/NA/23/H. J. Ranney/NL/$1.00/ Indisposition/2 Months/Single/NL/6 Days/NL/NR
823—Moses/Virginia/Slave/New Orleans/30 Years/February 13/NL/April 7/NA/41/Leeds & Co./NL/$1.00/ Delirium Tremens/1 Year/Single/NL/NL/NL/NR
824—Hannah/Louisiana/Slave/Centerville/4 Hours/February 17/NL/April 23/NA/33/Hall Rodd & Putman/ NL/$1.00/NL/5 Years/Single/NL/ NL/NL/NR
825—Frank/Virginia/Slave/Virginia/5 Years/February 18/NL/April 25/NA/32/T. J. Pipkin/NL/$1.00/ Indisposition/1 Day/Single/NL/8 Days/NL/NR
826—Charlotte & Child/Louisiana/Slave/Louisiana/1 Day/February 19/NL/March 5/NA/36/F. Foster/ NL/$1.00/ Indisposition/1 Day/Single/NL/15 Days/NL/NR
827—Baptiste/Louisiana/Slave/Louisiana/1 Day/February 19/NL/March 5/NA/10/F. Foster/NL/$1.00/ Indisposition/1 Day/Single/NL/15 Days/NL/NR
828—George/Louisiana/Slave/Louisiana/1 Day/February 19/NL/March 5/NA/5/F. Foster/NL/$1.00/ Indisposition/1 Day/Single/NL/15 Days/NL/NR
829—Maria/Louisiana/Slave/Louisiana/1 Day/February 19/NL//March 5/NA/3/F. Foster/NL/$1.00/ Indisposition/1 Day/Single/NL/15 Days/NL/NR
830—Charley/Kentucky/Slave/Kentucky/6 Years/February 22/NL/February 27/NA/29/T. J. Pipkin/NL/$1.00/ Dysentery/3 Days/Single/NL/6 Days/NL/NR

SLAVERY AND MEDICINE: ENSLAVEMENT AND MEDICAL PRACTICES IN ANTEBELLUM LOUISIANA

831—Abraham/Virginia/Slave/Virginia/20 Years/February 27/NL/March 7/NA/25/T. J. Pipkin/NL/$1.00/ Catarrh/1 Week/Single/NL/14 Days/NL/NR
832—Jim/South Carolina/Slave/South Carolina/3 Weeks/ February 27/NL/May 19/NA/NL/J. Boyd/NL/$1.00/ Bronchitis/ NL/Single/NL/NL/NL/NR
833—Nancy/Georgia/Slave/Montgomery/1 Day/February 25/NL/March 5/NA/32/McQueen/NL/$1.00/ Catarrh/NL/Single/NL/9 Days/NL/NR
834—Fanny/Georgia/Slave/Montgomery/1 Day/February 25/NL/ March 5/NA/4/McQueen/NL/$1.00/Catarrh/1 Day/Single/NL/9 Days/NL/NR
835—Sam Absolom/Alabama/Slave/Alabama/2 Weeks/February 26/NL/March 12/NA/35/F. Foster/NL/$1.00/ Measles/6 Days/Single/NL/15 Days/NL/NR
836—Ben/Maryland/Slave/Baltimore/3 Years/February 28/NL/March 21/NA/28/J. D. Brown/NL/$1.00/ Secondary Syphilis/10 Weeks/Single/NL/NL/NL/NR
837—Alfred/Alabama/Slave/Alabama/5 Years/March 1/NL/March 5/NA/24/T. J. Pipkin/NL/$1.00/ Variola/2 Days/Single/NL/5 Days/NL/NR
838—Horace/Alabama/Slave/Alabama/5 Years/March 1/NL/March 5/NA/24/T. J. Pipkin/NL/$1.00/ Variola/5 Days/Single/NL/5 Days/NL/NR
849?[839]—Joseph/New Orleans/Slave/New Orleans/NL/March 2/NL/March 9/NA/37/D. S. Graham/NL/$1.00/ Injury/1 Day/ Single/NL/8 Days/NL/NR
840—Bob/Louisiana/Slave/Louisiana/12 Years/March 2/NL/March 5/NA/32/T. J. Pipkin/NL/$1.00/NL/1 Day/Single/NL/4 Days/NL/NR
842—Solomon/South Carolina/Slave/South Carolina/3 Days/March 9/NL/March 13/NA/NL/F. Foster/NL/$1.00/Fever/18 Hours/Single/NL/5 Days/NL/NR

SLAVERY AND MEDICINE: ENSLAVEMENT AND MEDICAL PRACTICES IN
ANTEBELLUM LOUISIANA

843—Mooney/Georgia/Slave/Georgia/7 Days/March 9/NL/March 13/NA/NL/Foster/NL/$1.00/Fever/18 Hours/Single/NL/5 Days/NL/NR
844—Lucy/Alabama/Slave/Alabama/1 Week/March 9/NL/March 14/NA/15/F. Foster/NL/$1.00/Fever/12 Hours/Single/NL/6 Days/$6.00/NR
846—Lucinda/Georgia/Slave/Georgia/NL/March 10/NL/NL/March 17*/13/F. Foster/NL/$1.00/ Pleuropneumonia/1 Day/Single/NL/8 Days/$8.00/$12 Burial Expenses
847—Cyrus/South Carolina/Slave/Mobile/2 Weeks/March 11/NL/March 22/NA/24/F. Foster/NL/$1.00/ Tumour/3 Days/NL/NL/11 Days/$1.00/ NR
848—Tucker/Virginia/NL/Mississippi/2 Weeks/March 12/NL/ March 21/NA/33/G. R. King/NL/$1.00/Dysentery/3 Days/NL/10 Days/$10.00/NR
849—Ceasar/Georgia/NL/Mississippi/3 Years/March 12/NL/April 24/NA/30/H. B. Philips/NL/$1.00/ Indurated Gland/2 Weeks/NL/NL/NL/NL/NR
850—Sila/Alabama/Slave/Alabama/2 Months/March 13/NL/April 2/NA/NL/F. Foster/NL/$1.00/ Indispisition/NL/NL/NL/21 Days/$21.00/Metzger & Heinshfield
851—Alfred/Alabama/Slave/Alabama/2 Months/March 13/NL/April 2/NA/NL/F. Foster/NL/$1.00/Measles/3 Days/NL/NL/21 Days/$21.00/Metzger & Heinshfield
852—Alfred/Alabama/Slave/Alabama/2 Months/March 13/NL/April 2/NA/NL/F. Foster/NL/$1.00/Measles/5 Days/NL/NL/21 Days/$21.00/Metzgter & Heinshfield
853—Theresa & Infant/Louisiana/Slave/Louisiana/3 Weeks/March 13/NL/March 18/NA/NL/F. Foster/NL/ $1.00/Catarrh/NL/NL/NL/6 Days/$6.00/NR
854—Donelson/Louisiana/Slave/Louisiana/3 Weeks/March 13/NL/ March 18/NA/NL/F. Foster/NL/$1.00/ Fever/NL/NL/NL/6 Days/ $6.00/NR

SLAVERY AND MEDICINE: ENSLAVEMENT AND MEDICAL PRACTICES IN ANTEBELLUM LOUISIANA

855—Mary/Louisiana/Slave/Louisiana/3 Weeks/March 13/NL/March 18/NA/NL/F. Foster/NL/$1.00/Catarrh/NL/NL/Nl/6 Days/$6.00/NR
856—Frank/Louisiana/Slave/Louisiana/3 Weeks/March 13/NL/March 18/NA/NL/F. Foster/NL/$1.00/Catarrh/NL/NL/NL/6 Days/$6.00/NR
857—Clory/Georgia/Slave/Georgia/3 Weeks/NL/NL/March 22/NA/NL/F. Foster/NL/$1.00/Indisposition/NL/NL/NL/10 Days/$10.00/NR
858—March/Georgia/Slave/Georgia/3 Weeks/March 13/NL/March 22/NA/NL/F. Foster/NL/$1.00/Worms/NL/NL/NL/10 Days/$10.00/NR
859—Albert/Georgia/Slave/Georgia/3 Weeks/March 13/NL/March 18/NA/NL/F. Foster/NL/$1.00/Catarrh/NL/NL/NL/10 Days/$10.00/NR
860—Matt/South Carolina/Slave/Mississippi/3 Weeks/March 13/NL/March 18/NA/22/F. Foster/NL/$1.00/Inter. Fever/1 Day/Single/NL/6 Days/$6.00/NR
861—Frank/Louisiana/Slave/Louisiana/2 Weeks/March 14/NL/March 31/NA/19/F. Foster/NL/$1.00/Roseola/2 Days/Single/NL/18 Days/$18.00/NR
862—John/Virginia/Slave/New Orleans/16 Years/March 15/NL/March 20/NA/27/Pierce/NL/$1.00/Injury of Hand/8 Days/Single/NL/5 Days/$5.00/NR
863—William/Alabama/Slave/New Orleans/NL/NL/NL/April 6/NA/NL/McCann & Patterson/NL/$1.00/Pleuro Pneumonia/6 Day/Married/NL/21 Days/$21.00/NR
864—Sam Absolom/Alabama/Slave/Alabama/4 Weeks/March 17/NL/March 31/NA/35/F. Foster/NL/$1.00/Roseola/1 Day/Single/NL/15 Days/$15.00/NR
865—Abraham/Virginia/Slave/Virginia/2 Years/March 18/NL/NL/March 19*/25/T. J. Pipkin/NL/$1.00/Congestion of Brain/5 Days/Single/NL/2 Days/$2.00/Funeral Expenses $10.00

SLAVERY AND MEDICINE: ENSLAVEMENT AND MEDICAL PRACTICES IN ANTEBELLUM LOUISIANA

867—Aleck/New Orleans/Slave/New Orleans/30 Years/March 19/NL/March 21/NA/30/H. B. Philips/NL/$1.00/Dysentery/1 Day/Married/NL/3 Days/$3.00/NR
868—America/Kentucky/Slave/Arkansas/2 Weeks/March 22/NL/March 31/NA/22/F. Foster/NL/$1.00/Fever/3 Days/Married/NL/10 Days/$10.00/NR
869—Amanda/Virginia/Slave/Mississippi/3 Weeks/March 22/NL/April 23/NA/28/F. Foster/NL/$1.00/Measles/2 Weeks/Single/NL/NL/NL/NR
870—Sarah/Alabama/Slave/Alabama/3 Weeks/March 23/NL/April 7/NA/23/F. Foster/NL/$1.00/Catarrh/9 Days/Single/NL/NL/NL/NR
871—Lucy/Alabama/Slave/Alabama/2 Weeks/March 23/NL/April 19/NA/15/F. Foster/NL/$1.00/Fever/3 Days/Single/NL/NL/NL/NR
872—Judy/South Carolina/Slave/South Carolina/1 Week/March 23/NL/April 7/NA/15/F. Foster/NL/$1.00/Measles/2 Days/Single/NL/NL/NL/NR
874—Harriet/Kentucky/Slave/Kentucky/1 Year/March 26/NL/April 20/NA/24/C. M. Rutherford & Co./NL/$1.00/ Poisoned by Oak Vine/1 Week/Single/NL/NL/NL/NR
875—Aleck/Texas/Slave/Texas/1 Week/March 26/NL/April 19/NA/26/F. Foster/NL/$1.00/Pneumonia/4 Days/Single/ NL/NL/NL/NR
876—Coleman/Virginia/Slave/New Orleans/20 Years/March 28/NL/May 17/NA/69/H. J. Ranney/NL/$1.00/Pneumonia/2 Weeks/Married/NL/NL/NL/NR
877—George/Virginia/Slave/Virginia/3 Weeks/March 28/NL/April 16/NA/18/F. Foster/NL/$1.00/Dysentery/2 Weeks/Single/NL/NL/NL/NR
878—Jordan/North Carolina/Slave/North Carolina/NL/March 28/NL/April 16/NA/19/F. Foster/NL/$1.00/Pneumonia/2 Weeks/Single/NL/NL/NL/NR

SLAVERY AND MEDICINE: ENSLAVEMENT AND MEDICAL PRACTICES IN ANTEBELLUM LOUISIANA

879—Morning/Georgia/Slave/Georgia/4 Weeks/April 3/NL/April 25/NA/14/F. Foster/NL/$1.00/Measles/1 Day/Single/NL/NL/NL/NR
880—Austin/North Carolina/Slave/North Carolina/2 Years/April 6/NL/April 10/NA/28/H. M. Hays/NL/$1.00/ Dysentery/6 Days/Single/NL/NL/NL/NR
881—Claracy/Virginia/Slave/Louisiana/5 Hours/April 6/NL/April 5/NA/48/Col. R. A. Stewart/NL/$1.00/NL/2 Years/Married/NL/NL/NL/NR
882—Will Christian/Virginia/Slave/New Orleans/37 Years/April 7/NL/April 12/NA/64/H. J. Ranney/NL/$1.00/Intermittent/4 Days/Married/NL/6 Days/NL/NR
883—Flora/Virginia/Slave/Louisiana/15 Years/April 8/NL/April 12/NA/40/Col. R. A. Stewart/NL/$1.00/Phthisis/1 1/2 Years/Single/NL/5 Days/NL/NR
884—Chas. Phillips/Maryland/Slave/Mississippi/3 Years/April 9/NL/April 21/NA/40/H. M. Hays/NL/ $1.00/ Hydrocele/3 Months/Married/NL/12 Days/NL/NR
885—Edmund Brown/Virginia/Slave/Mississippi/15 Years/April 16/NL/June NL/NA/30/W. M. Stewall/NL/$1.00/ Fistula in Neck/2 1/2 Months/Married/NL/66 Days/NL/NR
886—Robert/Virginia/Slave/New Orleans/9 Years/April 19/NL/April 26/NA/23/H. J. Ranney/NL/$1.00/ Dislocation of the Arm/1 Day/Married/NL/8 Days/NL/NR
887—Mathilde/Louisiana/Slave/Louisiana/4 Years/April 19/NL/June 1/NA/15/Col. R. A. Stewart/NL/$1.00/NL /6 Months/Married/NL/44 Days/NL/NR
888—William/South Carolina/Slave/New Orleans/5 Years/April 21/NL/May 31/NA/30/John M. Bell/NL/$1.00/Tertiary Syphilis/2 Months/Single/NL/41 Days/NL/NR
889—Harriet/Kentucky/Slave/Kentucky/1 Year/April 22/NL/May 5/NA/24/Smith & Harris/NL/$1.00/ Fever/2 Days/Single/NL/14 Days/NL/NR

SLAVERY AND MEDICINE: ENSLAVEMENT AND MEDICAL PRACTICES IN
ANTEBELLUM LOUISIANA

891—John/Maryland/Slave/New Orleans/4 Years/April
25/NL/July 24/NA/26/J. Calder/$130.00/$1.00/Comp.
dislocation of Toe/3 Hours/Single/NL/91 Days/NL/NR
892—George/Alabama/Slave/New Orleans/NL/April
26/NL/May 29/NA/26/W. J. Poitevent/NL/$1.00/
Injury of Elbow Joint/1 Day/Single/NL/34
Days/NL/NR
893—Henry/Louisiana/Slave/New Orleans/24 Years/April
26/NL/June 1/NA/24/W. ?/NL/$1.00/Rhumatism/1
Week/ Single/NL/37 Days/NL/NR
894—Wolford/Maryland/Slave/New Orleans/10 Years/May
1/NL/May 4/NA/44/Maj. H. J. Ranney/NL/$1.00/
Diarrhea/2 Weeks/Single/NL/4 Days/NL/NR
895—Alice/Maryland/Slave/Louisiana/6 Years/May 3/NL/June
5/NA/35/Col. R. A. Stewart/NL/$1.00/Uterine
Disease/4 Weeks/Married/NL/34 Days/NL/NR
896—Aleck/Texas/Slave/Texas/1 Months/May 3/NL/June
11/NA/26/Edward Pillsbury/NL/$1.00/Pneumonia/2
Days/Married/NL/40 Days/NL/NR
897—Tom/Louisville/Slave/New Orleans/3 Years/May
4/NL/June 14/NA/24/W. Colter/NL/$1.00/Syphilis/3
Months/Married/NL/42 Days/NL/NR
898—Juliane/Virginia/Slave/Louisiana/1 Hour/May 8/NL/June
1/NA/30/Col. R. A. Stewart/NL/$1.00/
Dysmenorrhea/14 Months/Married/NL/24
Days/NL/NR
899—Willis/Louisiana/Slave/Louisiana/1 Hour/May 8/NL/June
1/NA/5/Col. R. A. Stewart/NL/$1.00/Chronic
Gastritis/4 Years/——/NL/24 Days/NL/NR
900—Nancy Ann/North Carolina/Slave/Arkansas/2 Weeks/May
8/NL/NL/July 25*/17/O. G. Cromwell/NL/$1.00/
Gonorrhea/6 Weeks/Single/NL/NL/NL/NR
901—Dick/North Carolina/Slave/Louisiana/22 Years/May
18/NL/May 19/NA/32/W. H. Carre' & Co./NL/$1.00/
Sprain/3 Weeks/Single/NL/4 Days/NL/NR

902—Reuben/Mississippi/Slave/Mississippi/3 Days/May
   18/NL/May 23/NA/24/W. H. Carre' & Co./NL/$1.00/
   Dysentery/4 Weeks/Single/NL/6 Days/NL/NR
904—Jack/North Carolina/Slave/Mississippi/1 Month/May
   21/NL/July 10/NA/37/W. J. Poitenvent/NL/$1.00/
   Secondary Syphilis/1 Week/Single/NL/51 Days/NL/NR
906—Anderson/Mississippi/Slave/New Orleans/4 Days/May
   22/NL/May 29/NA/24/W. J. Poitevent/NL/$1.00/
   Injury of Eye/1 Week/Single/NL/7 Days/NL/NR
907—Tom/Virginia/Slave/New Orleans/Several Years/May
   28/NL/May 30/NA/35/W. Levy/NL/$1.00/Diarrhea/1
   Day/Married/NL/3 Days/NL/NR
908—Thomas/Maryland/Slave/New Orleans/40 Years/May
   30/NL/NL/June 6*/48/John Turpin/NL/$1.00/
   Dropsy/6 Weeks/Married/NL/10 Days/NL/NR
910—Reuben/Mississippi/Slave/Mississippi/2 Days/June
   2/NL/June 9/NA/24/W. W. Carre' &
   Co./NL/$1.00/Diarrhea/4 Days/Single/NL/8
   Days/NL/NR
911—Henry/North Carolina/Slave/North Carolina/30
   Years/June 2/NL/June 17/NA/55/G. C. Bogart/NL/
   $1.00/Hemorrhoids/14 Days/Married/NL/16
   Days/NL/NR
912—Ann/Virginia/Slave/Virginia/14 Years/June 7/NL/June
   13/NA/40/Maj. H. J. Ranney/NL/$1.00/Pleuritis/4
   Days/Married/NL/7 Days/NL/NR
913—William/Virginia/Slave/Virginia/46 Years/June 8/NL/June
   26/NA/60/Capt. Cousin/NL/$1.00/Rheumatism/3
   Days/Married/NL/ 19 Days/NL/NR
914—Deacon/New Orleans/Slave/New Orleans/30 Years/June
   9/NL/June 28/NA/30/Will Batson/NL/$1.00/
   Ulceration of Rectum/9 Days/Married/NL/ 18
   Days/NL/NR
915—Fortune/Arkansas/Slave/Arkansas/2 Years/June
   10/NL/June 30/NA/22/Thos. McKnight/NL/$1.00/
   NL/6 Days/Single/NL/21 Days/NL/NR

SLAVERY AND MEDICINE: ENSLAVEMENT AND MEDICAL PRACTICES IN
ANTEBELLUM LOUISIANA

916—Henry/North Carolina/Slave/Louisiana/6 Months/June 11/NL/NL/June 17*/22/C. F. Hatcher/NL/$1.00/ Typhoid Fever/6 Weeks/Single/NL/7 Days/NL/NR
917—Charlotte/North Carolina/Slave/North Carolina/7 Months/June 22/NL/September 18/NA/23/Ms. Graham/NL/$1.00/ Epilepsy/2 Days/Single/NL/NL/NL/NR
918—William/South Carolina/Slave/New Orleans/5 Years/June 23/NL/October 7/NA/30/John M. Bell/NL/$1.00/ Tertiary Syphilis/3 Days/Single/NL/NL/NL/NR
919—Dock/Virginia/Slave/Louisiana/——/June 23/NL/NL/June 23*/NL/R. C. Cummings & Co./NL/$1.00/Dropsy/NL/ Single/NL/15 Days/NL/NR
920—John/New Orleans/Slave/Louisiana/16 Years/June 26/NL/June 30/NA/16/W. W. Carre' & Co./NL/$1.00/ Epilepsy/8 Days/Single/NL/5 Days/NL/NR
922—Edward/Missouri/Slave/New Orleans/20 Years/June 29/NL/July 15/NA/30/Mr. Yancy/NL/$1.00/Cut in Hand and Arm/NL/Single/NL/17 Days/NL/NR
926—William/North Carolina/Slave/New Orleans/3 Years/July 13/NL/July 19/NA/35/B. W. Huntington/NL/$1.00/ Diarrhea/1 Week/Single/NL/7 Days/NL/NR
927—Jim Leathers/Tennessee/Slave/New Orleans/NL/July 13/NL/July 19/NA/23/Capt. T. Leathers/NL/$1.00/ Diarrhea/1 Day/Single/NL/5 Days/NL/NR
929—Harriet/Florida/Slave/Texas/2 Weeks/July 16/NL/NL/ August 29*/17/R. Brenan/NL/$1.00/Secondary Syphilis/2 Weeks/Single/NL/NL/NL/NR
932—Jim/Virginia/Slave/Virginia/8 Years/July 19/NL/NL/July 24*/35/W. Colter/NL/$1.00/Chronic Dysentery/3 Weeks/Single/ NL/5 Days/NL/NR
933—Woolford/Maryland/Slave/New Orleans/24 Years/July 19/NL/July 27/NA/NL/Maj. H. J. Ranney/NL/$1.00/ Diarrhea/1 Day/Single/NL/9 Days/NL/NR

936—Jane/Virginia/Slave/Baton Rouge/15 Years/July
21/NL/August 6/NA/40/E. W. Rodd/NL/$1.00/
Neuralgia/3 Months/Married/NL/NL/NL/NR
943—William Thomas/Virginia/Slave/Baltimore/11 Years/July
23/NL/July 30/NA/22/H. J. Ranney/NL/$1.00/
Diarrhea/2 Days/Single/NL/8 Days/NL/NR
944—Patty Mussina/Baltimore/Slave/Mobile/6 Months/July
23/NL/NL/August 4*/65/J. Mussina/NL/$1.00/
Schirrus of Gland/6 Months/Single/NL/NL/NL/NR
945—York/South Carolina/Slave/South Carolina/20 Years/July
23/NL/July 30/NA/45/William Batson/NL/$1.00/
Remitt. Fever/4 Days/Single/NL/8 Days/NL/NR
948—Richard/South Carolina/Slave/Alabama/12 Years/July
27/NL/August 2/NA/27/William Batson/NL/$1.00/
Chronic Diarrhea/2 1/2 Days/Married/NL/7
Days/NL/NR
949—James/Virginia/Slave/Virginia/30 Years/July
27/NL/August 5/NA/43/W. J. Poitevent/NL/$1.00/
Chronic Diarrhea/4 Weeks/Single/NL/NL/NL/NR
950—Ben/Virginia/Slave/Virginia/16 Years/July 28/NL/August
3/NA/26/Jos. Stinson/NL/$1.00/NL Bilious Remitt./2
Days/Single/NL/NL/NL/NR
951—Basil/Maryland/Slave/Maryland/12 Years/July
28/NL/August 16/NA/28/H. J. Ranney/NL/$1.00/Cut
on the Arm/4 Days/Single/NL/6 Days/NL/NR
952—Joseph/Louisiana/Slave/Louisiana/22 Years/July
29/NL/August 2/NA/22/D. Graham/NL/$1.00/
Constipation/4 Days/Married/NL/5 Days/NL/NR
953—Horace/Virginia/Slave/Baltimore/7 Years/July
29/NL/August 6/NA/20/H. J. Ranney/NL/$1.00/
Epilepsy/1 Day/Single/NL/NL/NL/NR
959—Lisy Ann/North Carolina/Slave/Virginia/1 Year/August
3/NL/September 2/NA/NL/Thos. Wilbur/NL/$1.00/
Ulcer on Leg/3 Months/Single/NL/NL/NL/NR

960—Jack/North Carolina/Slave/Mississippi/2 Months/August 3/NL/September 2/NA/37/W. J. Poitevent/NL/$1.00/ Syphilitic Iretis/2 1/2 Days/Single/NL/NL/NL/NR

962—Jimmy/New Orleans/Slave/New Orleans/5 Years/August 3/NL/August 10/NA/5/Thos. F. Patton/NL/$1.00/ Convulsions/1 1/2 Days/Single/NL/7 Days/NL/NR

963—Richard/South Carolina/Slave/Alabama/12 Years/August 4/NL/NL/NA/27/William Batson/NL/$1.00/Chronic Diarrhea/1 Day/Married/NL/NL/NL/NR

964—Denis/Virginia/Slave/Mobile/3 Months/August 3/NL/August 12/NA/30/George Bates/NL/$1.00/ Chronic Diarrhea/1 Day/ Married/NL/8 Days/NL/NR

965—York/South Carolina/Slave/South Carolina/20 Years/ August 5/NL/August 23/NA/45/William Batson/NL/ $1.00/ Rheumatism/1 Day/Married/NL/NL/NL/NR

975—Lewis/Virginia/Slave/Virginia/NL/August 9/NL/NL/NA/ 40/Dr. Knapp/NL/$1.00/ Hemiplegia/2 Weeks/Single/NL/NL/NL/NR

976—Phil/Virginia/Slave/Virginia/3 Years/August 10/NL/NL/ August 21*/35/Adler Phillips/NL/$1.00/NL/2 Weeks/Single/ NL/NL/NL/NR

981—Colter/Virginia/Slave/Virginia/5 Years/August 14/NL/NL/ September 11*/30/John Gale/NL/$1.00/ Ulceration of Rectum/2 Years/Single/NL/NL/NL/NR

990—Alfred/Baltimore/Slave/Baltimore/2 Years/August 21/NL/ NL/September 11*/32/George Bates/NL/$1.00/Injury of Eyelid/4 Day/Single/NL/NL/NL/NR

993—Tom/Louisville/Slave/Vicksburg/3 Months/August 21/NL/ NL/August 24/NA/24/Capt. Leathers/NL/$1.00/NL/3 Days/Single/ NL/NL/NR

997—Joseph/Virginia/Slave/Virginia/5 Years/August 23/NL/ NL/August 30*/27/H. J. Ranney/NL/$1.00/NL/1 Day/Single/ NL/NL/NL/NR

1008—Jane/Virginia/Slave/Baton Rouge/15 Years/August 24/NL/ NL/September 17*/40/E. W. Rodd/NL/$1.00/NL/1 Week/NL/NL/NL/ NL/NR

SLAVERY AND MEDICINE: ENSLAVEMENT AND MEDICAL PRACTICES IN ANTEBELLUM LOUISIANA

1029—Fortune/Arkansas/Slave/Arkansas/2 Years/August 30/NL/September 6/NA/22/Thos. McKnight/NL/ $1.00/ Dysentery/ NL/Single/NL/NL/NL/NR

1062—Mathilda/North Carolina/Slave/Par of Catahoula (?)/2 Years/September 6/NL/September 19/NA/40/W. Van Benthayzen/ NL/$1.00/NL/1 Day/Single/NL/NL/ NL/NR

1066—Ann/Virginia/Slave/Virginia/3 Years/September 6/NL/ September 19/NA/35/Judge Bradford/NL/$1.00/Yellow Fever/1 Hour/Married/NL/NL/NL/NR

1070—Dover/Virginia/Slave/Opelousas/2 Years/September 8/NL/September 9/NA/20/Judge Bradford/NL/$1.00/ NL /15 Days/Single/NL/NL/NL/NR

1145—Deacon/New Orleans/Slave/New Orleans/28 Years/ September 20/NL/October 19/NA/28/William Batson/NL/ $1.00/NL/1 Day/Single/NL/NL/NL/NR

1147—Minerva Jane/Missouri/Slave/New Orleans/10 Years/ September 20/NL/September 27/NA/30/George Henderson (NL)/$5.00/$1.00/Yellow Fever/NL/ Married/ NL/NL/NL/NR

1150—Minerva/Louisville/Slave/Louisville/4 Years/September 20/NL/October 5/NA/19/David Bridwell/NL/$1.00 /Yellow Fever/NL/Single/NL/NL/NL/NR

1151—Charlotte/North Carolina/Slave/Red River/8 Years/ September 27/NL/October 2/NA/55/R. B. Post/NL/ $1.00/ Injury of Hand/1 Week/Married/NL/NL/ NL/NR

1165—Susan/Virginia/Slave/Texas/NL/September 15/NL/ September 29/NA/31/Capt. Huggins/NL/$1.00/Yellow Fever/NL/ Married/NL/NL/NL/NR

1195—Amos/Bayou Sara/Slave/Opelousas/2 Years/September 29/NL/NL/NA/22/Judge Bradford/NL/$1.00/Yellow Fever/1 1/2 Day/Single/NL/NL/NL/NR

1200—Nelson/NL/Slave/NL/NL/September 30/NL/October 11/NL/NA/NL/H. J. Ranney/NL/$1.00/Injury/ NL/NL/NL/NL/NR

SLAVERY AND MEDICINE: ENSLAVEMENT AND MEDICAL PRACTICES IN ANTEBELLUM LOUISIANA

1215—Ben/Virginia/Slave/Vicksburg/NL/October 8/NL/NL/ November 11*/NL/Col. Watson/NL/$1.00/ Consumption/1 Week/Single/NL/NL/NL/NR

1217—Harrison/Mississippi/Slave/Mississippi/2 Years/October 8/NL/October 12/NA/16/D. Bidwell/NL/$1.00/Yellow Fever/1 Day/Single/NL/NL/NL/NR

1218—Nathan/Maryland/Slave/Maryland/14 Years/October 9/NL/October 16/NA/34/H. J. Ranney/NL/$1.00/ Injury/1 1/2 Day/Single/NL/NL/NL/NR

1222—Lucinda/Kentucky/Slave/Louisville/13 Years/October 19/NL/October 14/NA/29/McKnight/NL/ $1.00/Yellow Fever/3 Days/Married/NL/NL/NL/NR

1225—Frank/Virginia/Slave/Arkansas/11 Months/October 13/NL/October 20/NA/24/T. S. Turner/NL/$1.00/ Yellow Fever/1/2 Day/Single/NL/NL/NL/NR

1226—Minerva/Georgia/Slave/Texas/2 Years/October 13/NL/ October 18/NA/32/L. N. Lane/NL/$1.00/Yellow Fever/1 Day/ Married/NL/NL/NL/NR

1236—William/North Carolina/Slave/North Carolina/4 Days/October 19/NL/October 38/NA/35/B. W. Huntington/NL/ $1.00/Yellow Fever/1 Week/Single/ NL/NL/NL/NR

1238—Herod/Virginia/Slave/Mobile/28 Years/October 21/NL/October 23/NA/43/William Brown/NL/$1.00/ Diarrhea/2 Weeks/Single/NL/NL/NL/NR

1241—Ann/Virginia/Slave/Coast/2 Years/October 22/NL/October 25/NA/40/H. J. Ranney/NL/$1.00/ Indisposition/5 Days/ Married/NL/NL/NL/NR

1242—Reid/New Orleans/Slave/New Orleans/5 Years/October 22/NL/October 25/NA/5/H. J. Ranney/NL/$1.00/ Intermittent Fever/5 Days/Single/NL/NL/NL/NR

1253—Simpson/Kentucky/Slave/Kentucky/11 Years/October 28/NL/November 1/NA/26/J. Morton/NL/$1.00/ Dysentery/1 Day/Married/NL/NL/NL/NR

1258—Louis/Virginia/Slave/Virginia/13 Years/November 3/NL/November 19/NA/40/Dennis Donnovan/NL/ $1.00/Gastro Enteritis/4 Days/Single/NL/NL/NL/NR

1263— William/NL/Slave/NL/NL/November/NL/NL/NL/NA/NL/H. J. Ranney/NL/$1.00/NL/NL /NL/NL/NL/NR

1267—John/NL/Slave/NL/NL/November 18/NL/November 29/NA/NL/ Thos. McKnight/NL/$1.00/NL/1 Week/ Single/NL/NL/NL/NR

1268—Frederick/Virginia/Slave/NL/NL/November 18/NL/NL / January 22*/65/R. A. Stewart/NL/$1.00/Dropsy/7 Months/ Married/NL/NL/NL/NR

1269—Zachariah/Virginia/Slave/NL/NL/November 18/NL/ November 25/NA/NL/H. J. Ranney/NL/$1.00/NL/1 Day/NL/NL/NL/NL/NR

1270—James/Virginia/Slave/Pearl River/1 Day/November 22/NL/ January 10/NA/40/W. J. Poitevent/NL/ $1.00/NL/3 Days/NL/NL/ NL/NL/NR

1273—Cyrus/Mississippi/Slave/NL/1 Day/November 27/NL/ January 10/NA/19/W. J. Poitevent/NL/$1.00/Hand Amputation/3 Days/Single/NL/NL/NL/NR

1274—Washington/Mississippi/Slave/Mississippi/3 Years/ November 28/NL/December 29/NA/50/R. A. Stewart/NL/$1.00/NL/3 Months/Married/ NL/NL/NL/NR

1276—John/NL/Slave/NL/NL/December 1/NL/December 15/NA/NL/ Thos. McKnight/NL/$1.00/ Dysentery/NL/Single/NL/NL/NL/NR

1277—Johnson/South Carolina/Slave/NL/NL/December 3/NL/December 28/NA/NL/W. O. Denegre/NL/$1.00/NL/NL/NL/NL/ NL/NL/NR

1278—Solomon/South Carolina/Slave/NL/NL/December /NL/NL/ December 18/NA/NL/Thos. McKnight/ NL/$1.00/NL/NL/NL/NL/NL/NR

SLAVERY AND MEDICINE: ENSLAVEMENT AND MEDICAL PRACTICES IN
ANTEBELLUM LOUISIANA

1279—John/Maryland/Slave/Maryland/11 Years/December/
NL/NL/ December 13/NA/NL/Dominic
Madden/NL/$1.00/NL/2 Days/NL/NL/ NL/NR
1280—Lethy Ann/North Carolina/Slave/Virginia/NL/December
NL/NL/January 22/NA/NL/H. M. Crookes/NL/$1.00/
Ulcer on Legs/NL/Single/NL/NL/NL/NR
1285—Richard/Virginia/Slave/NL/NL/December 9/NL/
December 16/NA/30/John Foster/NL/$1.00/NL/8
Days/Single/NL/NL/NL/NR
1287—Mary/Virginia/Slave/Opelousas/NL/December 12/NL/
December 23/NA/35/Judge Bradford/NL/$1.00/
NL/NL/Single/ NL/NL/NL/NR
1288—Henry/Kentucky/Slave/NL/NL/December 14/NL/
December 15/NA/30/Thos. McKnight/NL/
$1.00/Injury/1 Week/Single/ NL/NL/NL/NR
1289—Peter/Virginia/Slave/NL/NL/December 15/NL/
December 23/NA/33/H. J. Ranney/NL/$1.00/NL/1
Day/Married/NL/NL/NL/NR
1290—Archy/Virginia/Slave/Missouri/10 Years/December
15/NL/December 21/NA/44/T. D. Van Horn/
NL/$1.00/Rheumatism/1 Day/Married/NL/
NL/NL/NR
1291—John/Maryland/Slave/Maryland/3 Years/December
21/NL/January 6/NA/26/James Calder/NL/$1.00/NL/
1 Week/ NL/NL/NL/NL/NR
1292—Lewis/Virginia/Slave/Virginia/NL/December 21/NL/
December 23/NA/35/Capt. Poitevent/NL/$1.00/
NL/NL/NL/NL/ NL/NL/NR
1293—Jerry/Tennessee/Slave/Tennessee/NL/December
21/NL/ December 23/NA/22/Capt. Poitevent/NL/
$1.00/NL/2 Weeks/NL/NL/ NL/NL/NR
1295—Jack/North Carolina/Slave/Mississippi/NL/December
22/NL/December 23/NA/31/H. J. Poitevent/NL/
$1.00/NL/1 Week/Single/NL/NL/NL/NR

1297—Elsy/Alabama/Slave/Alabama/2 Weeks/December/NL/
NL/ January 20/NA/22/Jerry McClelland/NL/$1.00/1
Month/Single/ NL/NL/NL/NR

1298—Ben/Virginia/Slave/NL/NL/December 29/NL/January
4/NA/27/Jos. Stinson/NL/$1.00/NL/9 Days/Married
/NL/NL/NL/NR

1299—Henry/Virginia/Slave/NL/NL/December 30/NL/January
18/NA/31/Thos. McKnight/NL/$1.00/NL/1 Day/
Married/NL/NL /NL/NR

[1300/no notation in the record]

[1301/no notation in the record]

1859

1302—Ben/Maryland/Slave/NL/NL/January 3, 1859/NL/
January 11/NA/26/Henry Brocon/NL/$1.00/NL/1
Year/NL/NL/NL/NL/NR

1308—John/Virginia/Slave/Alabama/5 1/2 Years/January
12/NL/ January 25/NA/40/Mrs. Murphy/
NL/$1.00/NL/3 Months/Single/ NL/NL/NL/NR

1309—Jack/Virginia/Slave/NL/NL/January 12/NL/NL/January
14*/40/P. A. B. Delk/$25.00/$1.00/Pneumonia/2
Days/NL/NL/NL/ NL/NR

1312—Jane/Virginia/Slave/NL/NL/January 15/NL/February
3/NA/40/D. J. Ricardo/NL/$1.00/NL/1 Week/
Married/NL/NL/NL/NR

1313—Jim/Alabama/Slave/NL/NL/February 3/NL/NL/
February 4*/38/Scott Williams & Co./NL/$1.00/NL/6
Months/Married/ NL/NL/NL/NR

1314—Benjamin alias Louis/Alabama/Slave/NL/NL/February
5/NL/February 24/NA/34/Hardenbrook/NL/
$1.00/NL/NL/Married/ NL/NL/NL/NR

1316—Joshua/Florida/Slave/Tallahassee/3 Weeks/February
9/NL/February 12/NA/38/C. W. Lythle/NL/$1.00
/NL/2 Months/ Married/NL/NL/NL/NR

1317—Polly & Child/Louisiana/Slaves/Louisiana/—/February 15/NL/March 19/March 19*/20/Oakey & Hawkins/ NL/$1.00/NL/NL/ Married/NL/NL/NL/NR
1318—Susan/Mississippi/Slave/Mississippi/1 Day/February 22/NL/July 14/NA/45/G. P. Wooten/$60.00/$1.00/ NL/2 Years/ Married/NL/143 Days/$143.00/NR
1319—Toby/South Carolina/NL/Alabama/NL/February 22/NL/March 3/NA/53/H. P. Ranney/NL/$1.00/NL/2 Week/NL/NL/NL/NL/NR
1320—Lucy/Virginia/Slaves/Virginia/NL/February 23/NL/ March 28/NA/40/D. O. Sullivan/NL/$1.00/NL/1 Day/Married/NL/NL/ NL/NR
1321—Jim/Virginia/Slave/Virginia/NL/February 26/NL/NL/ March 25*/40/Capt. Poitevent/NL/$1.00 /NL/NL/Single/NL/NL/NL/NR
1322—Charlotte/Virginia/Slave/Virginia/NL/February 26/NL/ March 7/NA/25/Columbus Moise/NL/$1.00/NL/1 Month/Single/ NL/NL/NL/NR
1324—Peter/North Carolina/Slave/Missouri/15 Years/March 8/NL/April 5/NA/23/R. Miot/NL/$1.00/NL/5 Days/Single/ NL/NL/NL/NR
1325—Susan White/Missouri/Slave/Missouri/15 Years/March 8/ NL/April 5/NA/48/H. J. Ranney/NL/$1.00/NL/5 Years/Married/ NL/NL/NL/NR
1326—Dave/New Orleans/Slave/New Orleans/2 Months/March 11/NL/March 23/NA/8/Thos. Shields/NL/$1.00/ NL/12 Hours/ Single/NL/NL/NL/NR
1328—Robert/Alabama/Slave/Mississippi City/3 Days/March 11/NL/April 16/NA/20/Nimrod McGuire/NL/$1.00/ NL/3 Weeks/ Single/NL/37 Days/$37.00/$25.00 Extra Surgery
1329—Jerry/Maryland/Slave/Louisiana/1 Day/March 17/NL/ May 11/NA/26/Shaw & Gunts/NL/$1.00/NL/8 Months/Single/NL/NL/NL /NR

SLAVERY AND MEDICINE: ENSLAVEMENT AND MEDICAL PRACTICES IN ANTEBELLUM LOUISIANA

1330—Martin/North Carolina/Slave/Louisiana/12 Months/ March 24/NL/April 16/NA/25/D. S. Graham/NL/ $1.00/NL/1 Month/ Single/NL/NL/NL/NR
1333—Nathan Anderson/Baltimore/Slave/Louisiana/NL/March 29/NL/May 10/NA/32/H. J. Ranney/NL/$1.00/NL/1 Day/Single/ NL/NL/NL/NR
1334—Anna & Child/New Orleans/Slave/Louisiana/20 Years/ April 1/NL/April 11/NA/20/P. A. Beard & Co./ NL/$1.00/NL/NL/ Single/NL/NL/NL/NR
1335—Jeannette/Georgia/Slave/Georgia/10 Days/April 2/NL/ April 20/NA/22/P. A. Beard & Co./NL/$1.00/NL/NL/Single/NL/ NL/NL/NR
1336—Mitchell/Virginia/Slave/Virginia/6 Years/April 6/NL/ April 12/NA/26/Dominic Madden/NL/$1.00/NL/2 Day/Single/NL/ NL/NL/NR
1337—Diana/Texas/Slave/Texas/6 Years/April 7/NL/April 20/ NA/13/J. A. Beard & Co./NL/$1.00/ Measles/NL/ Single/NL/NL/ NL/NR
1339—Susan White/Missouri/Slave/Missouri/15 Years/April 9/NL/April 29/NA/48/H. J. Ranney/NL/$1.00/ NL/NL/Married/ NL/NL/NL/NR
1342—Dick/Tennessee/Slave/Tennessee/8 Days/April 19/NL/May 18/NA/24/G. E. Payne/NL/$1.00/NL/6 Months/Single/NL/NL/NL/NR
1350—Mary Ann/Memphis/Slave/Memphis/12 Years/May 5/NL/July 23/NA/25/N. F. Rice/NL/$1.00/NL/6 Months/Single/NL/NL/NL/NR
1351—Bob/Maryland/Slave/Alabama/9 Years/May 7/NL/May 10/NA/ 35/H. J. Ranney/NL/$1.00/NL/1 Week/ Married/NL/NL/NL/NR
1360—Toby/Charleston/Slave/Mobile/15 Years/May 30/NL/ June 12/NA/53/H. J. Ranney/NL/$1.00/NL/1 Week/ Married/NL/NL/NL/NR
1366—Zachariah/Virginia/Slave/Virginia/NL/June 20/NL/June 23/June 23*/60/H. J. Ranney/NL/$1.00/Typhoid Pneumonia/7 Days/Single/NL/NL/NL/NR

SLAVERY AND MEDICINE: ENSLAVEMENT AND MEDICAL PRACTICES IN
ANTEBELLUM LOUISIANA

1373—Susan White/Missouri/Slave/Missouri/15 Years/July 4/NL/July 14/NA/48/H. J. Ranney/NL/$1.00/NL/NL/Married/NL/ NL/NL/NR
1388—Ben/Maryland/Slave/Baltimore/4 Years/August 11/NL/August 14/NA/29/J. D. Brown/NL/$1.00/Secondary Syphilis/8 Weeks/Single/NL/NL/NL/NR
1392—George/Shreveport/Slave/Shreveport/15 Years/August 24/NL/October 5/NA/21/A. Brown & Co./NL/$1.00/Syphilis/2 Weeks/Single/NL/NL/NL/NR
1396—Toby/Charleston S.C./Slave/Mobile/15 Years/September 5/NL/September 13/NA/53/H. J. Ranney/NL/$1.00/Intermittent/1 Day/Married/NL/NL/NL/NR
1398—Amy/Virginia/Slave/Richmond/10 Years/September 12/NL/September 27*/25/James H. Wheeler/NL/$1.00/Anemia/5 Months/Married/NL/NL/NL/NL/NR
1399—Horace/Maryland/Slave/Norfolk/11 Years/September 13/NL/September 20/NA/30/H.J. Ranney/NL/$1.00/Intermittent/NL/Married/NL/NL/NL/NR
1400—Read & Mother/Louisiana/Slave/New Orleans/6 Years/September 13/NL/September 16/NA/6/H. J. Ranney/NL/$1.00/ Indisposition/1 Day/NL/NL/NL/NL/NR
1401—William/Virginia/Slave/New Orleans/21 Years/September 13/NL/October 3/NA/37/C. D. Yancy/NL/$1.00/Renal Hemorrhoids/4 Weeks/Married/NL/NL/NL/NR
1403—Joe/Virginia/Slave/Richmond/15 Years/September 14/NL/ September 21/NA/27/H.J. Ranney/NL/$1.00/Intermittent/8 Days/ Married/NL/NL/NL/NR
1408—Chester William/Maryland/Slave/Baltimore/7 Years/September 19/NL/NL/NA/30/J.E. ? /NL/$1.00/Fractured Thigh/2 Months/Married/NL/NL/NL/NR
1409—Viney/Louisiana/Slave/St. Barnard, Louisiana/3 Years/September 20/NL/NL/NA/45/C. H. Davis/NL/$1.00/General Debility/9 Months/Widow/NL/NL/NL/NR
1414—Susan White/Missouri/Slave/Missouri/15 Years/September 25/NL/October 28/NA/48/H. J. Ranney/

NL/ $1.00/ Intermittent/8 Weeks/Married/
NL/NL/NL/NR
1431—Sally/Virginia/Slave/Memphis/1 Day/October 11/NL/
December 21/NA/15/P. H. Wilson/NL/$1.00/
Gangrene/4 Weeks/ Single/NL/NL/NL/NR

APPENDIX C

SELECTED PHARMACOPOEIA USED BY ENSLAVED AFRICANS IN THE SOUTHEASTERN PARISHES OF ANTEBELLUM LOUISIANA

[General Properties and/or Functions attempt to represent antebellum ideas about the pharmacopoeia, but are not the only known properties or functions. The use of the post-bellum term "aromatic" is included because the medicine was used in either a poultice or asafetida bag, and the users of such also relied on the substance as a respiratory inhalant.]

Pharmacopoeia	General Properties and/or Functions	Uses Indicated by Enslaved Africans
Asafetida	Dried plant juice, anti-spasmodic, pungent aromatic, respiratory inhalant	Colds, teething, fever
Ashes	Residue from hearth or other fires	To stop bleeding (coagulator)
Basil	Aromatic	Divining (Good Luck)
Bleeding/ Cupping/ Leeching	Procedure for Extracting Blood from the body; Blood Transfusion	
Blue Mass	Powdered Mercury, Cathartic	General sickness, Jaundice
Calomel	Purgative, tonic, stimulant	General sickness
Castor Oil	Cathartic, Lubricant	Hoarseness of throat, Jaundice
Clay	Earth in the form of Hydrated (with Vinegar) Silicate of Aluminum	For Sprains, Poultice

SLAVERY AND MEDICINE: ENSLAVEMENT AND MEDICAL PRACTICES IN ANTEBELLUM LOUISIANA

Coal Oil	Kerosene (distilled hydrocarbons from crude petroleum)	Rheumatism
Cobwebs	Poultice	To stop bleeding (Coagulator)
Garlic	Aromatic, Bacterial retardant, diuretic, stimulant	Earache
Gris-Gris	Charm, amulet, powder	divining
Horseradish	Pungent Aromatic, Antiseptic, Diuretic	Hoarseness of throat
Indian Hemp (Indian Root)	Emetic, Cathartic, Tonic	Yellow Fever
Ipecac	Emetic, Alkaloid	General sickness, fever
Jimsonweed	Alkaloid (Toxic)	General sickness
Molasses	Raw cane or beet sugar liquor	Not Indicated
Pokeroot (Pokeweed) (Inkberry)	Stain, dye, poultice	"Seven year itch"
Pumpkinseed	Urinary tract tonic	(w/Indian Hemp) Yellow Fever
Quinine	Bitter Alkaloid, Malarial Infection tonic	General sickness
Rhubarb	Cathartic, bitter tonic	Not Indicated

SLAVERY AND MEDICINE: ENSLAVEMENT AND MEDICAL PRACTICES IN ANTEBELLUM LOUISIANA

Sage	Bitter Aromatic, Astringent, Expectorant	Flux
Sarsaparilla	Sweet essential oil	General sickness
Sassafras	Aromatic stimulant, Essential oil, blood tonic	Measles
Turpentine	Pine resin, essential oil	Fever
Vinegar	Acid liquid of alcohol, preservative, bacterial retardant	Womb, general pain

Definitions (Selected Terms Related to the Pharmacopoeia)

Alkaloid:	Nitrogen-containing substances from plants (e.g. morphine, codeine, nicotine, strychnine)
Antispasmodic:	Relaxes muscle spasms in bladder or intestines.
Aromatic:	Oils extracted from plants; olfactory stimulant.
Astringent:	Causes drying/shrinking of tissue, reduces water absorption.
Cathartic:	Stimulates bowel activity.
Emetic:	Causes vomiting, gastric irritant.
Poultice:	Substances (herbs) packed in layers of cloth/fabric; used on local pain, inflammation and circulation.
Purgative:	Causes cleansing, especially bowels; a Cathartic.

APPENDIX D

GLOSSARY

COMMON DEFINITIONS[3] FOR SELECTED MALADIES (MEDICAL HEALTH CONDITIONS) OF ENSLAVED AFRICANS IN THE ANTEBELLUM PERIOD

Abortion — A spontaneous or induced termination of a pregnancy.

Abscess — The formation of fluid in the form of pus, usually caused by bacterial infection. Abscesses can cause fever, site pain and inflammation.

Amenorrhea — The absence of the menstrual cycle. There are two types of amenorrhea, primary and secondary. Failure to menstruate by approximately age 16 is primary amenorrhea; periodic or the complete loss of the menstrual cycle is secondary amenorrhea.

Amputation — The surgical removal of a limb, usually due to the onset of gangrene.

Anasarca — Severe generalized edema (excessive tissue fluid). Another name for Dropsy.

Anemia — An abnormal concentration of oxygen-carrying hemoglobin; the most common form stems from an iron deficiency. Anemia generally can cause dizziness, heart palpitation and jaundice.

---

[3]Reflects ante- and post-bellum descriptions of the maladies; includes a selection of those maladies listed in the Touro Infirmary Admission Record, 1855–1860.

SLAVERY AND MEDICINE: ENSLAVEMENT AND MEDICAL PRACTICES IN
ANTEBELLUM LOUISIANA

Apoplexy
: An earlier term to describe a stroke (the interruption of blood flow within the brain); can cause paralysis or sudden loss of consciousness.

Arthritis
: The inflammation of a joint (or joints) which may produce stiffness, pain and swelling.

Ascites
: Excessive fluid of the peritoneal cavity (the space between the inside abdominal wall and the outside abdominal area); some symptoms are abdominal swelling and difficulty breathing.

Asthma
: Difficulty breathing in chronic periods of breathlessness. The two main types of asthma are extrinsic (caused by an allergy) and intrinsic (no external cause).

Bronchitis
: The inflammation of the bronchi (the air passages that connect the windpipe to the lungs); the symptoms are persistent cough which includes phlegm. The two types are acute and chronic bronchitis.

Burn
: Epidermal skin cell damage due to excessive heat. Various types of burns can cause pain, redness, peeling skin, blisters, etc.

Bubo
: Swollen lymph node in the groin or armpit in the early stages of bubonic plague.

Cachexia Africana
: A "Negro/Slave Disease" of the antebellum period. The main symptom of Cachexia Africana was dirt-eating; but it also included psycho-logical indicators such as loss of appetite, melancholia, nostalgia, etc. Cachexia Africana could bring on

	the intestinal disorder of hookworm disease. Also called Dirt-eating.
Cataract	A type of blindness (a diminished perception, acuity) that is the result of the loss of transparency of the lens of the eye; most non-injurial cataracts occur in old age.
Catarrh	Excessive secretion from an inflamed mucous membrane, especially of the air passages of the throat and head; the common cold.
Cholera	An acute, infectious, epidemic disease. A serious small intestinal disorder caused by bacterium. Victims of cholera usually experience profuse, watery diarrhea, dehydration, vomiting. Asiatic cholera—a malignant form is usually fatal.
Cholic	[Colic] Refers to chronic bowel irritability and pain.
Constipation	The difficult passage of hard, dry feces. Among other causes, a lack of dietary fiber, fluid, fruits, vegetable and whole grains. Symptoms are painful defecation, lower abdominal pain.
Consumption	A reference to pulmonary tuberculosis.
Convulsions	Violent, abnormal body contractions, also called seizure.
Cystitis	A bacterial condition of stagnant urine due to an inflammation of the inner lining of the bladder. Symptoms include frequent urges to pass urine, burning, stinging or bloody urine; inability to pass normal amounts of urine.

Slavery and Medicine: Enslavement and Medical Practices in Antebellum Louisiana

Debility	General weakness of the body; a lack of physical energy; can be physical or psychological.
Delirium Tremens	Considered a "confused" physical and psychological state whereby the individual trembles, has insomnia and experiences hallucinations. Often discussed in the context of chronic alcoholism.
Diarrhea	Abnormal bowel movements, usually increased fluid, frequency or volume; usually a symptom to another problem. There are two types of diarrhea, acute (caused by contaminated food or drinking water) and chronic (caused by intestinal disorders).
Dirt-Eating	Another name for Cachexia Africana; the condition involving the consumption of dirt or clay.
Dislocation	Occurs when the two bones in a joint are no longer in contact (displaced); the tearing of the ligaments causes pain and swelling.
Drapetomania	A "Negro/Slave Disease" of the antebellum period. It is specific described as the "disease causing negroes to run away" (Cartwright 1859, 331). It was psychological and physical. It was predominately thought to be an ailment related to the slaveowner's (or overseer's) ability to effectively manage enslaved Africans.
Dropsy	Another term for general edema (excessive tissue fluid); dropsy is an indication of another malfunction of the body. Dropsy (Ovarian), the swelling of the ovaries.

SLAVERY AND MEDICINE: ENSLAVEMENT AND MEDICAL PRACTICES IN ANTEBELLUM LOUISIANA

Dysaesthesia
Aethiopica   A "Negro/Slave Disease" of the antebellum period. Dysaesthesia Aethiopica was thought to be largely a mental disease among enslaved Africans, but also included lesions and blood disorders. The chief symptom, however, was "mischievous behavior" of enslaved Africans. Also called "Rascality."

Dysentery   A serious infection of the intestines which causes diarrhea; severe inflammation of the mucous membrane of the large intestines; includes fever, gripping pain and bloody evacuation. Also called the flux, and bloody flux.

Dysmenorrhea   Premenstrual or menstrual pain and/or discomfort felt in the lower abdomen. The two types of dysmenorrhea are primary (adolescent/young woman) and secondary (caused by another disorder, e.g. endometriosis).

Eczema   A skin inflammation which causes itching, rash, scaling and blisters.

Enteritis   The inflammation of the small intestines and usually brings on diarrhea.

Epilepsy   Caused by a malfunction of some areas of the brain which produces seizures. The two classifications of epileptic seizures are Generalized Seizures (loss of consciousness) and Partial Seizures (semi or full consciousness).

Erithema   [Erythema] A skin disease that causes abnormal redness.

SLAVERY AND MEDICINE: ENSLAVEMENT AND MEDICAL PRACTICES IN ANTEBELLUM LOUISIANA

Fever — (Pyrexia) Body temperature above 98.6 degrees Fahrenheit; additional symptoms include headaches, hot/cold flashes, sweating, dizziness. Fevers are either bacterial or viral.

Fistula — An abnormal hole (or passage) from an internal organ to the body's surface, or between two organs. Fistulas are congenital or acquired from tissue damage.

Flatulence — The expulsion of gas or air in the intestines; sometimes includes stomach pain and discomfort.

Fractures — A break in the bone(s) usually caused by sudden injury. The two main types are closed fractures (beneath the skin) and open fractures (projects through the skin).

Frostbite — The damage caused by tissues exposed to extremely cold temperatures (32 degrees Fahrenheit), especially affects extremities such as ears, nose, fingers and toes. Serious damage can result in gangrene.

Gangrene — The formation of dead tissue due to loss of blood supply; symptoms include blackening of skin, swelling and an unpleasant odor. There is dry and wet gangrene. Dry gangrene (no bacterial infection); Wet gangrene (bacterial infection); gas gangrene caused by bacteria and destroys muscle tissue.

Gastritis — In general an inflammation of the stomach lining, producing abdominal discomfort, nausea, vomiting.

Gastro Enteritis	An inflammation of the stomach and intestines. Among the characteristics are the loss of fluid and salt. Forms of gastroenteritis include cholera, diarrhea, dysentery and typhoid fever.
Gonorrhea	An infectious disease caused through sexual transmission; can also be transmitted from mother to new born during childbirth.
Hemiplegia	The condition of paralysis or general weakness in the muscles of the body. The muscles are either stiff (spastic) or limp/wasted (flaccid).
Hemorrhoids	An inflammation/enlargement of the veins in the lining of the anus; hemorrhoids can be internal, external or prolapsing. They are caused during or after pregnancy, are congenital or due to anal strain.
Hernia	Any protrusion of an organ or tissue through a weaker one; commonly refers to abdominal hernias (the intestine through the abdominal wall). Hernia Femoral (from the intestine, abdomen to the thigh), Hernia Inguinal (from the intestine through the passage that descends into the scrotum—scrotal hernia), Hernia Umbilical (from the intestines through the abdominal wall near the navel).
Hydrocele	Swelling, inflammation of the scrotum caused by the accumulation of fluid around the testis.
Hydro-Pericarditis	Inflammation of the membrane which surrounds and protects the heart (pericardium).

Hysteria	Physical and mental stress of a non-psychotic origin; may result in hallucinations and trance states.
Indigestion	General term denoting discomfort of the upper stomach region produced by eating. Symptoms include stomach pain, heartburn, flatulence and nausea.
Indisposition	Considered a general sickness, yet largely refers to a state of mental decline or a sudden change in attitude, behavior or disposition.
Injury	Any harm to the human body. Injuries can be caused by external physical factors such as environment, trauma, chemicals or internal malfunctions or abnormalities.
Itch	Irritation or abnormal skin sensation. Can be general (all over) or local (specific area). Generalized and local itching may be the cause of numerous underlying conditions.
Measles	A viral disease producing rash and a fever which is infectious and spreads airborne. Other symptoms include cough, runny nose and sore eyes.
Menorrhea	[Menorrhagia] The abnormal discharge (excessive) menstrual blood. Also described as a uterine hemorrhage; may or may not be accompanied by lower abdominal spasms/cramps.
Necrosis	Refers to the death of cell tissues; necrosis can be caused by lack of blood supply, infection or damage from external forces.

Slavery and Medicine: Enslavement and Medical Practices in Antebellum Louisiana

Negro Consumption	A "Negro/Slave Disease" of the antebellum period. A pulmonary disorder of enslaved Africans. Symptoms are both physical (mucous on gums, palpitations) and psychological (paranoia, a contrary disposition). Also called Struma Africana and "Negro Poison".
Neuralgia	Refers to acute or chronic nerve irritation causing pain.
Node on Tibia	A normal or abnormal small, round mass of tissue on the tibia.
Nostalgia	Considered a severe, prolonged, or even morbid fixation on home (homesickness), family, friends, etc.
Orchitis	Inflammation of the testis; may be caused by viral infection.
Paraplegia	The result of nerve damage to the brain or spinal cord; which causes weakness or paralysis of the legs or lower torso.
Pericarditis	Inflammation of the membrane that surrounds the heart (pericardium) and includes fever and chest pain; causes include bacterial, viral and fungal.
Peritonitis	Inflammation of the tissues that support the teeth (periodontium). The two types are Periapical Peritonitis (usually from dental neglect), Chronic Peritonitis (from inflamed gums).

Phthisis	Another term for pulmonary consumption, tuberculosis of the lungs, causes progressive emaciation.
Pleurisy	The inflammation of the membrane lining the lungs and chest cavity (pleura), usually caused by a lung infection.
Pneumonia	Inflammation of the lungs caused by virus or bacteria. Symptoms include chills, fever, a mucous cough and difficulty breathing.
Prolapses Uterus/Vagina	The displacement of the uterus from its normal position. Also called "Falling of the Womb."
Puncture Wound	A flesh wound caused by piercing with a sharp point.
Renal Hemorrhage	The discharge of blood from a rupture kidney.
Retention of Urine	Holding urine in the body which would normally be excreted.
Rheumatism	A general term for muscle/joint pain and stiffness.
Rubeola	Another term for measles.
Scirrhous of Gland	The hardening and development of fibrous tissue in a gland.

Scrofula	The development of tuberculosis in the lymph nodes of the neck, generally caused by the consumption of contaminated milk.
Scrofulous Tumor	The abscess formed in the lymph nodes, erupting and ultimately leaving scars on the neck.
Sprain	The inflammation and pain caused by torn and stretched ligaments that support the bones of a joint.
Syphilis	An infection that is sexually transmitted (or congenital in rare cases); there are four primary stages resulting from untreated syphilis: Primary (chancre sores), Secondary (skin rash, spotting, headaches, fatigue, loss of appetite,), Latent (appearance of remission), Tertiary (progressive tissue destruction, heart disease, brain damage, paralysis).
Syphilitic Eruption	Chancre sores and rashes resulting from primary syphilis.
Tetanus	The disease of the central nervous system caused by an infected wound. The infectious spores come from dirt and manure, enter the wound and multiply causing muscle stiffness including lockjaw.
Tonsillitis	Inflammation and soreness of the tonsils from infection.
Tumour	[Tumor] Any swelling or abnormal mass of tissue; the result of cells which reproduce at an increased

SLAVERY AND MEDICINE: ENSLAVEMENT AND MEDICAL PRACTICES IN
ANTEBELLUM LOUISIANA

	rate. Tumours are malignant (cancerous) or benign (non-cancerous).
Typhoid Fever	An infectious bacterial disease caused by contaminated food or drinking water. Bacteria is carried in human fecal matter of an infected person.
Ulcer	Generally an open sore on the skin or mucous membrane.
Ulcer on Leg	Most common form of skin ulcer.
Variola	Another term for smallpox.
Vesico-Vaginal Fistula	An abnormal hole emanating to/from the vagina. A major symptom/indicator of vesico-vaginal fistula(s) is the inability of the patient to control urination. The fistulas were closed using wire sutures or using a "button-hole" method. Other vaginal fistulas include recto-vaginal and urethra-vaginal.
Worms	The condition of hosting worm parasites in the human body acquired from meat, food, water or fecal matter which contain the worm larvae.
Yellow Fever	A viral infection transmitted by mosquitoes. The disease in its severe form causes jaundice, fever, headache, nausea, delirium, coma and in serious cases fatality.

BIBLIOGRAPHY

Adams, William Hampton. "Health and Medical Care on Antebellum Southern Plantations." *Plantation Society in the Americas* 2, No. 3 (1989): 259-278.

Adelman, David C. *Life and Times of Judah Touro* (Tercentenary Address Delivered Before the Officers and Members of The Touro Fraternal Association) Rhode Island: Touro Fraternal Association (May 13, 1936).

Admission Book of the Touro Infirmary 1855-1860. Touro Infirmary Archives, New Orleans, Louisiana.

Aimes, Hubert S. "African Institutions in America." *Journal of American Folklore* 18 (1905): 15-32.

Albert, Octavia V. Rogers. *The House of Bondage, or Charlotte Brooks and Other Slaves.* New York: Hunt and Eaton, 1890.

Alho, Olli. *The Religion of the Slaves.* Helsinki: Academia Scientiarium Fennica, 1976.

Allen, Lane. "Grandison Harris, Sr.; Slave, Resurrectionist and Judge." *Georgia Academy of Science Bulletin* X XXIV (April 1976):192–99.

Anderson, John Q. (ed.) "A Letter From a Yankee Bride in Ante-Bellum Louisiana." *Louisiana History* 1, No. 3 (Summer 1960): 245–250.

Anderson, L. H. "Report on the Disease of Sumterville and Vicinity." Medical Association of the State of Alabama, *Transactions* VII (January 1854): 61–66.

Ani, Marimba. *Yurugu.* Trenton: Africa World Press, Inc., 1994.

Armstrong, Orland Kay. *Old Massa's People: The Old Slaves Tell Their Story.* Indianapolis: The Bobbs-Merrill Co.: 1931.

Arsene v. Pigneguy, #459 June, 1847, La. Ann. 620, Supreme Court of Louisiana Collection of Legal Archives, University of New Orleans, E. K. Long Library Archives.

Asante, Molefi K. *Afrocentricity.* Trenton: Africa World Press, 1988.

Asante, Molefi K. *The Afrocentric Idea.* Philadelphia: Temple University Press, 1987.

Asante, Molefi K. *Kemet, Afrocentricity and Knowledge.* Trenton: Africa World Press, 1990.

Asante, Molefi K. *Malcolm X as Cultural Hero and Other Afrocentric Essays.* Trenton: Africa World Press, 1993.

Asante, Molefi and Kariamu W. Asante. *African Culture The Rhythms of Unity.* Trenton: Africa World Press, 1990.

Assumption Parish (La) Clerk of the Court. *Record of Slaves,* 1813–1844. Napoleonville, LA: Genealogical Society of Utah, 1971.

"Autobiography of James P. Thomas: A Slave and Free Negro in the Antebellum South." Moorland-Spingarn Research Center, Howard University, Washington, D.C.

Axelsen, Diana E. "Women as Victims of Medical Experimentation: J. Marion Sims' Surgery on Slave Women, 1845–1850." *Sage: A Scholarly Journal on Black Women* 2, No. 2 (1985): 10–12.

Azibo, Daudi Ajani ya. "Articulating the Distinction Between Black Studies and the Study of Blacks: The Fundamental Role of Culture and the African-centered Worldview." *The Afrocentric Scholar* 1, No. 1 (May 1992): 64–97.

Bailey, T. P. "Surgical Cases." *Charleston Medical Journal* 14, No. 5 (September 1859): 740–745.

Baldwin, Joseph A. "African (Black) Psychology." *Journal of Black Studies* 16, No. 3 (March 1986): 235–249.

Bandolph, Richard. (ed.) *The Civil Rights Record Black Americans and the Law 1849–1970.* New York: Thomas Y. Crowell Co., 1970.

Bankole, Katherine "A Critical Inquiry of Enslaved African Women and the Antebellum Hospital Experience," *Journal of Black Studies,* Vol. 31, No. 5, 517-538, May 2001.

Bankole, Katherine. *The Afrocentric Guide to Selected Black Studies Terms and Concepts.* New York: Whittier Publications, 1995.

Bankole-Medina, Katherine "Trust God...But Makin' Our Tea: The Slave Narratives and Indications of African Agency in the Treatment of Illness in Louisiana," *Synergy,* edited by

Elizabeth Clark-Lewis, Washington, D.C.: The A.P. Foundation Press, 2011.

Bascom, W. R. "'Secret Societies' Religious Cult Groups, and Kinship Units Among the West African Yoruba." Unpublished Doctor's Thesis, Northwestern University. 1939.

Berkeley, Edmund and Dorothy S. Berkeley. *Dr. Alexander Gordon of Charles Town*. Chapel Hill, NC., 1969.

Berquin-Duvallon (translated by John Davis). *Travels in Louisiana and the Floridas in the Year 1802*. New York, 1806.

"Bill for the Circus Street Hospital for the Medical Treatment and Attendance for Slave Joachin, 1856." MS., Kuntz Collection, Tulane University.

Billings, Edward Coke. *The Struggle between the Civilization of Slavery and that of Freedom, Recently and now going on in Louisiana; an address, delivered by Edward C. Billings, of New Orleans, at Hatfield, Mass., October 20, 1873*. Freeport, NY: Books for Libraries Press, 1971.

Billingslea, J.C. "An Appeal on Behalf of Southern Medical Colleges and Southern Medical Literature." *New Orleans Medical and Surgical Journal* 13 (1856–1857): 214–217.

Blake, John B. "Anatomy." in Ronald L. Numbers (ed.) *The Education of American Physicians: Historical Essays*. Los Angeles, 1980.

Blassingame, John W. *Black New Orleans*. Chicago: University of Chicago Press, 1973.

Blassingame, John W. *Slave Testimony, Two Centuries of Letters, Speeches, Interviews and Autobiographies*. Baton Rouge: Louisiana State University, 1977.

Blier, Suzanne Preston. *African Vodun*. Chicago: University of Chicago Press, 1994.

Bodin, Ron. *Voodoo Past and Present*. Lafayette, LA: Center for Louisiana Studies, 1990.

Boling, William M. "Experiments with Phosphorus, and Remarks upon it Dose and Action, when Given tin the Form of

Alcoholic Tincture or Solution." *New Orleans Medical and Surgical Journal* 10 (1853–1854): 726–738.

Boney, F. N. "Slaves as Guinea Pigs, Georgia and Alabama Episodes." *Alabama Review* 37, No. 1 (1984): 45–51.

Bostick, Clyde M. "Selected Aspects of Slave Health in Louisiana, 1804–1861." Master's Thesis, Louisiana State University, 1960.

Botkin, B. A. (ed.) *Lay My Burden Down*. Athens: University of Georgia Press, 1973.

Bozeman, Nathan. "Urethro-Vaginal Vesico-Vaginal, and Recto-Vaginal Fistulas; General Remarks; Report of Cases Successfully Treated with the Button Suture." *New Orleans Medical and Surgical Journal* XVII, No. 2 (March 1860): 180–199.

Bradley, Michael R. "The Role of the Black Church in the Colonial Slave Society." *Louisiana Studies* 14, No. 4 (Winter 1975): 413–421.

Breeden, James O. *Advice Among Masters. The Ideal in Slave Management in the Old South*. Connecticut: Greenwood Press, 1980.

Breeden, James O. "Body Snatchers and Anatomy Professors: Medical Education in Nineteenth-Century Virginia." *Virginia Magazine of History and Biography* LXXIII (July 1975): 321–345.

Brickell, D. Warren. "Epidemic Typhoid Pneumonia Amongst Negroes." *New Orleans Medical News and Hospital Gazette* II (February 1856): 548.

Brooks, R. "Extirpation of Tumors From the Neck." *New Orleans Medical and Surgical Journal* 11 (1854–1855): 457–460.

Burke-Gaffney, H.J.O'D. "The History of Medicine in the African Countries." *Medical History* 12 (1968): 31–44.

Burnett, Walter Mucklow. *Touro Infirmary*. Baton Rouge: Moran Publishing Corp., 1979.

Burns, Chester R. "Medical Ethics in the United States Before the Civil War." Ph.D. diss., Johns Hopkins University, 1969.

Burton, Annie L. *Memories of Childhood's Slavery Days*. 1919.

Bynum, Victoria E. *Unruly Women: The Politics of Social and Sexual Control in the Old South*. Chapel Hill: The University of North Carolina Press, 1992.

Cable, G. W. "New Orleans" in the Tenth Census of the United States. *Report on the Social Statistics of Cities.* XIX Washington, 1887.

Cable, G. W. "The Dance in Place Congo." *Century Magazine* 31 (1885–1886): 517–532.

Cade, John B. "Out of the Mouths of Ex-Slaves." *Journal of Negro History* (July 1935): 294–337.

"Calendar of Colonial Documents." *Louisiana Historical Society* 1, No. 1 (Series Two), (1973): 144–150

Callaway, George. "XVII. Case of a Remarkable Diseased Uterus." *Philadelphia Medical and Physical Journal* Part 1, 3 (1808): 138–142.

Cameron, Vivian K. "Folk Beliefs Pertaining to Health of the Southern Negro." Master's Thesis, Northwestern University, 1930.

Campbell, John. *Negro Mania: Being an Examination of the Falsely Assumed Equality of the Various Races of Men*. Philadelphia: Campbell and Power, 1851.

Carpenter, William. "Observations on the Cachexia Africana, or the Habit and Effects of Dirt-Eating in the Negro Race." *New Orleans Medical and Surgical Journal* 1 (1845): 146–168.

Carregen, Jo Ann. "Yellow Fever in New Orleans 1853: Abstractions and Realities." *The Journal of Southern History* 25, No. 3 (1959): 339–355.

Carregen, Jo Ann. "The Saffron Scourge: A History of Yellow Fever in Louisiana, 1796–1905." Ph.D. diss., Louisiana State University, 1961.

Cartwright, Samuel A. "Cartwright on Southern Medicine." New Orleans Medical and Surgical Journal 3, No. 2 (September 1846): 259–272.

Cartwright, Samuel A. "Dr. Cartwright on the Caucasian and the Africans." *De Bow's Review* XXV (July 1858): 45–56.

Cartwright, Samuel A. "Drapetomania, or the Disease Causing Negroes to Run Away: Dyaethesia Aethiopios, or Hebetude of the Mind and Obtuse Sensibility of Body—A Disease Peculiar to Negroes—Called by Overseers Rascality." *New Orleans Medical and Surgical Journal* 2 (1846): 694–731.

Cartwright, Samuel A. "Ethnology of the Negro or Prognathous Race." *New Orleans Medical and Surgical Journal* XIV (1857): 149–163.

Cartwright, Samuel A. "Philosophy of the Negro Constitution." *New Orleans Medical and Surgical Journal* IX (1853): 195–208.

Cartwright, Samuel A. "Remarks on Dysentery Among Negroes." *New Orleans Medical and Surgical Journal* XI, No. 2 (September 1854): 145–163.

Cartwright, Samuel A. "Report on the Diseases and Physical Peculiar-ities of the Negro Race." *New Orleans Medical and Surgical Journal* VII (May 1851): 331–336.

Cassidy, James H. *American Medicine and Statistical Thinking, 1800–1860*. Cambridge: Harvard University Press, 1984.

Castellanos, Henry C. *New Orleans as it Was, Episodes of Louisiana Life*. New Orleans: L. Graham and Son, Ltd. Printers, 1895.

Cates, Gerald. "Medical Schools in Ante-Bellum Georgia." Masters Thesis, University of Georgia, 1968.

Chatelain, Heli. "African Folk-Life." *Journal of American Folk-Lore* X, No. 36 (Jan-Mar. 1897): 21–34.

Child, Lydia Maria. *Incidents in the Life of a Slave Girl*. 1861.

Childs, St. Julien Ravenel. "Kitchen Physick Medical and Surgical Cases of Slaves on an 18th Century Rice Plantation." *Mississippi Valley Historical Review* 20, (1934): 549–54.

Civil Code of the State of Louisiana Preceded By the Treaty of Cession with France, the Constitution of the United States of America and of the State. New Orleans, Louisiana, 1825: 90–94.

Clayton, Ronnie W. *Mother Wit: The Exslave Narratives of the Louisiana Writers Project*. New York: Peter Lang, 1990.

Clayton, Ronnie W. "The Federal Writers' Project for Blacks in Louisiana." *Louisiana History* 19 (1978): 327–335.

Clinton, Catherine. "The Plantation Mistress: Another Side of Southern Slavery, 1780–1835." Ph.D. diss., Princeton University, 1980.

Clinton, Catherine. *The Plantation Mistress: Women's World in the Old South*. New York: Pantheon, 1983.

Coates, Benjamin H. "On the Effects of Secluded and Gloomy Imprisonment on Individuals of the African Variety of Mankind, in the Production of Disease." *New York Journal of Medicine* Part 1, 2 (January 1844): 91–95.

Code of Alabama, (Title 13, Chapter 3–4; Part II, Title 5 Chapter 4), 1852.

Cody Cheryll Ann. "A Note on Changing Patterns of Slave Fertility in the South Carolina Rice District, 1735–1865." *Southern Studies* 16 (1977): 457–463.

Coles, Harry L. "Some Notes on Slaveownership and Landownership in Louisiana, 1850–1860." *Journal of Southern History* 9 (1945): 381–394.

Collins, Dr. *Practical Rules for the Management and Medical Treatment of Negro Slaves, in the Sugar Colonies by a Professional Planter*. London: J. Barfield for Vernor and Hood, 1803.

Cook Charles Orson and James M. Poteet. "'Dem Was Black Times, Sure'Nough': The Slave Narratives of Lydia Jefferson and Stephen Williams." *Louisiana History* 20 (1979): 281–293.

Council of the First Municipality of the City of New Orleans, Journal, 1847, 3b.

Council of the Second Municipality of the City of New Orleans, Proceedings, March, 1847, City Archives, New Orleans Public Library.

Courlander, Harold. *A Treasury of Afro-American Folklore*. New York: Crown Publishers, Inc., 1976.

Cowdrey, Albert E. *War and Healing Stanhope Bayne-Jones and the Maturing of American Medicine*. Baton Rouge: Louisiana State University Press, 1992.

Craigin, F. W. "Observations on Cachexia Africana or Dirt-Eating." *American Journal of Medical Sciences* 17 (1836): 356–357.

Crete, Juliane (Translated by Patrick Gregory). *Daily Life in Louisiana 1815–1830*. Louisiana State University Press: Baton Rouge, 1978.

Cureau, Ad., *Les Societes Primitives de l'Afrique Equatoriale*. Paris, 1912.

Curtain, Philip D. *The Atlantic Slave Trade: A Census*. Madison, 1969.

Curtain, Philip D. "The Epidemiology of the Slave Trade," *Political Science Quarterly* 83 (1968): 190–216.

Curtain, Philip D. "'The White Man's Grave': Image and Reality 1780–1850." *Journal of British Studies* 1 (1951): 94–110.

Daily Picayune. "The Congo Dance: An Account Reported in New Orleans." New Orleans, Louisiana, October 18, 1843.

Darkis Jr., Fred R. "Madame Lalaurie of New Orleans." *Louisiana History* 23, No. 4 (Fall, 1982): 383–399.

Dart, Henry P. "Slavery in Louisiana, Editor's Chair." *Louisiana Historical Quarterly* 7, No. 2 (April 1924): 332–333.

d'Auvergne, Edmund. *Human Livestock, An Account of the Share of the English-speaking People in the Maintenance and Abolition of Slavery*. London: Grayson and Grayson, 1933.

Davies, Kenneth G. "The Living and the Dead: White Mortality in West Africa, 1684–1732." in Stanley Engerman and Eugene D. Genovese's *Race and Slavery in the Western Hemisphere*: Quantitative Studies. Princeton, 1975.

De Bow, J. D. B. *The Industrial Resources Etc. of the Southern and Western States*. 3 Vols., New Orleans, 1853.

"Department of Agriculture" ("Houses for Negroes"). *De Bow's Review* 3, No. 3 (November 1846): 325.

"Destrehan's Slave Roll." *Louisiana Historical Quarterly* 7, No. 2 (April 1924): 302–303.

Deutsch, Albert. "The First U.S. Census of the Insane (1840) and its Use as Pro-Slavery Propaganda." *Bulletin of the History of Medicine* 15 (1944): 469–482.

Digest of the Ordinances and Resolutions of the Corporation of New Orleans, New Orleans (1817): 222.
"Diseases and Peculiarities of the Negro Race." *De Bow's Review* 1, No. 1 (July 1851): 64–69.
Donaldson, Gary A. "A Window on Slave Culture: Dances at Congo Square in New Orleans, 1800–1862." *Journal of Negro History* 69, No. 2 (1984): 63–72.
Donegan, Jane B. *Hydropathic Highway to Health: Women and Water-Cure in Antebellum America*. New York: Greenwood, 1986.
Dorman, Dereic Daood. "Imhotep: The Symbol of African Medical Genius." *Imhotep: An Afrocentric Review* 2, No. 1 (January 1990): 1–6.
Dowler, Bennett. "The Vital Statistics of Negroes in the United States." *New Orleans Medical and Surgical Journal* 13 (1856–1857): 164–175.
Dowler, Bennett. "Obstetrical Cases and Physiological Remarks, &c." *New Orleans Medical and Surgical Journal* 11 (1854–1855): 18–21.
Dowling. "Case of Verminose Disease." *Transylvania Journal of Medicine and the Associate Sciences* II (May 1829): 250.
Drake, Daniel. "Diseases of the Negro Population." *New Orleans Medical and Surgical Journal* 1 (May 1845): 583–587.
Drew, Benjamin.. *The Refugee: or The Narratives of FugitiveSlaves in Canada, Related by Themselves*, Boston, 1856.
Drums and Shadows: Surviving Studies Among the Georgia Coastal Negroes, 1940.
Ducas, George (ed.) et. al. *Great Documents in Black American History*. New York: Praeger Publishers, 1970.
Du Pratz, M. Le Page. *The History of Louisiana*. (Translated from the French, *Histoire de la Louisiane*) 3 Vols., Paris, 1758.
Duffy, John. "A Note on Ante-Bellum Southern Nationalism and Medical Practice." *Journal of Southern History* 34 (May, 1968): 266–276.
Duffy, John. *The Healers A History of American Medicine*. New York: McGraw-Hill, 1976.

Duffy, John. "Slavery and Slave Health in Louisiana, 1766–1825." *Bulletin of the Tulane University Medical Faculty* 26 (February 1967): 1–6.

Duffy, John. *Sword of Pestilence: The New Orleans Yellow Fever Epidemic of 1853.* Baton Rouge: Louisiana State University Press, 1966.

Duffy, John. "Medical Practice in the Antebellum South," *The Journal of Southern History* 25, No. 1 (February 1959): 53–72.

Duffy, John. "One Hundred Years of the New Orleans Medical and Surgical Journal." *Louisiana Historical Quarterly* XL, No. 1 (January 1957): 3–24.

Duffy, John. "Sectional Conflict and Medical Education in Louisiana." *Journal of Southern History* 23, No. 3 (Aug. 1957): 289–306.

Duffy, John (ed.). *The Rudolph Matas History of Medicine in Louisiana.* (Vol. 1) Baton Rouge: Louisiana State University Press, 1958.

Dunbar, Gary S. "Elisee Reclus in Louisiana." *Louisiana History* 23, No. 4 (1982): 344–352.

Dunbar-Nelson, Alice. "People of Color in Louisiana." *Journal of Negro History* 1, No. 4 (October 1916): 361–376.

Eaken, Sue and Joseph Logsdon (eds.). *Twelve Years a Slave; Narrative of Solomon Northup, A Citizen of New York, Etc.* Baton Rouge: Louisiana State University Press, 1968.

Ebeyer, Pierre Paul. *Paramours of the Creoles: a Story of New Orleans and the Method of Promiscuous Mating Between White Creole Men and Negro and Colored Slaves and Freewomen.* New Orleans: Windmill Publishing Company, 1945.

Eccles, William John. *France in America.* New York, 1972.

Edwards, Paul (ed.). *The Encyclopedia of Philosophy.* New York: Macmillan, Inc. 1967.

Elkins, Stanley M. *Slavery, A Problem in American Institutional and Intellectual Life.* Chicago: The University of Chicago Press, 1959.

Ewing, A. "Wound of Abdomen—Followed by Hernia of Stomach and Strangulation—Contents of This Organ Discharged by Puncture—Reduction and Cure." *New Orleans Medical and Surgical Journal* 9, No. 6 (1853): 764–765.

Farrow, Stephen S. *Faith, Fancies and Fetich, or Yoruba Paganism.* London, 1926.

Faust, Drew-Gilpin. "Culture, Conflict and Community: The Meaning of Power on an Ante-Bellum Plantation." *Journal of Social History* 14, No. 1 (Fall 1980): 83–97.

Featherstonehaugh, George William. *An Excursion Through the Slave States.* New York: Harper, 1844.

Fike, Claude E. "Diary of James Oliver Hazard Perry Sessions of Rokeby Plantation on the Yazoo, January 1, 1862–June 1872." *Journal of Mississippi History* 39, No. 3 (1977): 239–254.

Finch, Charles S. *The African Background to Medical Science.* London: Karnak House, 1990.

Finkelman, Paul. *Slavery and the Founders.* New York: M. E. Sharpe, 1995.

Fisher, Walter "Physicians and Slavery in the Antebellum Southern Medical Journal." *Journal of the History of Medicine and Allied Sciences* 23 (1968): 36–49.

Fortier, Alcee. *Louisiana Studies.* New Orleans, 1894.

Fortes, M. "Ritual Festivals and Social Cohesion in the Hinterland of the Gold Coast." *American Anthropology* 38, (1936), 590–604.

Franklin, John Hope and Alfred A. Moss, Jr. *From Slavery to Freedom.* Seventh Edition. New York: McGraw-Hill, 1994.

Freeman, George W. *The Rights and Duties of Slave-Holders.* Charleston, 1837.

Freire, Paulo. *Pedagogy of the Oppressed.* New York: The Seabury Press, 1970.

Frost, William. "An Account of the Yellow Fever, As it appeared at Stabroek, in the Colony of Demarary, During the Principal Part of the Years 1803 and 1804." *Medical Repository* 1, No. 1 (May- July 1809): 29–35.

Fry, Gladys-Marie. *Night Riders in Black Folk History.* Knoxville, TN: University of Tennessee Press, 1975.

Fugate, V. H. "Practical Observations on Tetanus." *New Orleans Medical and Surgical Journal.* (1852): 193–195.

Gallay, Allan (ed.) *Voices of the Old South: Eyewitness Accounts, 1528–1861.* Athens: University of Georgia Press, 1994.

Garrett, Romeo B. "Imhotep-Father of Medicine." *Negro History Bulletin* 41, No. 5 (September-October 1978): 876–877.

Gates, Henry Louis (ed.) *The Classic Slave Narratives.* New York: Mentor Books, 1987.

Gaudet, Mary Marcia Gendron. "The Folklore and Customs of the West Bank of St. John the Baptist Parish." Ph.D. diss., University of Southeastern Louisiana, 1980.

Gayarre', Charles. *History of Louisiana*, 4 Vols. 1866: reprint ed., New Orleans, 1885.

Gary, Puckrein. "Climate, Health and Black Labor in the English Americas." *Journal of American Studies* (Great Britain) 13, No. 2 (1979): 179–193.

Gaudet, Marcia. "Bouki, the Hyena, in Louisiana and African Tales." *Journal of American Folklore* 105, No. 415 (1992): 66–72.

Genovese, Eugene. *Roll Jordan Roll: The World the Slaves Made.* New York: 1974.

Genovese, Eugene. "The Medical and Insurance Costs of Slaveholding in the Cotton Belt." *The Journal of Negro History* 45 (July 1960): 141–55.

Goodheart, Laurence B., et. al. (eds.) *Slavery in American Society.* Lexington, MA: D.C. Heath and Company, 1993

Goodson, Martia Graham. "The Medical and Botanical Contributions of African Slave Women to American Medicine." *The Western Journal of Black Studies* 11, No. 4 (1987): 198–203.

Goodwin, R. Christopher, Jill-Karen Yakubik and Cyd Heymann Goodwin. Elmwood: *The Historic Archeology of a Southeastern Louisiana Plantation.* Metarie, La.: Jefferson Parish Historical Commission, 1984.

Govan, Thomas P. "Was Plantation Slavery Profitable." *The Journal of Southern History* 8, No. 4 (November 1942): 513–535.

Greenwald, Bruce C. and Glasspiegel, Robert R. "Adverse Selection in the Market for Slaves: New Orleans, 1830–1860." *Quarterly Journal of Economics* 98, No. 3 (1983): 479–499.

Grier, S. L. "The Negro and His Diseases." *New Orleans Medical and Surgical Journal* X (May 1853): 759–60.

Griffith (Browne). *The Autobiography of a Female Slave*. 1858.

Grim, William E. *Ethno-botany of the Black Americans*. Algonac, MI: Reference Publications, 1979.

Guillory, James. "Southern Nationalism and the Louisiana Medical Profession, 1840–1860." Masters Thesis, Louisiana State University, Baton Rouge, 1965.

Guillory, James Denny. "The Pro-Slavery Arguments of Dr. Samuel A. Cartwright." *Louisiana History* 9, No. 3 (Fall 1968): 209–227.

Gutman, Herbert G. *Slavery and the Numbers Game a Critique of Time on the Cross*. Urbana: University of Illinois Press, 1975.

Hall, Julien A., "Negro Conjuring and Tricking." *Journal of American Folklore* 10 (1897): 241–243.

Hall, Mark. "The Proslavery Thought of J.D.B. De Bow: A Practical Man's Guide to Economics." *Southern Studies* 21, No. 1 (1982): 97–104.

Haller, John Jr. "The Negro and the Southern Physician: A Study of Medical and Racial Attitudes, 1800–1860." *Medical History* XVI (July 1972): 238–253.

Halley, Howard L. "Dr. Phillip Madison Shepard and His Medical School." *De Historia Medicinae* II (February 1958): 1–5.

Harland, R. "III. Observations on the Neglect of Supplying Vessels with Medical Assistance, in Long Voyages." *The American Medical Recorder* 1, No. 1 (January 1818): 8–11.

Hanger, Kimberly S. "Avenues to Freedom Open to New Orleans' Black Population, 1769–1779." *Louisiana History* 31, No. 3 (1990): 237–264.

Hardy, James, D. Jr. "A Slave Sale in Antebellum New Orleans." *Southern Studies* 23, No. 3 (1984): 306–314.

Harley, G. W. *Native African Medicine*. London: Frank Cass, 1970.

Harris, Joel Chandler. *Uncle Remus: His Songs and Sayings*. New York: D. Appleton, 1880.

Harris, Norma. "A Philosophical Basis for an Afrocentric Orientation." *The Western Journal of Black Studies* 16, No. 3 (1992): 154–159.

Harris, Robert P. "A Record of Cesarean Operations that have been Performed in the State of Louisiana during the Present Century." *New Orleans Medical and Surgical Journal* VI (1878–79): 933–942.

Harris, Robert P. "Twenty Cesarean Operations, with 15 Women Saved in Louisiana." *New Orleans Medical and Surgical Journal* VII (1879–80): 938–941.

Harrison, Ira E. "Health Status and Healing Practices: Continuations from an African Past." *Journal of African Studies* 2, No. 4 (1975–76): 547–560.

Harvey, W. M. and John Lindesay. "Account of the Cachexia Africana." *The Medical Repository* 2, No. 2 (1799): 282–284.

Haskins, James. *Witchcraft, Mysticism, and Magic in the Black World*. Garden City, NY: Doubleday, 1974.

Herron (Miss) and Bacon, A. M. "Conjuring and Conjure-Doctors in the Southern United States." *Journal of American Folklore* 9 (1896): 143–147, 224–226.

Herskovits, Melville. *The Myth of the Negro Past*. Boston: Beacon Press, 1968.

Herskovits, Melville. "African Gods and Catholic Saints in the New World." *American Anthropologist* 39 (1937): 635–643.

Hester, A. "List of Interments in the City of New Orleans from the 12th of February to the 28th of May, 1848, being 15 Weeks." *New Orleans Medical and Surgical Journal* 5, (1848–49): 136.

Hewlett and Bright, Announcement of Slave Sale, 1835. An original copy in the possession of Ms. Jermaine Jackson and Family, New Orleans, Louisiana.

Heustis, Jabez. *Physical Observations and Medical Tracts and Researches on the Topography and Disease of Louisiana.* New York: 1817.
Hicks, John R. "African Consumption." *Stethoscope* IV (November 1854): 625–629.
Hill, Henry B. and Larry Gara. "A French Traveler's View of Ante-Bellum New Orleans." *Louisiana History* 1, No. 1 (Fall 1960): 335–340.
"Historical Sketch of the New Orleans Charity Hospital." *New Orleans Medical and Surgical Journal* 1, No. 2 (May 1844): 72–77.
Holloway, Joseph E. (ed.). *Africanisms in American Culture.* Bloomington: Indiana University Press, 1990.
Holloway, Joseph E. "African Traditions and Cultures." *The Western Journal of Black Studies* 13, No. 3 (1989): 115–124.
Hughes, Charles and John M. Hunter. "Disease and 'Development' in Africa." *Social Science and Medicine* 3 (April 1970): 443–493.
Huhner, Leon. *The Life of Judah Touro (1775–1854).* Philadelphia: The Jewish Publication Society of America, 1946.
Humphrey, David C. "Dissection and Discrimination: The Social Origins of Cadavers in America, 1760–1915." *New York Academy of Medicine Bulletin* XLIX (September 1973): 819–827.
Hurmence, Belinda (ed.). *My Folks Don't Want Me to Talk About Slavery.* John F. Blair: Winston-Salem, North Carolina, 1984.
Hurston, Zora Neale. "Hoodoo in America." *Journal of American Folklore* 44 (1931): 317–417.
Hurston, Zora Neale. *Mules and Men.* Philadelphia, 1935.
Imperato, P. J., *African Gold Medicine.* Baltimore: York Press, 1979.
Ingersoll, Thomas. "Free Blacks in a Slave Society: New Orleans, 1718–1812." *William and Mary Quarterly* XLVIII, No. 2 (April 1991): 173–200.
Jackson, John G. *Introduction to African Civilizations.* New York: University Books, Inc. 1970.

Jacobs, Claude F. "Spirit Guides and Possession in New Orleans Black Spiritual Churches." *Journal of American Folklore* (1989): 45–67.

Jacobs, Claude F. and Andrew J. Kaslow. *The Spiritual Churches of New Orleans*. Knoxville: The University of Tennessee Press, 1991.

Jahn, Janheinz. *Muntu, African Culture and the Western World*. New York: Grove Weidenfeld, 1989.

Janzen, John M. *NGOMA: Discourses of Healing in Central and Southern Africa*. Berkeley: University of California Press, 1991.

Jenkins, George. "The Legal Status of Dissecting." *Anatomical Record* VII (November 1913): 387–88.

Jenkins, William Sumner. "Pro-Slavery Thought of the Old South." *Opportunity: A Journal of Negro Life* XV, No. 1 (January 1937): 8.

Johnson, Charles. *Unwritten History of Slavery*. Microcard Editions: Washington, D.C., 1968.

Johnson, Charles S. *Shadow of the Planation*. 1934.

Johnson, Jerah. "Marcus B. Christian and the WPA History of Black People in Louisiana." *Louisiana History* 20 (1979): 113–115.

Johnson, Jerah. "New Orlean's Congo Square: An Urban Setting for Early Afro-American Culture Formation." *Louisiana History* 32, No. 2 (1991): 117–157.

Jones, Jacqueline. *Labor of Sorrow, Labor of Love: Black Women, Work, and the Family from Slavery to the Present*. New York: Vintage of Random House, 1986.

Jordan, Weymouth F. "Plantation Medicine in the Old South." *The Alabama Reviews* 3 (1950): 83–107.

Jumonville, Florence M. *Bibliography of New Orleans Imprints 1764–1864*. New Orleans: The Historic New Orleans Collection, 1989.

Kahn, Catherine. "Directing Touro." *Tourovues* (Fall 1991): 4–5.

Kambon, Kobi Kazembe Kalongi. *The African Personality in America: An African-Centered Framework.* Florida: Nubian Nation Publications, 1992.

Kane, Harnett Thomas. *Plantation Parade: The Grand Manner in Louisiana.* New York: Morrow, 1945.

Karenga, Maulana. *Introduction to Black Studies.* Los Angeles: University of Sankore Press, 1993.

Karenga, Maulana. "Black Studies and the Problematic of Paradigm: The Philosophical Divisions." *The Journal of Black Studies* 18, 4 (June): 395–414.

Karenga, Maulana and Jacob H. Carruthers (eds). *Kemet and The African World View.* Los Angeles: University of Sankore Press, 1986.

Kaufman, Martin. "Medicine and Slavery: An Essay Review." *Georgia Historical Quarterly* 64, No. 3 (Fall 1979): 380–390.

Kelley, Jennifer O. and J. Lawrence Angel. "Life Stresses of Slavery." *American Journal of Physical Anthropology* 74, No. 2 (1987): 199–211.

Kemble, Frances Anne. "A Visit to the Infirmary on Butler's Island." in Willie Lee Rose's *A Documentary History of Slavery in North America.* New York: Oxford University Press, 1976.

Kendall, John S. "The Shawdow Over the City." *Louisiana Historical Quarterly* 22 (January 1939): 141–165.

Kendall, John S. "New Orleans Peculiar Institution." *Louisiana Historical Quarterly* XXIII (July 1940): 864–886.

Kenney, Elizabeth Barnaby. "Unless Powerful Sick: Domestic Medicine in the Old South." in Ronald Numbers and Todd Savitt's *Medicine in the Old South.* Baton Rouge: Louisiana State University Press, 1989: 276–294.

Kerrs, Gloria L. *Livingston Parish Louisiana Mortality and Slave Schedules 1850–1880.* Baker, Louisiana: Folk Finders, 1983.

Kershaw, Terry. "Afrocentrism and the Afrocentric Method." *Western Journal of Black Studies* 16, No. 3 (1992): 160–168.

Keto, C. Tsehloane. *The African Centered Perspective of History.* Blackwood: K. A. Publications, 1989.

Keto, C. Tsehloane. *Vision, Identity and Time.* Iowa: Kendall Hunt Publishing, Co., 1995.

Kilbourne, Richard Holcombe. *Debt, Investment, Slaves: Credit Relations in East Feliciana Parish, Louisiana, 1825–1885.* Tuscaloosa: University of Alabama Press, 1995.

Kiple, Kenneth F. and Virginia H. Kiple. "The African Connection: Slavery, Disease and Racism." *Phylon* XLI, No. 3 (1980): 211–222.

Kiple, Kenneth F and Virginia H. Kiple. "Slave Child Mortality: Some Nutritional Answers to a Perennial Puzzle." *Journal of Social History* 10 (1977): 284–306.

Kiple, Kenneth F. and Virginia H. Kiple. "Black Tongue and Black Men: Pellagra and Slavery in the Antebellum South." *Journal of Southern History* 43, No. 3 (1977): 411–428.

Knappert, Jan. *The Aquarian Guide to African Mythology.* England: The Aquarian Press, 1990.

Kolchin, Peter. *American Slavery 1619–1877.* New York: Hill and Wang, 1993.

Kreiger, Nancy. "Shades of Difference: Theoretical Underpinnings of the Medical Controversy on Black/White Differ- ences in the United States, 1830–1870." *International Journal of Health Services* 17, No. 2 (1987): 259–278.

Kunkel, Paul A. "Modifications in Louisiana Negro Legal Status under Louisiana Constitutions, 1812–1957." *Journal of Negro History* 44 (1959): 1–25.

Labb, Dolores Egger. "Mothers and Children in Antebellum Louisiana." *Louisiana History* 34, No. 2 (1993): 161–173.

Langridge, Leland A. "Asiatic Cholera in Louisiana 1832–1873." Masters Thesis, Louisiana State University, 1955.

Lathrop, Barnes Fletcher. "The Pugh Plantations, 1860–1865: A Study of Life in Lower Louisiana." Ph.D. diss., University of Texas, 1945.

Latrobe, Benjamin H. *Impressions Respecting New Orleans: Diary and Sketches, 1818–1820.* New York: Columbia University Press, 1951.

Leavitt, Judith Wolzer and Ronald L. Numbers (ed.) *Sickness and Health in America: Readings in the History of Medicine and Public Health.* Madison: University of Wisconsin Press, 1985.

Lee, Anne S. and Everett S. Lee. "The Health of Slaves and the Health of Freedmen: A Savannah Study." *Phylon* 38, No. 2 (1977): 170–180.

Levine, Laurence W. *Black Culture and Black Consciousness.* New York: Oxford University Press, 1977.

Lind, J. E. "Phylogenetic Elements in the Psychoses of the Negro." *Psychoanalytic Review* 4 (1917): 303–332.

Lowe, Richard and Randolph Campbell. "The Slave-Breeding Hypothesis: A Demographic Comment on the 'Buying' and 'Selling' States." *The Journal of Southern History* 42, No. 3 (August 1976): 401–412.

Lyell, Charles. *Selections. 1970* Life Letters, and Journals of Sir Charles Lyell.* England: Gregg International Publishers, 1970.

Maduell, Charles R. *The Census Tables for the French Colony of Louisiana from 1699 through 1732.* (Compiled and translated by Charles Maduell). Baltimore: Genealogical Publication, Co., 1972.

Mahorner, Howard. "The History of Medicine in Louisiana." *Louisiana Historical Quarterly.* 1, No. 1 (1973): 49–67.

Maisonneuve, M. "The Guinea-Worm-(Dranunuculus)." *New Orleans Medical and Surgical Journal* 2, No. 1 (July 1845): 78–79.

Malone, Ann Patton. *Sweet Chariot, Slave Family and Household Structure in Nineteenth Century Louisiana.* Chapel Hill: University of North Carolina Press, 1992.

Margo, Robert A. "The Heights of American Slaves: New Evidence on Slave Nutrition and Health." *Social Science History* 6, No. 4 (1982): 516–538.

Marshall, Mary L. "Planation Medicine." *Tulane Medical Faculty, Bulletin* I (May 1942): 52.

Marshall, Mary L. "Planation Medicine." *Bulletin of the Medical Library Association* 26 (1938): 116.

Martin, John M. "The People of New Orleans as Seen by Her Visitors, 1803–1860." *Louisiana Studies* VI, No. 4, (Winter 1967): 361–375.

Martin, Francois-Xavier. *History of Louisiana From The Earliest Period.* New Orleans: James A. Gresham, 1882.

Matas, Rudolph. "Francois Marie Prevost and the Early History of the Cesarean Section in Louisiana." *New Orleans Medical and Surgical Journal* LXXXIX (1937): 604–25.

Maxwell, James. "Pathological Inquiry into the Nature of Cachexia Africana." *Jamaica Phys. Journal* 2 (1935): 413–417.

May, Jude Thomas. "The Medical Care of Blacks in Louisiana During the Occupation and Reconstruction." Ph.D. diss., Tulane University, 1971.

Mayer, Brantz, *Captain Canot; or Twenty Years on an African Slaver.* New York: D. Appleton and Co., 1854.

Mbiti, John S. *African Religion and Philosophy*. New York: Anchor Books, 1970.

McDonald, Roderick. *The Economy and Material Culture of Slaves: Goods and Chattels on the Sugar Plantations of Jamaica and Louisiana*. Baton Rouge: Louisiana State University Press, 1993.

McElrath, J. J. "Art. III—Surgical Memoranda." *New Orleans Medical and Surgical Journal* 16 (1859): 195–197.

McGinty, Garnie William. *A History of Louisiana*. New York: Exposition Press, 1951.

McGregor, Deborah Kuhn. "Silver Sutures: The Medical Career of J. Marion Sims." Ph.D. diss., State University of New York at Binghamton, 1986.

McLaurin, Melton A. *Celia: A Slave: A True Story of Violence and Retribution in Antebellum Missouri*. Athens, GA: University of Georgia Press, 1991.

McMillen, Sally G. "Antebellum Southern Fathers and the Health Care of Children." *The Journal of Southern History* LX, No. 3 (August 1994): 513–532.

McTyeire, H. N. et. al. *Duties of Masters of Servants: Three Premium Essays*, Charleston, 1851.

Mellon, James (ed.) *Bullwhip Days The Slaves Remember.* New York: Avon Books, 1988.
Menn, Joseph Karl. *The Large Slaveholders of Louisiana*. New Orleans, 1964.
Midlo-Hall, Gwendolyn. *Africans in Colonial Louisiana.* Baton Rouge: Louisiana University Press, 1993.
Miller, Kelly. "The Historic Background of the Negro Physician." *The Journal of Negro History* 1 (April 1916): 99–109.
Miller, Randall M. (ed.) *Dear Master Letters of a Slave Family.* Athens: University of Georgia Press, 1990.
Milligan, R. H. *The Fetish Folk of West Africa.* New York, 1912.
Mitchell, Martha Carolyn. "Health and the Medical Profession in the Lower South, 1845–1860." *The Journal of Southern History* X, No. 4 (November 1944): 424–446.
Moody, Vernie A. "Slavery on Louisiana Sugar Plantations." *Louisiana Historical Quarterly* 2 (1924): 191–301.
Morais, Herbert M. *The History of the Negro in Medicine.* New York: Association for the Study of Negro Life and History, 1967.
Morgan, John. "An Essay on the Causes of the Production of Abortion among Our Negro Population." *Nashville Journal of Medicine and Surgery* 19 (1860): 117–118.
Morris, James P. "An American First: Blood Transfusion in New Orleans in the 1850s." *Louisiana History* 16, No. 4 (Fall 1975): 341–360.
Mulira, Jessie Gaston. "The Case of Voodoo in New Orleans." in Joseph E. Holloway's *Africanisms in American Culture.* Bloomington: Indiana University Press, 1990.
Myers, Linda James. *Understanding the Afrocentric Worldview.* Dubuque, Iowa: Kendall-Hunt, 1988.
Nadel, S. F. "Witchcraft and Anti-Witchcraft in Nupe Society." *Africa* 8 (1935): 423–447.
Neeley, Bobby Joe. "Contemporary Afro-American Voodooism (Black Religion): The Retention and Adaptation of the Ancient African-Egyptian Mystery System." Ph.D. diss., University of California—Berkeley, October, 1989.
New Orleans Bee. (*L'Abeille*) April 11, 1834.

Newman, Debra. "Slave Manifests." *Journal of the Afro-American Historical and Genealogical Society* 3, No. 1 (1982): 40–44.

Newsome, Frederick. "Black Contributions to the Early History of Western Medicine." in Ivan Van Sertima's *Blacks in Science: Ancient and Modern Journal of African Civilizations.* New Brunswick: Transaction Books, 1986: 127–139.

Ngubane, Jordan. *Conflict of Minds, Changing Power Dispositions in South Africa.* New York: Books in Focus, Inc., 1979.

Numbers, Ronald L. and Todd L. Savitt (eds.) *Science and Medicine in the Old South.* Baton Rouge: Louisiana State University Press, 1989.

Olmsted, Frederick Law. *The Cotton Kingdom: A Traveller's Observations on Cotton and Slavery in the American Slave States.* (2 Vols.) New York, 1861.

Olmsted, Frederick Law. *A Journey in the Seaboard Slave States.* New York: Mason, 1856.

Oppenheim, Leonard. *Louisiana Civil Law Treatise.* (Vol. 10). St. Paul, MN: West Publishing, Co., 1973.

Osofsky, Gilbert (ed.). *Puttin on Ole Massa: The Slave Narratives of Henry Bibb, William Wells Brown and Solomon Northup.* New York, 1969.

Otto, John Solomon and Augustus Marion Burners, III. "Black Folks and Poor Buckras: Archeological Evidence of Slave and Overseer Living Conditions on an Antebellum Plantation." *Journal of Black Studies* 14, No. 2 (1983): 185–200.

Owen, Nicholas. *Journal of a Slave-dealer.* Boston, 1930.

Ownby, Ted (ed.) *Black and White Cultural Interaction in the Antebellum South.* (Chancellor's Symposium Series.) Jackson: University Press of Mississippi, 1993.

Owsley, Douglas W., et. al. "Demography and Pathology of an Urban Slave Publication From New Orleans." *American Journal of Physical Anthropology* 74, No. 2 (1987): 185–197.

Oyebade, Bayo. "African Studies and the Afrocentric Paradigm a Critique." *Journal of Black Studies* 21, No. 2 (December 1990): 233–238.

Parrinder, E. G. *African Traditional Religion.* London, 1954.
Paxton, John Adam, *The New Orleans Directory and Register.* New Orleans, 1822.
Pelton, Robert W. *The Complete Book of Voodoo.* New York: Arco, 1972.
Pendleton, E. M. "On the Susceptibility of the Caucasian and African Races to the Different Classes of Disease." *Southern Medical Reports* I (1849): 336–37.
Pendleton, Louis. "Negro Folk-Lore and Witchcraft in the South." *Journal of American Folklore* 3 (1890): 201–207.
Pfeiffer, Carl J. *The Art and Practice of Western Medicine in the Early Nineteenth Century.* Jefferson, N.C.: McFarland, 1985.
Phillips, Ulrich Bonnell. *American Negro Slavery.* New York: D. Appleton, 1929.
Phillips, Ulrich Bonnell. *The Slave Economy of the Old South.* Baton Rouge: Louisiana State University Press, 1968.
Picayune, The. Vol. 1, 1837; Vol. 2, 1838.
Pickett, Albert. *Eight Days in New Orleans* (n.p., 1847).
Police Code, or Collection of the Ordinances of Police Made by the City Council of New Orleans. New Orleans, 1808.
Porteus, Laura L. "The Gri Gri Case: A Criminal Trial in Louisiana During the Spanish Regime, 1773." *Louisiana Historical Quarterly* XVII (1934): 48–63.
Postell, William D. *The Health of Slaves on Southern Plantations.* Baton Rouge: Louisiana State University Press, 1951.
Pritchett, Jonathan B. and Freudenberger, Herman. "A Peculiar Sample: The Selection of Slaves for the New Orleans Market." *Journal of Economic History* 52, No. 1 (1992): 109–127.
Puckett, N. N. *The Magic and Folk Beliefs of the Southern Negro.* New York: Dover Publications, Inc., 1969.
Puckrein, Gary. "Climate, Health and Black Labor in the English Americas." *American Studies* (Great Britain) 13, No. 2 (1979): 179–193.
Quarles, Benjamin. *The Negro in the Making of America.* New York: Collier Books, 1964.

Raboteau, Albert J. *Slave Religion: The "Invisible Institution" in the Antebellum*. Oxford University Press, 1978.

Ralston, Robert. "A Few Observations on a Case of Mania." *The Medical Repository* 3, No. 1 (May - July 1811): 142–147.

Ramsay, W. G. "The Physiological Differences Between the European (or White Man) and the Negro." *Southern Agriculturalists and Register of Rural Affairs* XII (June 1839): 286–294.

Rankin, David C. "The Tannenbaum Thesis Reconsidered: Slavery and Race Relations in Antebellum Louisiana." *Southern Studies* XVIII (Spring 1979): 5–31.

Rawick, George P. (ed). *The American Slave: A Composite Autobiography*. (19 volumes). Westport, CT, 1972.

Redard, Thomas E. "The Port of New Orleans: An Economic History, 1821–1860." Ph.D. diss., Louisiana State University, 1985.

Reddick, Laurence D. "The Negro in the New Orleans Press, 1859–1860: A Study in Attitudes and Propaganda." Ph.D. diss., University of Chicago, 1941.

"Regulations, Edicts, Declarations and Decrees Concerning the Commerce, Administration of Justice, and Policing of Louisiana and other French Colonies in America Together with the Black Code." (1685) Translated from the French by Olivia Blanchard, Survey of Federal Archives in Louisiana, Works Projects Administration, 1940.

Reilly, Timothy F. "Le Ligerateur: New Orleans' Free Negro Newspaper." *Gulf Coast Historical Review* 2, No. 1 (1986): 5–24.

Rice, C. Duncan. *The Rise and Fall of Black Slavery*. Baton Rouge: Louisiana University Press, 1975.

Rice, Mitchell F. "On Assessing Black Health Status: A Historical Overview." *Urban League Review* 9, No. 2 (1985–86): 6–12.

Richards, Dona Marimba (Marimba Ani). "The Implications of African-American Spirituality." in Molefi K. Asante and Karimu Welsh-Asante's *African Culture: The Rhythms of Unity*. New Jersey: Africa World Press, 1990.

Richards, Dona Marimba. (Marimba Ani). *Let the Circle Be Unbroken, The Implications of African Spirituality in the Diaspora.* New York, 1980.
Riddell, William R. "Le Code Noir." *Journal of Negro History* 10, No. 3 (July 1925): 321–329.
Robb, Bernard. *Welcum Hinges.* New York: E. P. Dutton, 1942.
Robinson, Beverly J. "Africanisms and the Study of Folklore." in Joseph E. Holloway's *Africanisms in American Culture.* Bloomington: Indiana University Press, 1990.
Robinson, Jean Wealmont. "Black Healers During the Colonial Period and Early 19th Century America." Ph.D. diss., Southern Illinois University—Carbondale, 1979.
Rose, Willie Lee (ed.). *A Documentary History of Slavery in North America.* New York: Oxford University Press, 1976.
Rosengarten, Theodore. *Tombee: Portrait of a Cotton Planter.* New York: William Morrow and Co., Inc., 1986.
Rousseve, Charles Barthelemy. *The Negro in Louisiana: Aspects of His History and His Literature.* New Orleans: Xavier University Press, 1937.
Salvaggio, John. *New Orleans Charity Hospital: A Story of Physicians, Politics and Poverty.* Baton Rouge: Louisiana State University Press, 1992.
Saxon, Lyle. *Fabulous New Orleans.* New York: The Century Publishing Co., 1928 (Gretna: Pelican Publishing Co., 1988).
Saxon, Lyle. *Old Louisiana.* New York: The Century Publishing Co., 1929 (Gretna: Pelican Publishing Co., 1988).
Saxon, Lyle, Edward Dreyer and Robert Tallant. *Gumbo Ya-Ya.* Louisiana Library Commission, 1945 (Gretna: Pelican Publishing, Co., 1987).
Savitt, Todd. *Medicine and Slavery: The Disease and Health Care of Blacks in Antebellum Virginia.* Urbana: University of Illinois Press, 1978.
Savitt, Todd L. "Smothering and Overlaying of Virginia Slave Children: A Suggested Explanation." *Bulletin of History of Medicine* 49 (1975): 402.

Savitt, Todd L. "Black Health on the Plantation: Masters, Slaves, and Physicians." in Ronald Numbers and Todd Savitt's, *Science and Medicine in the Old South*. Baton Rouge: Louisiana State University Press, 1989: 327–355.

Savitt, Todd L. "The Use of Blacks for Medical Experimentation and Demonstration in the Old South." *Journal of Southern History* 48, No. 3 (1982): 331–348.

Scarborough, William Kauffman. *The Overseer: Plantation Management in the Old South*. Baton Rouge: Louisiana State University Press, 1966.

Schafer, Judith Kelleher. "'Guaranteed Against the Vice and Maladies Prescribed by Law': Consumer Protection, the Law of Slave Sales, and the Supreme Court in Antebellum Louisiana." *The American Journal of Legal History* XXXI (1987): 306–321.

Schafer, Judith Kelleher. "New Orleans Slavery in 1850 as Seen in Advertisements." *The Journal of Southern History* XLVII, No. 1 (February 1981): 33–56.

Schafer, Judith Kelleher. "'Open and Notorious Concubinage': The Emancipation of Slave Mistresses by Will and the Supreme Court in Antebellum Louisiana." *Louisiana History* 28, No. 2 (Spring 1987): 165–182.

Schafer, Judith Kelleher. *Slavery, The Civil Law, and The Supreme Court of Louisiana*. Baton Rouge: Louisiana State University Press, 1993.

Schweninger, Loren. "A Negro Sojourner in Antebellum New Orleans." *Louisiana History* 20, No. 3 (1979): 305–314.

Setiloane, Gabriel. *African Theology*. Capetown: Skotaville Publishers, 1986.

Sheridan, Richard. *Doctors and Slaves: a Medical and Demographic History of Slavery in the British West Indies, 1680–1834*. New York: Cambridge University Press, 1985.

Shryock, Richard H. "Medical Sources and the Social Historian." *American Historical Review*. 41 (1936): 458–473.

Sims, J. Marion. *The Story of My Life* (ed. by H. Marion-Sims). New York, 1884.

Simons, J. Hume. *The Planter's Guide and Family Book of Medicine.* Charleston, 1848.
Sitterson, Carlyle. "The William J. Minor Plantations: A Study in Ante-Bellum Absentee Ownership." *Journal of Southern History.* (1967): 59–74.
Skipper, Ottis Clark. "J.D.B. De Bow, the Man." *The Journal of Southern History* X, No. 4 (November 1944): 404–423.
"Slave Laws at the South." *De Bow's Review* 2, No. II, N.S. (February 1850): 182–185.
Smart, Ninian. *The Religious Experience of Mankind.* New York: Charles Scribner's Sons, 1984.
Some, Malidoma Patrice. *Of Water and the Spirit. Ritual, Magic, and Initiation in the Life of an African Shaman.* New York: Tarcher/Putnam Books, 1994.
Soniat, Meloney C. "The Tchoupitoulas Plantation." *Louisiana Historical Quarterly* 7, No. 2 (April 1924): 308–315.
Stampp, Kenneth. *The Peculiar Institution: Slavery in the Antebellum South.* New York: Vintage Books, 1956.
Starobin, Robert S. (ed.). *Blacks in Bondage: Letters of American Slaves.* New York, 1974.
Steckel, Richard. "Sante Et Mortalite Des Esclaves Americains, Nouveaux Resultats." (Health and Mortality of American Slaves: New Findings). *Bulletin d'Information de la Societe de Demographic Historique* (France). 53 (1988): 44–49.
Steckel, Richard H. "A Dreadful Childhood: The Excess Mortality of American Slaves." *Social Sciences History* 10, No. 4 (1986): 427–466.
Steckel, Richard H. "A Peculiar Population: The Nutrition, Health, and Mortality of American Slaves From Childhood to Maturity." *Journal of Economic History* 46, No. 3 (1986): 721–741.
Stephens, Lester D. "Scientific Societies in the Old South: The Elliott Society and the New Orleans Academy of Sciences." in Ronald Numbers and Todd Savitt's *Science and Medicine in the Old South.* Baton Rouge: Louisiana State University, 1989: 55–78.

Sterling, Dorothy (ed.). *We Are Your Sisters.* New York: W. W. Norton and Co., 1984.

Steward, Austin. *Twenty-two years a Slave.* Rochester, 1857.

Still, William. *The Underground Rail Road: A Record of Facts, Authentic Narratives, Letters, &c., Narrating the Hardships Hair-breadth Escapes and Death Struggles of the Slaves in Their Efforts for Freedom, as Related by Themselves and Others, or Witnessed by the Author.* 1872.

Sutherland, Daniel E. and Lisa Roberts. "Looking for De Bow." *Louisiana History* 27, No. 1 (Winter 1986): 69–75.

Tallent, Robert. *Voodoo in New Orleans.* New York: Macmillan, 1946.

Tannenbaum, Frank. *Slave and Citizen: The Negro in the Americas.* New York, 1946.

Tansey, Richard. "Bernard Kendig and the New Orleans Slave Trade." *Louisiana History* 23, No. 2 (Spring 1982): 159–178.

Tate, Gayle T. "Black Nationalism and Spiritual Redemption." *The Western Journal of Black Studies* 15, No. 4 (1991): 213–222.

Taylor, Joe Gray. *Negro Slavery in Louisiana.* Louisiana Historical Association, 1963.

Thompson, Robert Ferris. *Flash of the Spirit.* New York: Vintage Books, 1984.

Thomson, James. *Treatise on the Diseases of Negroes.* Jamaica: Alex Aikman, 1820.

Thrasher, Albert. "On To New Orleans." *Unpublished paper.* New Orleans, Louisiana, 1994.

Tidyman, P. "A Sketch of the most Remarkable Diseases of the Negroes of the Southern States." *Philadelphia Journal of the Medical and Physical Sciences* 12 (1826): 306–338.

Touchstone, Blake. "Voodoo in New Orleans." *Louisiana History* 13, No. 4 (1972): 371–386.

U.S. Seventh Census 1850. *Slave Inhabitants*, Louisiana, IV.

Usner, Daniel H. "From African Captivity to American Slavery: The Introduction to Black Laborers to Colonial Louisiana." *Louisiana History* 20 (1979): 25–48.

Wade, Richard C. *Slavery in the Cities, the South 1820–1860.* New York: Oxford University Press, 1968.

Waite, Frederick C. "Grave Robbing in New England." *Medical Library Association, Bulletin* XXXIII (July 1945): 283–284.

Walker, Samuel. *"The Diary of a Louisiana Planter, Elia Plantation."* Typescript, Tulane University Library.

Walker, Sheila. "African Gods in the Americas: The Black Religious Continuum." *The Black Scholar* 11, No. 8 (November-December 1980): 25–36.

Wells, Bennett H. *Louisiana: A History.* Arlington Heights, IL: Forum Press, Inc. 1990.

Warner, John Harley. "The Selective Transport of Medical Knowledge: Antebellum American Physicians and Parisian Medical Therapies." *Bulletin of the History of Medicine* 59, No. 2 (1985): 213–231.

Watson, Wilbur H. *Black Folk Medicine.* New Brunswick: Transaction Books, 1984.

Wax, Darold D. "A Philadelphia Surgeon on a Slaving Voyage to Africa, 1749–1751." *Pennsylvania Magazine of History and Biography* 92, No. 4 (1968): 465–493.

Webb, Allie Bayne Windham. *Mistress of Evergreen Plantation, Rachel O'Connor's Legacy of Letters 1823–1845.* Albany: State University of New York Press, 1983.

Wegener, Vernon A. "Negro Slavery in New Orleans." Master's Thesis, Tulane University, 1935.

Weld, Theodore Dwight (ed.). *American Slavery As it Is: Testimony of a Thousand Witnesses.* New York, 1839.

Whitten, David O. "Medical Care of Slaves: Louisiana Sugar Region and South Carolina Rice District." *Southern Studies* 16, No. 2 (1977): 153–180.

Whitten, David O. "Slave Buying in 1835 Virginia as Revealed by Letters of a Louisiana Negro Sugar Planter." *Louisiana History* 11, No. 3 (Summer 1970): 231–244.

Whitten, David O. *Andrew Durford: A Black Sugar Plantation Owner in Antebellum Louisiana.* Louisiana: Northwestern State University Press, 1981.

Wilson, Robert. "Their Shawdowy Influence Still Hovers About Medical College." *Charleston Sunday News Courier* (April 13, 1913).

Wilson, Samuel, Jr. "Plantation of the Company of the Indies." *Louisiana History* 31, No. 2 (1990): 161–191.

Wilson, Theodore Brantner. *The Black Codes of the South.* University: University of Alabama Press, 1965.

Wilson, Thomas Woodrow. "Ancient Environments and Modern Disease: The Case of Hypertension Among Afro-Americans." Ph.D. diss., Bowling Green State University, 1987.

Winsell, Keith A. "Black Identity: The Southern Negro, 1830–1895." Ph.D. diss., University of California—Los Angeles, 1971.

Woessner, Herman C., III. "New Orleans Slavery, 1840–1860 a Study in Urban Slavery." Masters Thesis, Louisiana State University, 1967.

Wooster, Ralph A. "The Structure of Government in Late Antebellum Louisiana." *Louisiana Studies* 14 (1975): 361–78.

Wooten, H. V. "Dysentery Among Negroes." *New Orleans Medical and Surgical Journal* 11 (1854–1855): 448–456.

Yandell, Lunsford P. "Remarks on Struma Africana, or the Disease Usually Called Negro Poison, or Negro Consumption." *Transylvania Journal of Medicine and the Associate Sciences* IV (February 1831): 83–103.

"Yellow Fever at New Orleans." *New York Journal of Medicine.* 1, No. 2 (September 1843): 288.

Yetman, Norman R. "Ex-Slave Interviews and the Historiography of Slavery." *American Quarterly* 36 (1984): 181–210.

Ziegler, Dhyana (ed.). *Molefi Kete Asante and Afrocentricity.* Nashville: James C. Winston Publishing Co., Inc. 1995.

INDEX

A

Admission Book of the Touro Infirmary, 96, 100, 107, 189, 207-270
African Living Belief System, 151, 152, 153, 154, 155, 156, 157, 160, 167,180, 182
Afrocentricity, 156
Amenorrhea, 19, 74, 76, 106, 118, 218, 219, 220, 229, 275
Amputation, 23, 47, 106, 109, 111, 120, 122, 241, 264, 275
Anarcha, 115, 116
Asafetida, 146, 166, 271

B

Babalawo, iii, 163
Basil, 171, 260, 271
Black Bottle Men, 114
Black Codes, 7, 20, 21, 49, 51, 183, 187, 188
Bleeding/Blood-letting, 43, 74, 132, 133, 148, 271, 272
Blue Mass Pills, 31, 131, 146, 147, 148, 162, 190, 271
Breeding/Concubinage, iii, 55, 64, 65, 66, 69, 72, 73, 74, 145, 178, 205

C

Cachexia Africana, 19, 123, 125, 126, 127, 130, 177, 185, 189, 276
Cartwright, Samuel, 5, 57, 83, 86, 117, 125, 127, 128, 129, 131, 132, 139, 140, 141, 145, 185, 186, 189, 278
Castor Oil, 31, 89, 114, 147, 165, 190, 271
Cesarian Section, 19, 118, 119, 189, 197
Cholera, 19, 34, 92, 93, 106, 123, 131, 132, 133, 134, 140, 141, 177, 210, 219, 221, 228, 241, 277, 281
Cistern Water, 134
Coal Oil, 165, 272
Code Noir, 2, 21, 177
Congo Square, 49, 168
Conjurers/Conjuring, 140, 141, 143, 159, 199

D

De Bow, J. D. B., 5, 23, 123, 124, 125
De Bow's Review, 23, 124, 125
Defective Slave, 54, 184, 195
Diarrhea, 19, 104, 106. 123, 130, 131, 133, 134, 177, 184, 209, 210, 211, 214, 217, 218, 219, 220, 222, 223, 224, 227, 230, 231, 232, 233, 234, 235, 236, 237, 238, 240, 242, 243, 244, 245, 246, 249, 257, 258, 259, 260, 261, 263, 277, 278, 279, 281
Dispensers, iii, 162, 163, 174, 180, 201
Diviners, iii, 162, 163, 170, 171, 180
Drapetomania, 19, 123, 127, 128, 129, 130, 177, 186, 189, 278
Dysaesthesia Aethiopica, 123, 128, 129, 130, 177, 279
Dysentery, 19, 33, 34, 99, 104, 106, 123, 130, 131, 133, 134, 145, 177, 207, 211, 214, 220, 221, 224, 226, 234, 236, 238, 239, 241, 243, 244, 245, 246, 247, 248, 251, 253, 255, 256, 258, 259, 262, 263, 264, 279, 281
Dysmenorrhea, 19, 74, 76, 104, 106, 208, 257, 279

E

Effective, Non-Effective Hands, 63
Enslavement (defined), 3-4

F

Falling of the Womb, 19, 75, 284
French Code, 54,

G

Gens de la couleur libre, 2, 21, 62, 175, 207
Gris-Gris, 142, 173, 272

SLAVERY AND MEDICINE: ENSLAVEMENT AND MEDICAL PRACTICES IN ANTEBELLUM LOUISIANA

H

Half Hands/Full Hands, 47, 63, 97
Hookworm Disease, 126, 127, 277
Horseradish, 166, 272
Hysteria, 19, 106, 128, 130, 210, 218, 219, 222, 230, 239, 245, 282

I

Indisposition, 19, 106, 128, 130, 247, 250, 251, 254, 263, 269, 282
Ipecac, 146, 162, 190, 272

L

Las Siete Partidas, 21,
Louisiana Writer's Project, 26, 190
Louisiana Historical Quarterly, 10

M

Maafa (Middle Passage), 12, 205
Ma'at, 153, 160, 200
Menorrhagia, 75, 114, 282
Morphine, 121, 122, 273

N

Negro Consumption, 123, 124, 125, 127, 130, 177, 185, 186, 283
Negro Folklorists, 141, 142, 199
Negro/Slave Diseases, 4, 123-134, 177, 191, 194, 276, 278, 279, 283,
New Orleans Medical and Surgical Journal, 23, 112, 113, 116, 189,
Night Doctor, 22, 114
Nommo, 154, 199, 201
Northup, Solomon, 15, 32, 35, 47, 48, 68

O

Onishegun, iii, 163
Ovarian Dropsy, 76, 106, 243, 278

P

Pentateuch, The, 127
Peritoneum, 47,
Phosphorus, 112,
Post-mortem Examinations, 79, 111-122, 179, 181
Prolapses of the Uterus, 74, 75, 76, 104, 106, 108, 213, 284

Q

Quinine, 165, 166, 272

R

Raw Head and Bloody Bones, 142
Rhubarb, 148, 190, 272

S

Seasoning, 14, 32, 205
Small Pox, 19, 34
Sulphur, 94, 121, 122

T

Tinc. Iodine, 121
Touro Infirmary, 74, 75, 76, 94, 95, 96, 97, 98, 99, 100, 101, 102, 104, 105, 106, 107, 108, 127, 128, 130, 131, 132, 133, 188, 189, 207-270, 275
Two-Headed Person, 149, 171, 172

U

Uqobo, 152, 153
Urtica Urains, 113, 114

V

Vagico-fistula (Vesicovaginal, Vaginal Fistulas), 74, 76, 116, 117, 118, 119, 196, 286
Vinegar, 165, 166, 271, 273
Voodoo, 25, 142, 151, 154, 159, 160, 167, 168, 169, 173, 179, 180, 199

W

Wet Nursing, 64
Whipping, 15, 38, 42, 54, 128, 206
"Whipping Hole," 44, 45, 46
Whipping logs, 9, 15
Works Progress Administration, 11, 73, 136, 137, 165

Y

Yellow Fever, 18, 19, 33, 34, 99, 104, 106, 123, 130, 132, 133, 164, 173, 177, 193, 211, 212, 213, 262, 263, 272, 286

ABOUT THE AUTHOR

Dr. Katherine Bankole-Medina joined Coppin State University's department of History, Geography and Global Studies as Professor of History and Chair of the Department in August 2008. She is a Distinguished Faculty Researcher at CSU. Before coming to CSU, she was a tenured Associate Professor of History in the Department of History at West Virginia University (Morgantown, WV). While holding a joint tenure-track faculty appointment, she also served as the administrative Director of the Center for Black Culture and Research; and Coordinator (and 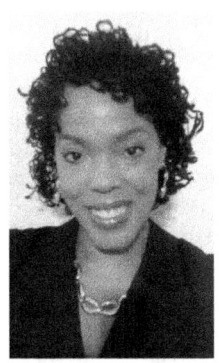 Interim-Coordinator) of the Africana Studies Program at WVU. In addition, Dr. Bankole-Medina was employed at several notable research institutions including: Xavier University (Department of History, New Orleans, LA), the University of Virginia (Luther Porter Jackson Black Culture Center, Charlottesville, VA), and Kean University (Africana Studies, Human Relations Center, Union, NJ).

Dr. Bankole-Medina is the author of many scholarly publications including the groundbreaking text *Slavery and Medicine: Enslavement and Medical Practices in Antebellum Louisiana* (New York: Garland Publishing, Inc., 1998). Her paper, "In the Age of Malcolm X: Social Conflict and the Critique of African American Identity Construction" appears in James L. Conyers, Jr. and James Smallwood's, *Malcolm X A Historical Reader* (Baltimore, MD: Carolina Academic Press, 2008). She published several entries in the *Encyclopedia of African Religion* (edited by Molefi Kete Asante and Ama Mazama), and book reviews including a review of slavery and botanical medicine for the *Journal of Southern History*. Building on her previous work as the Historical Consultant for *Caminho De Sao Tome: A Documentary on Cape Verde*, she published the chapter "Mulheres Africanas Nos Estados Unidos," in *Afrocentricidade: Uma Abordagem Epistemologica Inovadora* (Sankofa: Matrizes Africanas Da Cultura Brasileira 4 by Elisa Larkin Nascimento, Sao Paulo, Brasil: Selo Negro Edicoes, 2009.) In twentieth century African American history, her articulation of the life and legacy of Charles Hamilton Houston was published in one book edited by James L. Conyers Jr., and another scholarly paper on Houston appears in a CSU conference proceeding.

Dr. Bankole-Medina is founding editor of *Africalogical Perspectives* a scholarly journal and senior editor of *Women of African Descent and Justice in World Societies* (with Dr. Abena Lewis-Mhoon and Prof. Stephanie

SLAVERY AND MEDICINE: ENSLAVEMENT AND MEDICAL PRACTICES IN
ANTEBELLUM LOUISIANA

Yarbough). Currently, articles on Malcolm X and the history of antebellum diagnostic racism are pending peer review. Furthermore, Dr. Bankole-Medina is also author of the first book published on the Baltimore Uprising, entitled *World to Come: The Baltimore Uprising Militant Racism and History* (2016). In addition, she published *Self-Emancipated and Unforgotten Women* with Dr. Abena Lewis-Mhoon; and a paper in the prestigious journal *Phillis* (edited by Dr. Claudia Nelson) on the life and legacy of Fanny Jackson Coppin.

Dr. Bankole-Medina has received numerous awards and grants for research and scholarship in higher education. In 2009 she received the Distinguished Faculty Researcher Award at CSU. Further, in 2007 she received the WV Humanities Council Grant for her research on Africana Women. In 2006 Bankole-Medina was named the Judith Gold Stitzel Endowment Teacher for her research addressing instructional themes, gender and enslavement. In 2004-2005 Bankole-Medina was named Humanities Scholar for the West Virginia Humanities Grant Project "Segregation and Integration of High School Sports in West Virginia" (Project Coordinators Drs. Dana Brooks and Ronald Althouse). Dr. Niyi Coker featured her in the documentary *Black Studies USA* and she served as Historical Consultant and Television Show Host for Dreamcatchers Productions and the Dolphi Media Group (2004-2006). In 2003 she was recognized for her contributions to the state at the West Virginia Black Heritage Festival; and received the "Living the Dream" Award for Scholarship, an honor from the state of West Virginia's Martin Luther King, Jr. Holiday Commission. Twice cited among West Virginia's "most influential" people, Dr. Bankole-Medina is moderator of "History is a State of Mind," an independent and facilitated faculty discourse (blog and YouTube video podcasts) on history, race, culture and the African American experience. In 2016 Dr. Bankole-Medina was awarded the Chester W. Gregory Colloquium Scholarship and Research Award for "her commitment to scholarly research and publication along with her efforts to promote History at Coppin State University."

For more than twenty years, Dr. Bankole-Medina has taught an extensive selection of courses in history and Africana Studies including: African American Cultural and Intellectual History, African American History (I&II), African American Women's History, United States History (I&II), History of Black Nationalism, History of Enslavement in the United States, History of Science, Medicine and Technology, and graduate (master's and doctoral candidates) seminars in history and Black Studies.

A sought after lecturer, Dr. Bankole-Medina delivered major addresses

SLAVERY AND MEDICINE: ENSLAVEMENT AND MEDICAL PRACTICES IN ANTEBELLUM LOUISIANA

(The Merze Tate, Carter G. Woodson and African American History Month lectures) on such topics as "The Historical Legacy of the Nadir and the Moral-Jurisprudential Principles of Charles Hamilton Houston," "Evidence of Africans in the Vanguard of American Citizenship: The Primacy of the Fourteenth Amendment to the Constitution," and "Slavery and Antebellum Medicine: Historical Perspectives on the Study of the Science of Healing."

History faculty and students recognized Dr. Bankole-Medina with the Founder's Leadership Award from the Fanny J. Coppin Branch of ASALH. She is a member of several national women's and professional historical organizations. She is a life member of several professional organizations including: the Association for the Study of African American Life and History, the Association of Black Women Historians, and the African American Intellectual History Society. Dr. Bankole-Medina is also a founding member (with noted Cuban Linguist and Latin American Studies scholar Caridad Morales-Nussa) of the Tau Epsilon Chapter of Zeta Phi Beta Sorority, Inc. In addition, she was named a fellow to the Molefi Kete Asante Institute in Philadelphia.

Dr. Bankole-Medina earned a B.A. in History with a concentration in African American and United States history from Howard University in Washington, D.C. and an M.A. and PhD in African American Studies with concentrations in history from Temple University in Philadelphia, PA (the first university in the nation to grant a doctorate in African American Studies). Dr. Bankole-Medina has also received certification and training in Conflict Resolution (mediation and racial/ethnic conflict) and Teaching with Technology (especially in the area of online instruction). She has extensive technology training and has completed The Online Learning Consortium's Certificate (formerly The Sloan-C Certificate) for Teaching and Improving Online Courses.

Twitter: @KBankoleMedina

SLAVERY AND MEDICINE: ENSLAVEMENT AND MEDICAL PRACTICES IN ANTEBELLUM LOUISIANA

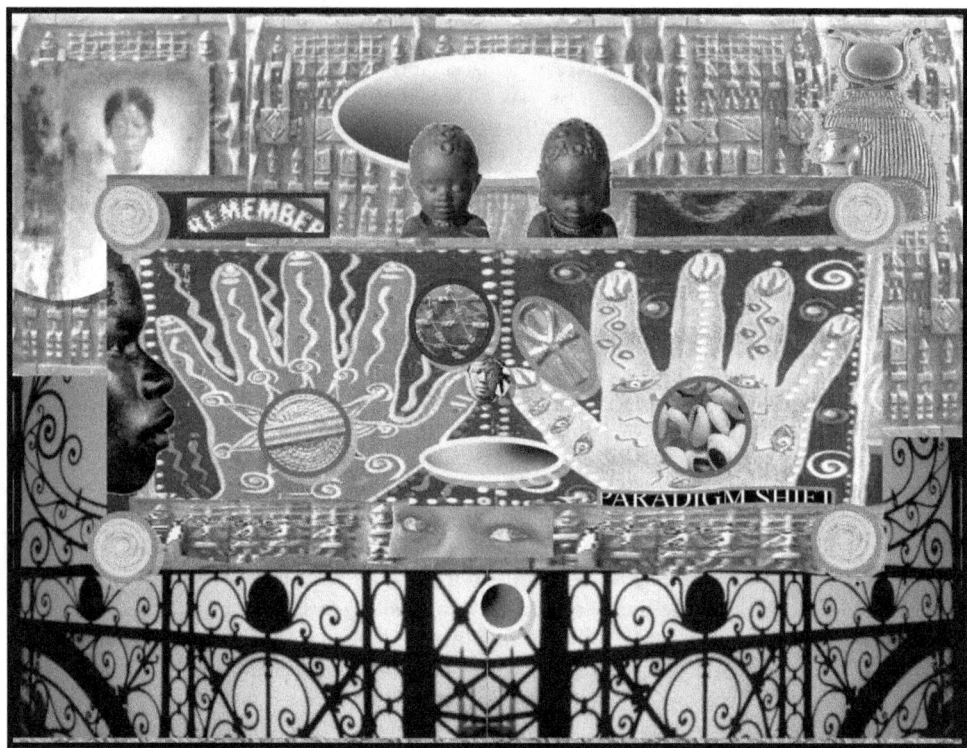

Back Cover Art: "Angie's Gate"

www.ingramcontent.com/pod-product-compliance
Lightning Source LLC
Chambersburg PA
CBHW071016240426
43661CB00073B/2326